AF803091

60

Intercellular and intracellular communication

General Editor: Professor B. Cinader

Receptors and ligands in neurological disorders

Intercellular and intracellular communication

1 Hormones, receptors and cellular interactions in plants
Edited by C. M. Chadwick and D. R. Garrod
2 Receptors in tumour biology
Edited by C. M. Chadwick
3 Receptors and ligands in psychiatry
Edited by A. K. Sen and T. Lee
4 Receptors and ligands in neurological disorders
Edited by A. K. Sen and T. Lee

Receptors and ligands in neurological disorders

EDITORS

AMAR K. SEN

Professor, Department of Pharmacology, University of Toronto, Toronto, Canada

TYRONE LEE

Assistant Director, Psychopharmacology Unit, Clarke Institute of Psychiatry and Assistant Professor, Departments of Pharmacology and Psychiatry, University of Toronto, Toronto, Canada

The right of the University of Cambridge to print and sell all manner of books was granted by Henry VIII in 1534. The University has printed and published continuously since 1584.

CAMBRIDGE UNIVERSITY PRESS

Cambridge

New York   New Rochelle   Melbourne   Sydney

Published by the Press Syndicate of the University of Cambridge
The Pitt Building, Trumpington Street, Cambridge CB2 1RP
32 East 57th Street, New York, NY 10022, USA
10 Stamford Road, Oakleigh, Melbourne 3166, Australia

© Cambridge University Press 1988

First published 1988

Printed in Great Britain at The Bath Press, Avon

British Library cataloguing in publication data

Receptors and ligands in neurological disorders
– (Intercellular and intracellular
communication, 4).
1. Nervous system – Diseases
2. Neurotransmitter receptors
I. Sen, Amar K. II. Lee, Tyrone
III. Series
616.8′047 RC347

Library of Congress cataloguing in publication data

Receptors and ligands in neurological disorders.
(Intercellular and intracellular communication; 4)
Includes bibliographies and index.
1. Central nervous system – Diseases. 2. Neurotransmitter receptors. 3. Neuromuscular diseases.
4. Alzheimer's disease. I. Sen, Amar K. II. Lee, Tyrone. III. Series. [DNLM: 1. Ligands. 2. Nervous System Diseases – physiopathology. 3. Receptors, Endogenous Substances – physiology. W1 IN669H v.4/ WL 100 R2955]
RC361.R43 1988 616.8′047 87-17659

ISBN 0 521 30720 1

BS

CONTENTS

CONTRIBUTORS

Bassel Abou-Khalil
Department of Neurology, University of Michigan School of Medicine, Ann Arbor, Michigan 48109, USA

George M. Anderson
Department of Pediatrics, Yale Child Study Center, Neurology and Laboratory Medicine, Yale University, New Haven, Connecticut 06510, USA

Anders Björklund
University of Lund, Department of Histology, S-22101 Lund, Sweden

R. J. Boegman
Department of Pharmacology and Toxicology, Queen's University, Kingston, Ontario K7L 3N6, Canada

W. M. Burnham
Department of Pharmacology, Medical Sciences Building, University of Toronto, Toronto, Ontario M5S 1A8, Canada

J. M. Candy
MRC Neuroendocrinology Unit, Newcastle General Hospital, Newcastle upon Tyne NE4 6BE, UK

C. J. Carter
Laboratoires d'Etudes et de Recherches Synthelabo (L.E.R.S.), 31 Ave. P.V. Couturier, 92220 Bagneux, France.

Donald J. Cohen
Department of Pediatrics, Yale Child Study Center, Neurology and Laboratory Medicine, Yale University, New Haven, Connecticut 06510, USA

Ted M. Dawson
Department of Psychiatry, University of Utah School of Medicine, Salt Lake City, Utah 84132, USA

Stephen B. Dunnett
Department of Experimental Psychology, University of Cambridge, Cambridge CB2 3EB, UK

Caleb E. Finch
Andrus Gerontology Center and Department of Biological Sciences, University of Southern California, Los Angeles, California 90089, USA

Arnold J. Friedhoff
Department of Psychiatry, New York University School of Medicine, Millhauser Laboratories, New York, New York 10016, USA

Menek Goldstein
New York University Medical Center, Department of Psychiatry, Neurochemistry Research Laboratories, New York, New York 10016, USA

Harold L. Klawans
Department of Neurological Sciences, Rush Presbyterian–St. Luke's Medical Center, Chicago, Illinois 60612, USA

James F. Leckman
Department of Pediatrics, Yale Child Study Center, Neurology and Laboratory Medicine, Yale University, New Haven, Connecticut 06510, USA

K. G. Lloyd
Laboratoires d'Etudes et de Recherches Synthelabo (L.E.R.S.), 31 Ave. P. V. Couturier, 92220 Bagneux, France

Mortimer Mamelak
Sunnybrook Medical Center, Department of Psychiatry, University of Toronto, Toronto, Ontario M4N 3M5, Canada

Patrick C. May
Andrus Gerontology Center and Department of Biological Sciences, University of Southern California, Los Angeles, California 90089, USA

D. R. Crapper McLachlan
Departments of Physiology and Medicine, Faculty of Medicine, University of Toronto, Toronto, Ontario, M5S 1A8, Canada

Emanuel Meller
New York University Medical Center, Department of Psychiatry, Millhauser Laboratories, New York, New York 10016, USA

David G. Morgan
Andrus Gerontology Center and Department of Biological Sciences, University of Southern California, Los Angeles, California 90089, USA

E. K. Perry
Department of Pathology and MRC Neuroendocrinology Unit, Newcastle General Hospital, Newcastle upon Tyne NE4 6BE, UK

Thomas L. Perry
Department of Pharmacology and Therapeutics, University of British Columbia, Vancouver, British Columbia V6T 1W5, Canada

Lisa A. Raskin
Amherst College, Psychology Department, Amherst, Massachusetts 01002, USA

J. Chris Sackellares
Department of Neurology, University of Michigan, School of Medicine, Ann Arbor, Michigan 48109, USA

Jack W. Schweitzer
Department of Psychiatry, New York University School of Medicine, Millhauser Laboratories, New York, New York 10016, USA

Bennett A. Shaywitz
Department of Pediatrics, Yale Child Study Center, Neurology and Laboratory Medicine, Yale University, New Haven, Connecticut 06510, USA

Sally E. Shaywitz
Department of Pediatrics, Yale Child Study Center, Neurology and Laboratory Medicine, Yale University, New Haven, Connecticut 06510, USA

George J. Siegel
Department of Neurology, University of Michigan, School of Medicine, Ann Arbor, Michigan 48109, USA

Caroline M. Tanner
Department of Neurological Sciences, Rush Presbyterian–St. Luke's Medical Center, Chicago, Illinois 60612, USA

James K. Wamsley
Department of Psychiatry, University of Utah School of Medicine, Salt Lake City, Utah 84132, USA

K. K. Wan
Department of Biochemistry, University of Toronto, Toronto, Ontario M5S 1A8, Canada

PREFACE

The books of this series are dedicated to a survey of modern biology in terms of a linguistic concept of ligand receptor interactions and of pathological processes in terms of malfunctions of the communication system. In this context, autoimmune disease, cancer, some neurological diseases and many psychiatric abnormalities can be analyzed as failures of this communication system.

Interlocking ligand-receptor networks of communication constitute an intercellular language, in which molecules, e.g. growth factors, lymphokines and hormones, serve as words and convey signals – messages – through combination with membrane molecules, i.e. receptors. These signals can give rise to the production of other factors which can combine with receptors and thus form the sentences of the intercellular language. In the immune system, macromolecules of the external world cause distortions of the internal communication. The resulting change in the balance of molecular communication constitutes the immune response. Factors of the immune system interact with receptors of the immune as well as the neural system and so do factors of the neural system.

The analogy between verbal and molecular communication is supported by the existence of superfamilies of molecules, designed with a common two-chain structure and involved in recognition of different ligands. Members of these families show homologies in a variety of cell types among cells of different animals from invertebrates to vertebrates.

Cell communication involves sequential molecular interactions between receptors and ligands, which are either cell-bound or are secreted by one cell and taken up by surface structures (receptors) of another cell. A succession of these interactions at the membranes of cells and organelles coordinates cell metabolism within the same and between different organs.

Receptors can be activated at a distance, or by receptor–ligand interaction between membranes of different cell types, i.e. via adhesion molecules which guide the structural development of organs, as exemplified by neural cell adhesion and embryological development under the influence of 'master' cells. Recognition and, thus, receptor–ligand interaction directs homing of cells in development, differentiation and cell migration.

Receptor–ligand communication plays various roles in the initiation of, and resistance to, infectious disease. Antigen recognition by B and T cells is one aspect of this process, the ability of a particular parasite to attach to a cell receptor is an example of another. In short, the interaction of the cellular milieu with external molecular occurs through receptors of the lymphoid system and through receptors of other cells, which control the ability of parasites to attach to special membrane sites, e.g. malarial merozoites to the *N*-terminal sugar *N*-acetyl glucosamine.

Interaction between ligand and receptor activates cells for a limited time. This limitation is achieved by endocytosis or receptor, or by dissociation of the complex in which the receptor is contained, resulting in decreased affinity for ligand.

Malfunction of a single step in cell communication results in disease and contributes to neoplastic transformation. Proliferation of neoplastic cells and spread of metastases may be promoted by the disappearance or blockage of receptors through which growth and metastatic spread are controlled.

The analysis of molecular language represents a major stream in biology of the twentieth century. This book is a part of a series in which we shall examine intercellular communication within and between organs, comparative as well as evolutionary aspects of this communication, and, finally, as in this volume – the effect on initiation and progression of disease.

This volume is dedicated to an examination of neurological disorders as malfunction in cell communication. It should contribute to insight into the relation between disease and intra as well as intercellular communication.

B. Cinader

INTRODUCTION

Receptors play a very important and integral part in cell-to-cell communication in all living organisms. For example, in the mammalian central nervous system, neurotransmitter receptors located on cell membranes primarily respond to transmitter substances that are released in the course of impulse propagation, eliciting a chain of events that leads to physiologically effective conduction of the impulse. In recent years, research into the nature, function and regulation of various types of receptors has been vigorous. Joint effort by scientists of various disciplines has been focused on the localization, isolation and purification of receptors, receptor response to lesions or drugs, and cloning of receptor subunits to permit more detailed analysis of gene expression. In spite of the tremendous amount of research done on the nature and function of receptors, many aspects of the subject are still in the dark. Many of the CNS disorders which are thought to be of biochemical origin have not yet been proven to be so.

The aim of this book is to summarize the current studies involving receptors and their ligands in various neurological disorders. These studies emphasize the importance of exploring the mechanisms of action of pharmacological agents used in neurology, with the ultimate goal of finding the origins of central nervous system disease and subsequently developing better or more effective therapeutic treatment for such disease.

Movement disorders can be classified as idiopathic or iatrogenic. Idiopathic movement disorder stems from an organic origin which usually is in a form of degeneration of certain types of nerve cells. Huntington's disease and Parkinson's disease are examples. Iatrogenic disorders are usually caused by exogenous factors such as drugs. In the case of tardive dyskinesia, the onset of abnormal involuntary oral-buccal movements is brought about by long-term administration of neuroleptic drugs in schizophrenic patients.

Huntington's disease is characterized by choreatic abnormal movements and mental deterioration accompanied by massive neuronal degeneration in the cortex and basal ganglia of the affected brain. Chapter 1 described the dysfunction of cholinergic neuronal system that is thought to be responsible for Huntington's disease. The authors emphasized that because the neuronal loss in Huntington's disease is massive, it is naive to think of a single neuronal system deficit being responsible for the disorder. Chapter 1 also contains a discussion on the therapeutic strategies in treating Huntington's disease with pharmacological agents that affect the cholinergic system.

Thomas Perry in Chapter 2 discusses his findings of reduced Gamma-aminobutyric acid (GABA) content in basal ganglia and other areas of autopsied brains from Huntington's disease patients. The reduced GABA is accompanied by deficient glutamic acid decarboxylase activity. However, Perry is aware that reduced GABA content can also be found in other neurological disorders such as dialysis encephalopathy, dominantly inherited olivopontocerebellar atrophies and Hallervorden-Spatz disease. Treatment strategies aiming at replenishing the loss of GABA in Huntington's disease have not been very successful. The author suggests the presence of a neurotoxin in the serum of Huntington's disease patients which may be responsible for the reduced GABA content. This neurotoxin, once identified, could lead to a treatment for delaying or preventing onset of symptoms in carriers of the Huntington's disease gene.

The role of dopamine in movement disorders is discussed in chapter 3. The chapter enlisted a dopamine dysfunction in Parkinson's disease and possibly Lesch-Nyhan patients. Using primate models for Parkinson's disease and Lesch-Nyhan syndrome the authors describe the action of a series of dopaminergic agents and proposed the possible mechanism at the receptor level.

Tardive dyskinesia is an abnormal movement disorder caused by long-term administration of neuroleptic drugs. Chapter 4 contains a thorough review on the historical aspects of this iatrogenic disease. A brief description of animal studies as well as recent clinical studies is pertinent here as investigators are trying to determine the pathogenesis of the disease in order to develop effective prevention of treatment protocols.

Chapter 5 carries a detailed description of Gilles de la Tourette's syndrome in which the authors pointed out that the clinical symptomatology of the disorder is not compatible with any known localized CNS lesion.

However, they have elaborated on five neurotransmitter systems, each one of which may be responsible for causing episodic irregularity in speech and motor functions. The systems discussed are dopamine, serotonin, GABA, noradrenaline and acetylcholine. In the hope of finding the marker for this disorder, the authors suggest using recombinant DNA technologies to look at restriction fragment length polymorphisms in the human genome.

With the availability of better health care and nutrition, the average life expectancy of the human population is steadily increasing. However, along with increasing life spans, we are also facing the problems of old age diseases. Alzheimer's disease is one such problem that is receiving much attention recently. As it is common with other psychiatric and neurological disorders the etiology and pathogenesis of Alzheimer's disease is poorly understood. It is thought that the disease is brought about by either infectious agents, or an immunological defect along with an error in gene expression. It is also believed that the neurotoxic properties of aluminum might be the causative factor in the production of the disease. In chapter 6, Dr McLachlan has extensively discussed the problem with particular reference to the role which aluminum plays in Alzheimer's disease. The next two chapters (7 and 8) deal with the involvement of neurotransmitter receptors in the process of normal human aging and Alzheimer's disease. It is apparent that no definite conclusions could be reached about any specific receptors to the disease process. However, it appears likely that both the noradrenergic and cholinergic receptors may be involved in the process. Thus, it is suggested that both adrenergic agonists and cholinomimetics might be beneficial in the treatment of the disease.

Chapter 9 deals with the acetylcholine receptor in myasthenia gravis. It has been suggested that myasthenia gravis is an autoimmune disease which primarily affects the nicotinic acetylcholine receptor located in the neuromuscular junction. In this chapter, Boegman and Wan discuss very thoroughly the possible etiology of the disease along with the rational therapy.

Epilepsy which affects one out of 200 people is one of the most common CNS disorders. It is therefore highly pertinent that the disorder be discussed thoroughly in a book that deals with the neurological diseases. Dr Burnham in chapter 10 has done so using the kindling model of epilepsy. Using this model it has been demonstrated that almost all putative neurotransmitter systems are affected in the abnormality. However, so far, a definite cause-effect relationship has not been established. In this chapter, Dr Burnham discusses the present state of the art with the kindling phenomenon in relation to biochemical changes in the brain.

Chapter 11 by Siegel and co-workers deals with regional cerebral metabolism and blood flow in epilepsy. The authors point out that in the late 19th century it was postulated that, on occasion, excessive liberations of energy with paroxysmal excessive discharges in the brain result in unstable equilibrium. Thus, it is postulated that there is a relationship between neuronal activity, metabolism and blood flow. With the advent of modern techniques such as positron emission tomography, it is now possible to examine the brain metabolism of glucose as well as blood flow by non-invasive techniques. With the use of these techniques it is now possible to examine the differences in these parameters in different types of epilepsy. Further studies such as these hold promise to a better understanding of these processes in disease state.

Attention deficit disorder of the childhood is a common disorder and is believed to affect the boys more than the girls. In this chapter (chapter 12) Dr Raskin *et al.* have dealt with the neurochemical basis of this disorder and has attempted to elucidate the etiology of the disease which may lead to the discovery of new and safe medications for the treatment of attention deficit disorder.

Normal sleep wakefulness cycles are regulated by activity of various neuronal systems of the CNS, as the author in chapter 13 has indicated. Receptors of these neurotransmitter systems are therefore invariably involved in the process. The author summarizes such involvement of the receptors from the adrenergic, cholinergic, serotonergic and dopaminergic systems.

Since the benzodiazepines are often used as hypnotics it is suggested that a number of benzodiazepine derivatives might influence sleep via the benzodiazepine receptors. The action of caffeine in causing disturbance in sleep is due to adenosine receptor blockade and therefore analogs of adenosine are being used to study their effect on sleep. Finally, narcolepsy, a disorder of sleep, is briefly discussed in association with the CNS metabolite gammahydroxybutyrate and its receptor.

A recent advancement in receptor studies is the use of autoradiographic techniques for receptor localization in the CNS. The authors in chapter 14 described the technique in detail. They emphasized that the technique can be used quantitatively to analyze the density and distribution of neurotransmitter and drug receptors in very small regions of the brain. This in turn will determine receptor alterations in response to long-term drug administration, lesions by toxins, genetic aberrations and disease studies, as the authors have indicated.

Another advancement in neurology research is the successful implantation studies in laboratory animals whereby healthy embryonic donor brain tissues can be transplanted to degenerative brain areas in the adult host to develop new neurons in the host animal in order to restore the functional deficit before the transplantation. As the authors in chapter 15 have pointed out, implication of such techniques can be tremendous. Patients suffering from Parkinsonian movement disorders can benefit surgically if they are not responsive to medication. Chapter 15 also contains several important issues: the extent and limitations of regeneration capacity in the adult CNS, the conditions that the grafts will ameliorate functional impairments, the use of transplant to generate animal models of neurological disorders and finally to determine the conditions under which transplants can provide viable clinical treatment of neurological disorders.

With improved technologies currently available we are beginning to see the light of the tunnel and hopefully in the near future, we will be able to understand the nature and etiology of the diseases discussed in this book for better and perhaps more effective treatments.

Finally we would like to express our sincere thanks to all colleagues for their participation and valuable contribution to this book. We also appreciate the cooperation of Cambridge University Press in the preparation of this volume.

A. K. Sen
T. Lee

1

Cholinergic neurons in Huntington's disease

K. G. Lloyd and C. J. Carter

1.1 Introduction

Huntington's disease is an autosomal dominant inherited disorder whose symptoms of choreatic abnormal movements and mental deterioration usually appear in middle age but may appear as early as 15 years of age. The mutant gene has been localized to chromosome 4 (Gusella *et al.*, 1983), but so far its identity has eluded detection. The effects of this deficit are revealed by massive neuronal degeneration, primarily affecting the cortex and basal ganglia, although other regions are by no means unscathed. Recent studies suggesting loss of the corticostriatal glutamatergic innervation (Wong *et al.*, 1982) as well as the earlier documented loss of striatal interneurons and striatal efferent pathways (for reviews see Bruyn, 1968; Hayden, 1981; Sanberg & Coyle, 1984; Carter, 1986), suggest that degeneration of a particular system, in this case the voluntary motor control system, may represent the neuropathological core of the disease. This is not surprisingly responsible for the bizarre motor symptomatology of the disease.

Among the neurotransmitter systems damaged by the mutant gene are possibly the corticostriatal excitatory amino acid projections, and the γ-aminobutyric acid (GABA, see T. L. Perry, Chapter 2) and acetylcholine (ACh) neuronal systems primarily in the basal ganglia. This review centres on the effects of Huntington's disease on the brain's cholinergic system, on the possible links this may have with the symptomatology of the disease, and with the clinical attempts to remedy the cholinergic dysfunction.

1.2 Central cholinergic synapses in Huntington's disease

1.2.1 *Choline acetyltransferase (CAT)*

Biochemical indices of central cholinergic synaptic function have been widely studied in Huntington's disease brains, with at least a dozen reports existing on this subject (Table 1.1). Consistently major changes are observed in the striatum (caudate nucleus and putamen) with more variable alterations occurring in other basal ganglia regions. As summarized in Table 1.1, most studies show that CAT (which is localized to cholinergic terminals and cell bodies) is reduced by 50–60% in the caudate nucleus and putamen of Huntington's disease patients, as compared to controls. The changes in the putamen exhibit a greater degree of variability (from almost total absence to normal levels) than in the caudate. This occurs not only between studies, but between patients in the same study, as Bird & Iversen (1974) reported that 14 of 37 patients had normal CAT activity in the putamen although glutamate decarboxylase activity was low in all patients. This may be a reflection of the sampling technique as CAT losses are reported to be very 'patchy' within the striatum with some areas having almost normal values. The rostral portion of the striatum has the greatest loss (Aquilonius *et al.*, 1975). In patients without Huntington's disease a considerable variation also occurs in the striatal distribution of CAT activity, but the low levels of Huntington's brain are not observed (Aquilonius *et al.*, 1975). In other basal ganglia regions in Huntington's disease (Table 1.1) CAT activity is either much more variable (pallidum) or is within the control range in most studies (substantia nigra).

In a study (apparently reported twice: Bird & Iversen, 1974; Spokes, 1980) of a large number of Huntington's patients, the relationship of CAT activity to disease form or medication was investigated (Table 1.2). Both the rigid and non-rigid forms of the disease had similar CAT levels in the different areas studied. Furthermore, both those patients receiving neuroleptic medication and medication-free patients exhibited CAT levels within the same range.

Within the limbic system, the hippocampus appears to have lost some cholinergic function, but this is generally less severe than that observed in the striatum and in most reports the differences do not reach statistical significance. In one study (Spokes, 1980) in which significantly low hippocampal CAT was observed (72% of control), a similar (63% of control) significant decrease in septal enzyme activity was reported. Thus, the septal–hippocampal cholinergic pathway may be hypofunctional in Huntington's disease. Sorbi *et al.* (1982) found no change in hippocampal or amygdaloid CAT activity in Huntington's disease, although there

Table 1.1. *Biochemical indices of cholinergic synaptic activity in the basal ganglia and selected other brain regions in Huntington's disease*

Caudate nucleus			Putamen			Pallidum			Substantia nigra			Accumbens			Neocortex			Hippocampus		
% control	No. patients	Ref.	% control	No. patients	Ref.	% control	No. patients	Ref.	% control	No. patients	Ref.	% control	No. patients	Ref.	% control	No. patients	Ref.	% control	No. patients	Ref.
(a) Choline acetyltransferase activity																				
32*	5	a	5*	3	e	20*	3	b	60	3	i	83*	30	l	64	—	n	40	3	e
38*	3	b	20*	3	b	34*	5	a	73	3	b	83*	30	k	67	3	o	58	3	i
38*	6	c	39*	5	a	60	8	f	83	14	f	106	5	c	93	3	i	67	11	f
40*	7	d	41*	42	f	75	3	e	96(C)	28	l	141	3	i	100	11	g	72*	23	l
41*	3	e	44*	37	g	76	32	l	113(R)	28	l				101	4	j	75	6	a
45*	64	f	48*	7	m				123	6	a				102	27	l	97	12	d
46*	37	g	50	6	c										105	10	d	113	3	b
48*	15	h	50*	6	d										117	11	f			
50*	3	i	58*	—	n										130	3	e			
53	2	j	65*	52	l										141	3	b			
57*	52	k	68	2	j										145	5	a			
57*	52	l	92	3	o															
66	11	m	97	3	i															
(b) Acetyl cholinesterase activity																				
108	3	i	134	3	i	—	—	—	98	3	i	138*	5	c	85	6	j	210	3	i
186	2	j	201	2	j							180	3	i	188	3	i			
															250*	4	c			
(c) Muscarinic receptor binding																				
33*	5	a	26* Q	6	b	47* Q	17	p	95 Q	3	a	—	—	—	88 Q	15	h	94 Q	3	b
35*	3	b	35* Q	3	a	52* Q	3	b	107 Q	4	b				117 Q	3	b	95 Q	6	a
49* Q	15	h	46* Q	17	p	55 Q	5	a							120 Q	5	a			
63* Pr	11	m	46* Pr	6	m															

*$P < 0.05$ vs controls. For substantia nigra, R = reticulata; C = compacta. For muscarinic receptor binding, Q = [^{3}H]quinuclidinylbenzylate; Pr = [^{3}H]propylbenzylcholine mustard.

References: (a) Wastek & Yamamura, 1978; (b) Wastek *et al.*, 1976b; (c) McGeer & McGeer, 1976; (d) Sorbi *et al.*, 1982; (e) Reisine *et al.*, 1977; (f) Bird & Iversen, 1977; (g) Bird & Iversen, 1974; (h) Enna *et al.*, 1976a; (i) McGeer *et al.*, 1973; (j) Stahl & Swanson, 1974; (k) Bird, 1980; (l) Spokes, 1980; (m) Hiley & Bird, 1974; (n) Wu *et al.*, 1979; (o) Walker *et al.*, 1984; (p) Enna *et al.*, 1976b.

was a significant reduction in pyruvate dehydrogenase activity in the hippocampus (see below). This enzyme may be concentrated in cholinergic neurons to provide the additional acetyl coenzyme A needed for ACh synthesis (Blass *et al.*, 1980). Such hippocampal deficits could of course contribute to the cognitive disturbances in Huntington's disease. However, it must be emphasized that the hippocampal deficit in CAT is not as marked as that seen in Alzheimer's disease (Bird *et al.*, 1983) nor, as in the latter, are there marked cortical cholinergic deficits. In contrast to the caudate nucleus and putamen the nucleus accumbens (often termed the limbic striatum) has CAT activity essentially within the normal range, although a small (17%) but significant decrease has been observed (Bird & Iversen, 1974; Spokes, 1980).

Possible variations of ACh synthesis have been studied in other brain regions. Neocortical (frontal cortex, motor cortex, unidentified cortical areas) CAT activity falls within normal limits, or may even be slightly elevated in the brains of Huntington's disease patients (Table 1.1). This is consistent with a normal anatomy of the nucleus basalis in Huntington's disease (Clark *et al.*, 1983), which provides most of the cholinergic input to the cerebral cortex (Johnston *et al.*, 1979). Other areas have CAT activity mostly within the normal range. It has been reported that enzyme activity is low in the cerebellar dentate nucleus and vermis (Wastek

Table 1.2. *Choline acetyltransferase activity in Huntington's disease: influence of different forms of the disease and medication*

	Choline acetyltransferase activity (% control)				
			Substantia nigra		
Huntington patients	Caudate nucleus	Putamen	Compacta	Reticulata	Nucleus accumbens
All patients	57 ± 6 (52)	65 ± 5 (56)	96 ± 10 (28)	113 ± 13 (28)	83 ± 7 (30)
Rigid patients	58 ± 13 (11)	68 ± 7 (13)	114 ± 22 (7)	113 ± 25 (7)	94 ± 13 (6)
Non-rigid patients	57 ± 7 (41)	65 ± 7 (43)	90 ± 11 (21)	113 ± 15 (21)	87 ± 11 (24)
Medicated (neuroleptic) patients	59 ± 7 (43)	66 ± 6 (46)	103 ± 13 (20)	121 ± 15 (20)	91 ± 12 (21)
Non-medicated patients	47 ± 14 (9)	61 ± 10 (10)	82 ± 14 (8)	92 ± 19 (8)	81 ± 13 (9)

Values represent the means and SEMs expressed as percentage of the control mean. The number of patients is given in parentheses.
From Bird & Iversen, 1974; Spokes,1980.

et al., 1976a) but this was not observed in another study (Bird & Iversen, 1974). Similarly the low enzyme activity in the olfactory tubercle reported by Simpson *et al.* (1984) was not noted in the earlier report by Bird & Iversen (1974). Low CAT activity (40% of control) was observed by McGeer & McGeer (1976) in the locus coeruleus of three Huntington's patients. This region has apparently not been examined in other studies, but may indicate an altered cholinergic control of cerebral noradrenergic neuron activity in Huntington's disease.

1.2.2 *AcetylcholineEsterase activity (AChE)*

As shown in Table 1.1, AChE activity has not been found to be decreased in any of the brain areas studied, including the striatum, substantia nigra, nucleus accumbens, hippocampus and neocortex. In fact, a generalized increase in AChE activity (up to 200% of control) has been noted in different studies; however, this reached statistical significance ($p < 0.05$) for only one study (McGeer & McGeer, 1976) in the temporal cortex, the accumbens and the lateral geniculate body (162% of control).

As AChE activity is not specifically localized to cholinergic neurons, it is difficult to evaluate these changes. However, it is possible that such increases in AChE activity would exacerbate the cholinergic deficit present subsequent to the reduced CAT activity, at least in the striatum.

1.2.3 *Pyruvate dehydrogenase activity*

Pyruvate dehydrogenase is a three enzyme complex catalysing the conversion of pyruvate to acetyl coenzyme A (AcCoA). This is the rate-limiting step for the entry of pyruvate into the Krebs cycle, and the enzyme complex is of necessity present in all cells in the brain. However, it is believed to be additionally concentrated in cholinergic neurons in order to provide the extra AcCoA needed for ACh synthesis (Tucek & Cheng, 1974; Jope & Blass, 1976). It has been shown that there is a close correlation between CAT and pyruvate dehydrogenase activities in the brain (Sorbi *et al.*, 1982). Pyruvate dehydrogenase activity is reduced in the caudate, putamen and hippocampus in Huntington's disease (Sorbi *et al.*, 1982; Carter, 1984; Butterworth *et al.*, 1985). This loss is quite substantial in the caudate and putamen ($\approx$70%) and possibly greater than could be expected solely as a result of neuronal loss, which is generally estimated at about 50% in these areas. Sorbi *et al.* (1982) found reduced pyruvate dehydrogenase activity in the hippocampus in the absence of reduced CAT activity, and suggested that reduced pyruvate dehydrogenase activity might be involved in the pathophysiology of neuronal death. Pyruvate dehydrogenase activity is under feedback control by the products of Krebs cycle metabolism (Jope & Blass, 1976; Reed, 1981) and in normal brain a possible consequence of this is an inverse correlation between pyruvate dehydrogenase and Krebs cycle enzyme (2-oxoglutarate dehydrogenase) activities (Carter, 1985a). This relationship was not observed in Huntington's disease brain samples (Carter, 1985b), suggesting that this metabolic feedback control may be defective in Huntington's disease (Carter, 1986). As pyruvate dehydrogenase is heavily concentrated in cholinergic neurons, this could explain the vulnerability of cholinergic neurons in this state, although the triggering factors behind such changes are not understood.

1.2.4 *Muscarinic receptor binding*

Complementary to pre-synaptic indices of central cholinergic activity, post-synaptic receptor densities can be estimated by the use of specific radioligands. Two different ligands for muscarinic receptors ([^{3}H]quinuclidinylbenzylate, QNB, and [^{3}H]propylbenzylcholine mustard, Pr) have been used to quantitate receptor densities in membranes prepared from different regions of Huntington's disease brains (Table 1.1).

Both QNB and Pr provide similar results: a decrease in muscarinic binding sites in the basal ganglia but not in other brain regions. In the putamen, the loss of muscarinic receptor varied from 50–75%, thus the receptor loss is more homogeneous than the variable decreases in CAT observed in this structure. In the caudate nucleus, the decreases in muscarinic receptor binding were in the same range as those observed for CAT. Decreases in muscarinic binding, again quantitatively similar to those observed for CAT, also occur in the pallidum.

For most of these studies, the binding assays were performed only at one concentration of [^{3}H]ligand, due to the limited amounts of tissue available. Wastek & Yamamura (1978) performed a Scatchard analysis of [^{3}H]QNB binding on membranes from the putamen of Huntington's disease patients, which demonstrated that the binding changes were due to a decreased receptor number as the affinity for [^{3}H]QNB did not differ between Huntington's and control brains.

Thus, both pre- and post-synaptic elements are greatly diminished in the striatum in Huntington's disease. These changes are similar for those observed for glutamate decarboxylase and [^{3}H]GABA binding (cf. Lloyd, 1980a,b) and correlate with the neuronal pathology of the striatum in Huntington's disease (Bruyn *et al.*, 1979). This loss of intrinsic cholinergic and intrinsic and efferent GABAergic neurons likely accounts for much of the massive cell loss observed in the Huntington's striatum.

Certain striatal afferents (e.g. serotonin, dopamine and noradrenaline) are intact in Huntington's disease (Bernheimer & Hornykiewicz, 1973; Barbeau, 1979), although it has been suggested that the corticostriatal glutamatergic inputs may degenerate (Wong *et al.*, 1982). It would appear that their target cells (e.g. striatal cholinergic and GABAergic neurons) are either greatly diminished or absent. This latter observation that the target cells of striatal afferents are absent would imply that therapy predicated upon a striatal site of action, or upon neurons impinging upon these structures, would have *a priori* a very limited possibility for success, except perhaps in early stages of the disease. This is the case for GABAmimetics (cf. Lloyd *et al.*, 1983, and below) and likely also for cholinomimetics (see below).

1.2.5 *Cerebrospinal fluid levels of choline and ACh in Huntington's disease*

There is a rather surprising paucity of data using cerebrospinal fluid in the study of cholinergic function in Huntington's disease. This can at least be partially explained by the ambiguous interpretation of CSF ACh and choline levels, as to their origin, reflection of CNS synthesis and levels, and relevance to function and pathology. In one study by Welch *et al.* (1976) ACh and choline levels in the lumbar fluid were found to be very similar to those from control subjects (71% and 87% of controls, respectively). Consolo *et al.* (1977) also found no difference in lumbar CSF choline or acetylcholineEsterase between control and Huntington's disease patients.

1.3 Clinical pharmacology of central cholinergic synapses in Huntington's disease

1.3.1 *Rationale*

To date there is no remarkable therapy of Huntington's disease, although neuroleptics are the standard medication (Shoulson, 1979). A rational basis for the pharmacotherapy of Huntington's disease would appear to exist for the use of neuroleptics, GABAmimetics and cholinomimetics. This rationale is based upon the known neurotransmitter interactions in the basal ganglia (cf. Lloyd, 1977, 1978). Thus, the nigrostriatal dopaminergic neurons appear to have a functional hyperactivity in Huntington's disease, although such increased activity is difficult to demonstrate biochemically in postmortem samples (cf. Bernheimer &

Hornykiewicz, 1983; Barbeau, 1979; Lloyd, 1980c). GABAergic neurons normally inhibit the synthesis and release of dopamine from the nigrostriatal dopamine terminals (Lloyd *et al.*, 1980; Scatton *et al.*, 1982). As GABAergic function is severely diminished in Huntington's disease (Lloyd, 1978, 1980b), GABAmimetic replacement therapy would appear logical in order to overcome this deficit and to restore neurotransmitter interactions. Unfortunately, of diverse GABA agonists (progabide, muscimol, THIP) and mimetics (sodium valproate, aminooxyacetic acid, γ-acetylenic GABA), none have provided satisfactory results in clinical trials (cf. Pearce *et al.*, 1977; Symington *et al.*, 1978; Shoulson *et al.*, 1978; Perry *et al.*, 1980; Tell *et al.*, 1981; Foster *et al.*, 1983; Lloyd *et al.*, 1983).

The nigrostriatal dopamine neurons normally inhibit striatal ACh synthesis and release (Bartholini *et al.*, 1976; Lloyd, 1978) and in the case of Huntington's disease this inhibition would be exaggerated. When combined with the severe striatal cholinergic hypofunction in Huntington's disease, the logic for cholinomimetic therapy is clearly evident.

1.3.2 *Cholinomimetics in Huntington's disease*

A variety of approaches have been used to augment central cholinergic activity in Huntington's patients: precursor loading techniques, inhibition of ACh metabolism, and direct receptor stimulation with a muscarinic agonist.

Precursor loading

Dimethylaminoethanol (deanol) increases ACh levels by metabolism to choline, which is the precursor for ACh synthesis (Goldberg, 1977). The literature reports a total of 49 Huntington's patients treated with this compound (Table 1.3). A total of six patients responded, five of them in one trial (Walker *et al.*, 1973). Two trials persisted for 3–6 months and in one trial a deterioration of symptoms was noted, although this may have been due to the previous cessation of tetrabenazine (Laterre & Fortemps, 1985).

Clinical trials with choline, the direct precursor of ACh, have also been conducted in Huntington's disease (Table 1.3), at doses up to 20 g/day. In spite of these high levels (which were reputed sufficient to give a 'fishy' odor to the patients), only five patients of a total of 25 were considered to exhibit a therapeutic response. In one trial (Growden *et al.*, 1977) some patients demonstrated an apparent initial response which was not maintained with time.

Another precursor of choline (lecithin, phosphatidylcholine) was reported to have therapeutic benefit in two of three patients after a slow dose increase to 16 g/day (Barbeau, 1978). To the authors' knowledge, clinical trials with lecithin have not yet been reported for larger patient populations.

One obvious problem with precursor loading with choline or its precursors is that choline only provides one half of the ACh molecule, the acetyl moiety being derived from AcCoA through the action of pyruvate dehydrogenase. As the activity of this enzyme is also severely compromised in Huntington's disease (Sorbi *et al.*, 1982; Carter, 1984, 1987) it is perhaps not surprising that choline therapy is ineffectual. Perhaps we should also be looking at ways to provide, in addition, the acetyl portion of ACh or of boosting cerebral glucose metabolism to allow a greater leeway for synthesis not only of ACh, but also of GABA and glutamate.

AcetylcholineEsterase inhibitors

The centrally acting AChE inhibitor physostigmine is the most-studied cholinomimetic in Huntington's disease (eight trials), although the total number of patients (45) is slightly less than for deanol. Four of these trials report success rates of greater than 50% patients responding to an acute i.v. injection of the compound. However, the largest study (12 patients) reported that only two patients benefited whereas six had symptoms exacerbated by physostigmine (Table 1.2).

It is difficult to compare these apparently more positive results (although the overall response rate is only 36%) with those obtained with precursor therapy, as the latter trials were performed on the basis of chronic oral administration with subsequent long-term results. It is impossible to predict if these positive effects of physostigmine would be maintained on long-term therapy. Such trials are unlikely, due to the inherent toxicity of cholinesterase inhibitors.

Two quaternary AChE inhibitors (neostigmine and edrophonium) which therefore have a poor rate of entry into the brain, were inactive in a limited number of Huntington's patients (Table 1.3).

Administration of a muscarinic agonist, arecoline

The effects of the muscarinic agonist arecoline in Huntington's chorea have been published in two reports (Table 1.3). In one double-blind trial a dose-dependent exacerbation of choreic movements was reported. In the other trial the growth hormone response to arecoline was similar in controls and Huntington's patients, suggesting normal pituitary muscarinic receptor sensitivity in these patients.

Table 1.3. *Activity of cholinomimetics in Huntington's disease: literature review*

Mimetic	Mechanism	Reference	Dose (mg/day)	No. patients	Response rate (%)	Comments
Dimethylamino-ethanol (Deanol)	ACh precursor	a	Unstated	9	0	6 month trial
		b	300–1000 po	7	71	—
		c	300–1200 po	17	0	Some subjective response
		d	1200 po	1	100	3 month trial
		e	1000 po	9	0	Several weeks
		f	225–900 po	6	0	—
Choline	ACh precursor	g	20 000 po	6	50	Slow build-up 1 month study
		h	20 000 po	4	50	Slow build-up 2 month study
		i	20 000 po	10	0	Increased CSF choline Transient effect Slow build-up
		j	3000–15 000 po	5	0	Slow build-up
Lecithin	ACh precursor	k	16 000 po	3	67	Slow build-up
Arecoline	ACh agonist	l	5–20 sc	6	0	Dose dependent Exacerbation
		m	5 sc	8	0	No correlation with symptoms Unchanged growth hormone response
Physostigmine	AChE inhibitor	n	1–2 iv	12	17	50% exacerbated
		o	1 iv	6	83	Ameliorate chorea and coordination
		h	0.5 iv	3	67	—
		g	3–4 iv	5	60	—
		p	1–2 iv	4	0	No effect on dyskinesia or coordination

		q	0.04/kg iv	4	100	—
		r	1 iv	4	0	—
		s	1 iv	7	0	No effect on memory
Neostigmine	Peripherally acting AChE inhibitor	q	0.04/kg iv	3	0	—
Edrophonium	Peripheral mimetic and AChE inhibitor	o	10	4	0	

References [for Table 1.3]: (a) Bird & Iversen, 1977; (b) Walker *et al.*, 1973; (c) Reibling *et al.*, 1975; (d) Amsterdam & Dubin, 1978; (e) Caraceni *et al.*, 1978; (f) Laterre & Fortemps, 1975; (g) Davis & Berger, 1978; (h) Davis *et al.*, 1976; (i) Growden *et al.*, 1977; (j) Aquilonius & Eckernäs, 1977; (k) Barbeau, 1978; (l) Nutt *et al.*, 1978; (m) Durso *et al.*, 1983; (n) Tarsy *et al.*, 1974; (o) Klawans & Rubovits, 1972; (p) Caraceni *et al.*, 1977; (q) Aquilonius & Sjöström, 1971; (r) Eckernäs, 1977; (s) Weingartner, 1979.

1.3.3 *Antimuscarinic compounds in Huntington's disease*

Following the rationale outlined in Section 1.3.1, cholinergic function in Huntington's patients can be investigated also by means of anticholinergic compounds. Although such trials have the *a priori* disadvantage that an exacerbation of the disease state is to be expected, a clear advantage is that several anticholinergics are available with well-known clinical profiles and considerably lower toxicity than for cholinomimetics.

Benztropine (Table 1.4) worsened the chorea and diminished coordination and motor function in some patients in the three trials reported in the literature. In one trial improvement was seen in two of the four patients studied. However, a confounding factor in studies with benztropine is that the compound is also a dopamine uptake inhibitor. As increased dopamine synaptic activity would also be expected to exacerbate Huntington's disease, the relevance of the results with benztropine to striatal cholinergic function are difficult to interpret.

Scopolamine is an anticholinergic without the potential for dopamine uptake inhibition. In one trial paradoxical results of decreased chorea together with a worsening of coordination were reported (Table 1.4). The marked sedation observed with the relatively high dose of scopolamine used is the likely explanation. In a trial with a lower dose of scopolamine, Huntington's symptoms were apparently unaltered by this antimuscarinic agent (Table 1.4).

Table 1.4. *Activity of anticholinergics in Huntington's disease: literature review*

Compound	Reference	Dose (mg, i.v.)	No. patients	Response rate (%)	Comments
Benztropine	a	2	4	100% Exacerbation	Increased chorea Decreased coordination
	b	2	4	50% Exacerbation 50% Slight improvement	Marked sedation
	c	2	6	16% Exacerbation	
Scopolamine	b	2	4	0	Worsen coordination but decrease chorea
	d	0.8	7	0	Marked sedation is likely explanation
Glycopyrrolate	b	0.1	4	0	Peripheral Anticholinergic

References: (a) Klawans & Rubovits, 1972; (b) Nutt, 1983; (c) Fahn *et al.*, 1973; (d) Weingartner, 1979.

In four patients the peripheral anticholinergic glycopyrrolate was without evident effect (Table 1.4).

1.3.4 *Does the clinical pharmacology of central cholinergic synapses provide evidence for cholinergic hypofunction in Huntington's chorea?*

As summarized in Table 1.5, clinical evidence suggests that the biochemical deficits observed in the striatum in Huntington's disease, while quantitatively large, are without a major functional correlate. Thus, of 136 patients reported in the literature in trials with various cholinomimetics, only 21% respond positively to the drugs. The AChE inhibitor physostigmine seems to induce a somewhat higher rate of response, but as discussed above this is a very acute (1–2 h) response to i.v. administration.

These observations on the lack of response to cholinomimetics are supported by the studies with anticholinergics in a smaller patient population ($N = 25$), where only 28% of patients had their symptoms exacerbated. These effects may rather be due to increased striatal dopamine activity rather than to a blockade of muscarinic receptors.

Table 1.5. *Overall response rates in clinical trials with agents altering central cholinergic transmission: lack of evidence for a critical role of muscarinic synapses in Huntington's disease*

Mechanism	Compound	Total no. patients	No. patients	Response rate (%)
(a) Cholinomimetics			(Amelioration)	
1. ACh precursors	Deanol	49	6	12
	Choline	25	5	20
	Lecithin	3	2	67
Total:		77	13	17
2. Agonist	Arecoline	14	0	0
3. AcetylcholineEsterase inhibitor	Physostigmine	45	16	36
Total cholinomimetics		136	29	21
(b) Antimuscarinic			(Exacerbation)	
	Benztropine	14	7	50
	Scopolamine	11	0	0
Total antimuscarinic		25	7	28

Several factors could contribute to this apparent dissociation between function and biochemical observations. The most evident is the severe degree of degeneration of the striatum; thus the cells containing the cholinergic receptors may themselves be dysfunctional and incapable of providing a physiological response to receptor stimulation. Additionally, the decreased number of muscarinic receptors provides fewer sites of action for endogenous ACh or administered agonists, although a sufficient number of sites would appear to remain. Another possible consideration is that precursor loading or AChE inhibition are insufficient due to the severe loss of ACh synthetic capacity, or, although unlikely, that it is actually nicotinic synapses which are important for Huntington's chorea. If this were to be the case, then a muscarinic agonist such as arecoline would have little activity.

1.4 The validity of the kainic acid model of Huntington's disease with respect to cholinergic neurons

The local injection of kainic acid into the striatum of the rat has been proposed as a laboratory model for Huntington's disease (Coyle & Schwarcz, 1976). Kainic acid induces neuronal death without damaging axons traversing or terminating in the striatum. The neuropathological changes following the intrastriatal injection of kainic acid resemble the neuropathology of Huntington's disease, with a severe degeneration of small and medium sized striatal and pallidal neurons, while sparing large striatal neurons, the nucleus basalis and the pars compacta of the substantia nigra (Bruyn *et al.*, 1979; Krammer, 1980). It appears that kainic acid may induce its neurotoxic effects via the release of excitatory amino acids (glutamate, aspartate) from the corticostriatal nerve terminals (Coyle *et al.*, 1978; Ferkany & Coyle, 1983; Coyle, 1983).

Intrastriatal kainic acid induces alterations in GABA synapses which are similar to those observed in the striatum in Huntington's disease (cf. Lloyd, 1980a,b,c), with large decreases in glutamic acid decarboxylase, GABA levels and [^{3}H]GABA receptor binding (cf. Coyle *et al.*, 1978; Zaczek *et al.*, 1978).

As shown in Table 1.6, the low CAT activity observed in Huntington's disease is reproduced by intrastriatal kainic acid injection, although the rat model seems to involve a more severe destruction of striatal cholinergic neurons than actually occurs in the human pathological condition. One report (Sanberg *et al.*, 1978) reported a much smaller loss of CAT activity in the rat after intrastriatal kainic acid, although marked striatal atrophy and behavioral changes were noted. A major methodological difference exists between this study and the others in that most of the latter studies were of an acute (up to 21 days) nature whereas in the Sanberg *et al.* (1978) study sacrifice occurred several months after kainic acid. The authors suggested that due to tissue atrophy and fluid and dead tissue loss, the changes in CAT activity (on a mg/tissue or protein basis) would become apparently less with time as the surviving neurons would exist in a smaller tissue mass. However, in Huntington's chorea the striatal tissue is severely atrophied, yet in the caudate nucleus the CAT losses are usually of a large magnitude. Thus if the reasoning of Sanberg *et al.* (1978) is correct, the acute kainic acid model does not provide a good reflection of the striatal cholinergic biochemistry in Huntington's disease. Coyle *et al.* (1978) come to a similar conclusion based on the observation that after delays of 5–9 months the kainic acid biochemistry is closer to that of Huntington's disease than after short-term periods.

The data available on muscarinic receptor binding ([^{3}H]QNB and [^{3}H]Pr in man, [^{3}H]QNB in the rat) indicate a somewhat more severe loss in the human condition than after intrastriatal kainic acid. However, in the rat model such binding data must be treated with caution as they may vary considerably with the delay to sacrifice post-kainic acid. Thus, [^{3}H]GABA binding is apparently elevated when the striata are studied with short time periods (1–30 days) post-kainic acid. However, when longer delays are attained (5–9 months) a decrease in [^{3}H]GABA binding

Table 1.6. *Comparison of biochemical indices in the striatum of Huntington's disease patients and rats after intrastriatal kainic acid injection*

Parameter	Huntington's disease (caudate–putamen)	Intrastriatal kainic acid – rat (5–12 nM)
Choline acetyltransferase		
% control	30–60	20–30; 78
(References)	(Table 1.1)	(a–c) (d)
Muscarinic receptor binding		
% control	30–50	55–60
(References)	(Table 1.1)	(c, e, f)
AcetylcholineEsterase		
% control	100–200	40
(References)	(Table 1.1)	(g)

References: (a) Beaumont *et al.*, 1979; (b) Coyle & Schwarcz, 1976; (c) Coyle, 1979; (d) Sanberg *et al.*, 1978; (e) Schwarcz & Coyle, 1977a; (f) Schwarcz & Coyle, 1977b; (g) Coyle *et al.*, 1978.

is obtained (16% of control, Zaczek *et al.*, 1978) which is slightly greater than that observed in Huntington's chorea (20–60% of control, Lloyd *et al.*, 1977; Iversen *et al.*, 1979; Reisine *et al.*, 1979; Beaumont *et al.* 1979; Olsen *et al.*, 1979).

That intrastriatal kainic acid induces more severe and non-specific lesions than those which occur in Huntington's disease is supported by the observation that AChE is decreased by 60% in the rat striatum after kainic acid (Coyle *et al.*, 1978) whereas in the Huntington's patients AChE activity is either normal or increased (Tables 1.1 and 1.6). Choline uptake (Coyle & Schwarcz, 1976), ACh levels (Coyle & Schwarcz, 1976) and AChE (Frankhuyzen & Mulder, 1977) activity are decreased 60–80% in the rat striatum after local kainic acid administration, confirming the severe loss of cholinergic neurons induced by the neurotoxic agent.

Thus, the kainic model for Huntington's disease does not produce a faithful quantitative representation of the altered striatal cholinergic biochemistry observed in Huntington's disease. This is not surprising as Huntington's disease is of slow onset with changes occurring over a span of decades whereas the major alterations are observed in the rat 3–5 days after intrastriatal injection of the neurotoxin. It should be noted that other excitatory amino acid receptor stimulants including *N*-methyl-D-aspartate (Zaczek *et al.*, 1981) are also capable of producing neurotoxic lesions. There has also recently been much emphasis on the ability of the endogenous neurotoxin quinolinic acid to mimic more faithfully the lesions produced in Huntington's disease. The neurotoxic effects of this agent in the laboratory are blocked by *N*-methyl-D-aspartate receptor antagonism (Schwarcz *et al.*, 1983; Beal *et al.*, 1986).

1.5 Conclusions

It is evident that cholinergic neurons within the basal ganglia are among those that are particularly susceptible to the effects of the genetic deficit in Huntington's chorea. However, this disease cannot be regarded as fundamentally a cholinergic deficit, as seen for example in Alzheimer's disease. In fact compared to other susceptible neuronal systems, particularly basal ganglia GABA neurons, the cholinergic deficit might even be regarded as incidental. The extent of neuronal loss in Huntington's disease is massive, and any symptomatology resulting from such damage is best regarded in the context of the loss of integrative capacity of a number of brain regions or systems rather than in terms of any single neurotransmitter deficit. In this context, it is perhaps not surprising that neurotransmitter replacement therapy, either with

GABAmimetics or cholinomimetics has been so fruitless in Huntington's disease. One additional problem with regard to the cholinergic system is that both the cholinergic neurons and their target cells are destroyed in this condition. Thus, even if an effective means can be found to elevate striatal cholinergic function, there is nothing much left of the striatum upon which ACh can act.

The choice of therapeutic strategies in central degenerative disorders has been heavily influenced by the success of l-DOPA therapy in Parkinson's disease, and by the resulting notion that once the deficit is known the patient should respond to replacement of the missing neurotransmitter. This unfortunately is not always the case, as has been shown by the overt failure of GABAmimetics and cholinomimetics in Huntington's disease, and of cholinomimetics in Alzheimer's disease. The difference may lie in the distinction between the roles of certain transmitters (or modulators) such as dopamine, which are diffusely organized but need to be present to allow the efficient passage of impulses through other more finely organized point-to-point fast transmitter systems, and the transmitters more specifically involved in this more organized circuitry. Evidently, the pathology of the disease is also important as GABAmimetics are therapeutically useful in epilepsy (cf. Bartholini *et al.*, 1984; Lloyd, 1986), but not in Huntington's disease.

Although pharmacological replacement strategies have to date met with little success in Huntington's disease, it is possible that the process of cell death may be retarded by use of pharmacological measures. This is a relatively new concept in pharmacology, and stems from studies with excitatory amino acid neurotoxins and from research aimed at characterizing the various neurotoxic factors responsible for the damage produced by such insults as hypoglycaemia, anoxia, ischaemia or epilepsy. Although the primary deficit in Huntington's disease is unknown, there is some evidence that the effects of this deficit are manifest as a disruption of cerebral energy metabolism and regulatory control. It has been suggested that this leads to destruction of neurons which are relatively more dependent upon glucose in the brain. These neurons primarily include those which use glucose as a neurotransmitter precursor (glutamate, GABA, ACh) which logically would be the first to react to changes in glucose metabolism (for review see Carter, 1986). If this is the case in Huntington's disease, it is possible that the same principles as have been applied in the laboratory to retard the neurotoxic consequences of ischaemia or hypoglycaemia may be applicable to Huntington's disease. During such conditions, a number of factors (additional or consequent to the initial energy failure) combine to reinforce the neurotoxic process. Briefly, these include the production of glutamate and or aspartate in excessive quantities, and, for reasons not yet fully understood, a build-up of intracellular calcium to neurotoxic levels (for reviews see Siesjo, 1978; Meldrum, 1985; Schwarcz & Meldrum, 1985; Godfraind *et al.*, 1985). It has been shown in both hypoglycaemia and ischaemia that neurotoxicity can be reduced by *N*-methyl-D-aspartate receptor antagonism (Simon *et al.*, 1984; Wieloch, 1985). There are currently no clinically available NMDA antagonists, nor are their overall effects yet clearly understood. However, in relation to the destruction of striatal cholinergic neurons in Huntington's disease, it is worth considering that these cells are believed to be innervated by corticostriatal excitatory amino acid projections (Hassler *et al.*, 1978), and that the receptors which control striatal ACh release are of the NMDA type (Scatton & Lehmann, 1982). This approach is currently only a theoretical proposition, but one that is likely to be applied to neurodegenerative diseases in the near future. It also remains to be seen whether centrally active calcium antagonists are of any use in such conditions.

One further factor that might be considered is that cholinergic neurons are susceptible in Huntington's disease because certain aspects of cholinergic metabolism are closely coupled to cerebral glucose metabolism, the AcCoA used for ACh synthesis being derived from pyruvate via pyruvate dehydrogenase. The idea that cholinergic neurons contribute to their own demise assumes that synthesis of ACh from glucose exacerbates potentially toxic situations involving compromised energy metabolism, i.e. those neurons diverting glucose to neurotransmitter synthesis from intermediary metabolism are less able to cope with potential reductions in glucose availability. Whether there are any chemical means of reducing the dependence of cholinergic neurons on cerebral glucose metabolism (and thus increasing the pool for intermediary metabolism) is not known, but this might be a subject for future research, particularly in terms of providing precursors for the acetyl portion of ACh.

References

Amsterdam, J. D. & Dubin, W. (1978). Huntington's chorea and dimethylaminoethanol (Deanol). *The Journal of Clinical Psychiatry*, **39**, 626–8.

Aquilonius, S.-M. & Eckernäs, S. A. (1977) Choline therapy in Huntington's chorea. *Neurology*, **27**, 887–9.

Aquilonius, S.-M., Eckernäs, S. A. & Sundwall, A. (1975). Regional distribution of choline acetyltransferase in the human brain: changes in Huntington's chorea. *Journal of Neurology, Neurosurgery and Psychiatry*, **38**, 669–77.

Aquilonius, S.-M. & Sjöström, R. (1971). Cholinergic and dopaminergic mechanisms in Huntington's chorea. *Life Sciences*, **10,** 405–14.

Barbeau, A. (1978). Phosphatidylcholine (lecithin) in neurologic disorders. *Neurology*, **28,** 358.

Barbeau, A. (1979). Update on the biochemistry of Huntington's chorea. In *Huntington's Disease, Advances in Neurology*, vol. 23, ed. T. N. Chase, N. S. Wexler & A. Barbeau, pp. 449–62. New York: Raven Press.

Bartholini, G., Bossi, L., Lloyd, K. G. & Morselli, P. L. (1984). *Epilepsy and GABA Receptor Agonists*. New York: Raven Press.

Bartholini, G., Stadler, M., Gadea-Ciria, M. & Lloyd, K. G. (1976). The use of the push–pull cannula to estimate the dynamics of acetylcholine and catecholamines within various brain areas. *Neuropharmacology*, **15,** 515–9.

Beal, M. F., Kowall, N. W., Ellison, D. W., Mazurek, M. F., Swartz, K. & Martin, J. B. (1986). Duplication of the neurochemical characteristics of Huntington's disease by quinolinic acid. *Nature*, **321,** 168–71.

Beaumont, K., Maurin, Y., Reisine, T. D., Fields, J. Z., Spokes, E., Bird, E. D. & Yamamura, H. I. (1979). Huntington's disease and its animal model: alterations in kainic acid binding. *Life Sciences*, **24,** 809–16.

Bernheimer, H. & Hornykiewicz, O. (1973). Brain amines in Huntington's chorea. In *Huntington's Chorea: 1872–1972, Advances in Neurology*, vol. 1, ed A. Barbeau, T. N. Chase & G. W. Paulson, pp. 525–32. New York: Raven Press.

Bird, E. D. (1980). Chemical pathology of Huntington's disease. *Annual Reviews of Pharmacology and Toxicology*, **20,** 533–51.

Bird, E. D. & Iversen, L. L. (1974). Huntington's chorea. Post-mortem measurement of glutamic acid decarboxylase, choline acetyltransferase and dopamine in basal ganglia. *Brain*, **97,** 457–72.

Bird, E. D. & Iversen, L. L. (1977). Neurochemical findings in Huntington's chorea. In *Essays in Neurochemistry and Neuropharmacology*, vol. 1, ed. M. B. H. Youdim, W. Lovenberg, D. F. Sharman & J. R. Lagnado, pp. 177–95. New York: Wiley.

Bird, T. D., Stranahan, S., Sumi, S. M. & Roskind, M. (1983). Alzheimer's disease: choline acetyltransferase activity in brain tissue from clinical and pathological subgroups. *Annals of Neurology*, **14,** 284–93.

Blass, J. P., Gibson, G. F. & Phimada, M. (1980). Brain carbohydrate metabolism and dementias. In *Biochemistry of Dementia*, ed. P. J. Roberts, pp. 121–34. New York: Wiley.

Bruyn, G. W. (1968). Huntington's chorea: Historical clinical and laboratory synopsis. *Handbook of Clinical Neurology*, **6,** 298–378.

Bruyn, G. W., Bots, G. T. A. M. & Dom, R. (1979). Huntington's chorea: Current neuropathological status. *Huntington's Disease, Advances in Neurology*, vol. 23, ed. T. N. Chase, N. S. Wexler & A. Barbeau, pp. 83–94. New York: Raven Press.

Butterworth, J., Yates, C. M. & Reynolds, G. P. (1985). Distribution of phosphate-activated glutaminase, succinic dehydrogenase, pyruvate dehydrogenase and γ-glutamyltranspeptidase in post-mortem brain from Huntington's chorea and agonal cases. *Journal of the Neurological Sciences*, **67,** 161–71.

Caraceni, T., Giovannini, P., Girotti, F. & Avanzini, G. (1977). Pharmocology of Huntington's chorea. *European Neurology*, **16,** 42–50.

Caraceni, T. A., Girotti, F., Celano, I., Parati, E. & Balboni, L. (1978). 2-Dimethylaminoethanol (Deanol) in Huntington's chorea. *Journal of Neurology, Neurosurgery and Psychiatry*, **41,** 1114–18.

Carter, C. J. (1984). Reduced pyruvate and 2-oxoglutarate dehydrogenase activity in the Huntington's disease putamen. *Journal of Physiology* **358,** 37.

Carter, C. J. (1985a). Enzymes of carbohydrate and amino acid metabolism in the human brain. *Biochemical Society Transactions*, **13,** 957–8.

Carter, C. J. (1985b). Abnormal carbohydrate and amino acid metabolism in the Huntington's disease brain. *Biochemical Society Transactions*, **13,** 958–9.

Carter, C. J. (1986). The biochemical pathology of Huntington's disease. *Reviews in the Neurosciences*, **1,** 1–34.

Clark, A. W., Prahad, I. M., Folstein, S. E., Whitehouse, P. J., Hedreen, J. C., Price, D. L. & Chase, G. A. (1983). The nucleus basalis in Huntington's disease. *Neurology*, **33,** 1262–7.

Consolo, S., Ladinsky, H., Bianchi, S. & Caraceni, T. (1977). The cerebrospinal fluid choline levels in patients with Huntington's chorea. Negative effect of halperidol treatment. *Archiv der Psychiatrie und Nervenkranken*, **223,** 265–70.

Coyle, J. T. (1979). An animal model for Huntington's disease. *Biological Psychiatry*, **14,** 251–76.

Coyle, J. T. (1983). Neurotoxic action of kainic acid. *Journal of Neurochemistry*, **41,** 1–11.

Coyle, J. T., McGeer, E. G., McGeer, P. L. & Schwarcz, P. (1978). Neostriatal injections: A model for Huntington's chorea. In *Kainic Acid as a Tool in Neurobiology*, ed. E. G. McGeer, J. W. Olney & P. L. McGeer, pp. 139–59. New York: Raven Press.

Coyle, J. T. & Schwarcz, R. (1976). Lesion of striatal neurones with kainic acid provides a model for Huntington's chorea. *Nature*, **263,** 244–6.

Davis, K. L. & Berger, P. A. (1978). Pharmacological investigations of the cholinergic imbalance hypothesis of movement disorders and psychosis. *Biological Psychiatry*, **13,** 23–49.

Davis, K. L., Hollister, L. E., Barchas, J. D. & Berger, P. A. (1976). Choline in tardive dyskinesia and Huntington's disease. *Life Sciences*, **19,** 1507–16.

Durso, R., Tamminga, C. A., Denaro, A., Ruggeri, S. & Chase, T. N. (1983). Plasma growth hormone and prolactin response to dopaminergic, GABAmimetic and cholinergic stimulation in Huntington's disease. *Neurology*, **33,** 1229–32.

Eckernäs, S. A. (1977). Plasma choline and cholinergic mechanisms in the brain. *Acta Physiologica Scandanavica, Supplementum*, **449,** 8–62.

Enna, S. J., Bennett, J. P., Bylund, D. B., Snyder, S. H., Bird, E. D. & Iversen, L. L. (1976b). Alterations of brain neurotransmitter receptor binding in Huntington's chorea. *Brain Research*, **116**, 531–7.

Enna, S. J., Bird, E. D., Bennett, J. P., Bylund, D. B., Yamamura, H. I., Iversen, L. L. & Snyder, S. H. (1976a). Huntington's chorea. Changes in neurotransmitter receptors in brain. *The New England Journal of Medicine*, **294,** 1305–9.

Fahn, S., Mishkin, M. M. & Hoffman, R. R. (1973). Pharmacologic and radiologic investigations in Huntington's chorea. In *Huntington's Chorea, 1872–1972, Advances in Neurology*, vol. 1, ed. A. Barbeau, T. N. Chase, & G. W. Paulsen, pp. 581–98. New York: Raven Press.

Ferkany, J. W. & Coyle, J. T. (1983). Kainic acid selectively stimulates the release of endogenous excitatory acidic amino acids. *The Journal of Pharmacology and Experimental Therapeutics*, **225,** 399–406.

Foster, N. L., Chase, T. N., Renaro, A., Hare, T. A. & Tamminga, C. A. (1983). THIP treatment of Huntington's disease. *Neurology*, **33,** 637–9.

Frankhuyzen, A. L. & Mulder, A. H. (1977). Release of radiolabeled dopamine, serotonin, acetylcholine and GABA from slices of rat brain after intrastriatal kainic acid injections. *Brain Research* **135,** 368–73.
Godfraind, T., Vanhoutte, P. M. Govoni, S. & Paoletti, R. (1978). *Calcium Entry Blockers and Tissue Protection.* New York: Raven Press.
Goldberg, A. M. (1977). Is deanol a precursor of acetylcholine? *Diseases of the Nervous System*, **38,** 16–20.
Growden, J. H., Cohen, E. L. & Wurtman, R. J. (1977). Huntington's disease: Clinical and chemical effects of choline administration. *Annals of Neurology*, **1,** 418–22.
Gusella, J. F., Wexler, N. S., Conneally, P. M., Naylor, S. L., Anderson, M. A., Tanzi, R. F., Watkins, P. C., Otlina, K., Wallace, M. R., Sakaguchi, A. Y., Young, A. B., Shoulson, I., Bouilla, E. & Martin, J. B. (1983). A polymorphic DNA marker genetically linked to Huntington's disease. *Nature*, **306,** 234–9.
Hassler, R., Chung, J. W., Rinne, U. & Wagner, A. (1978). Selective degeneration of two out of the nine types of synaptic in cat caudate nucleus after cortical lesions. *Experimental Brain Research*, **31,** 67–80.
Hayden, M. R. (1981). *Huntington's Chorea.* New York: Springer Verlag.
Hiley, C. R. & Bird, E. D. (1974). Decrease muscarinic receptor concentration in post-mortem brain in Huntington's chorea. *Brain Research*, **80**, 355–8.
Iversen, L. L., Bird, E., Spokes, E., Nicholson, S. H. & Suckling, C. J. (1979). Agonist specificity of GABA binding sites in human brain and GABA in Huntington's disease and schizophrenia. In *GABA Neurotransmitters*, ed. P. Krogsgaard-Larsen, J. Scheel-Kruger & H. Kofod, pp. 179–90. Copenhagen: Munksgaard.
Johnston, M. V., McKenney, M. & Coyle, J. T. (1979). Evidence for a cholinergic projection to neocortex from neurons in basal forebrain. *Proceedings of the National Academy of Sciences, USA*, **76**, 5392–6.
Jope, R. & Blass, J. P. (1975). A comparison of the regulation of pyruvate dehydrogenase in mitochondria from rat brain and liver. *Biochemical Journal*, **150,** 397–403.
Klawans, H. L. & Rubovits, R. (1972). Central cholinergic anticholinergic antagonism in Huntington's chorea. *Neurology*, **22,** 107–16.
Krammer, E. B. (1980). Anterograde and transynaptic degeneration 'en cascade' in basal ganglia induced by intrastriatal injection of kainic acid: An animal analogue of Huntington's disease. *Brain Research*, **196,** 209–21.
Laterre, E. C. & Fortemps, E. (1975). Deanol in spontaneous and induced dyskinesias. *Lancet*, I, 1301.
Lloyd, K. G. (1977). Neurotransmitter interactions related to central dopamine neurons. In *Essays in Neurochemistry and Neuropharmacology*, vol. 3, ed. M. B. H. Youdim, W. Lovenberg, D. F. Sharman, & R. Lagnado, pp. 130–207. Chichester: Wiley.
Lloyd, K. G. (1978). Observations concerning neurotransmitter interactions in schizophrenia. In *Cholinergic–Monoaminergic Interactions in the Brain*, ed. L. L. Butcher, pp. 363–92. New York: Academic Press.
Lloyd, K. G. (1980a). The neuropathology of GABA neurons in extrapyramidal disorders. *Journal of Neural Transmission, Supplement*, **16,** 217–27.
Lloyd, K. G. (1980b). Indication for GABA neuron dysfunction in mental disease. In *Enzymes and Neurotransmitters in Mental Disease*, ed. E. Usdin, T. L. Sourkes & M. B. H. Youdin, pp. 329–44. Chichester: Wiley.

Lloyd, K. G. (1980c). Chemical pathology of the extrapyramidal system. In *Synaptic Constituents in Health and Disease*, ed. M. Brzin, D. Sket & H. Bachelard, pp. 725–40. Oxford: Pergamon.

Lloyd, K. G. (1986). La théorie GABAergique de l'épilepsie. *La Révue du Praticien*, **36**, 243–54.

Lloyd, K. G., Dreksler, S. & Bird, E. D. (1977). Alterations in ^{3}H-GABA binding in Huntington's chorea. *Life Sciences*, **21**, 747–54.

Lloyd, K. G., Worms, P., Zivkovic, B., Scatton, B. & Bartholini, G. (1980). Interaction of GABA mimetics with nigro-striatal dopamine neurons. *Brain Research Bulletin*, **5**, *Supplement 2*, 439–45.

Lloyd, K. G., Morselli, P. L., Depoortere, H., Fournier, V., Zivkovic, B., Scatton, B., Broekkamp, C. L. E, Worms, P. & Bartholini, G. (1983). The potential use of GABA agonists in psychiatric disorders: Evidence from studies with progabide in animal models and clinical trials. *Pharmacology, Biochemistry and Behaviour*, **18**, 957–66.

McGeer, P. L. & McGeer, E. G. (1976). Enzymes associated with the metabolism of catecholamines, acetylcholine and GABA in human controls and patients with Parkinson's disease and Huntington's chorea. *Journal of Neurochemistry*, **26**, 65–76.

McGeer, P. L., McGeer, E. G. & Fibiger, H. C. (1973). Choline acetylase and glutamic acid decarboxylase in Huntington's chorea. *Neurology*, **23**, 912–7.

Meldrum, B. (1985). Possible therapeutic applications of antagonists of excitatory amino acid neurotransmitters. *Clinical Science*, **68**, 113–22.

Nutt, J. G. (1983). Effect of cholinergic agents in Huntington's disease: A reappraisal. *Neurology*, **33**, 932–5.

Nutt, J. G., Rosin, A. & Chase, T. N. (1978). Treatment of Huntington's disease with a direct cholinergic agonist. *Neurology*, **28**, 358.

Olsen, R. W., VanNess, P. C. & Tourtelotte, W. C. (1979). Gamma-aminobutyric acid receptor binding curves for human brain regions: comparison of Huntington's disease and normal. In *Huntington's Disease, Advances in Neurology*, vol. 23, ed. T. N. Chase, N. S. Wexler & A. Barbeau, pp. 697–704. New York: Raven Press.

Pearce, I., Heathfield, K. W. G. & Pearce, J. M. S. (1977). Valproate sodium in Huntington's chorea. *Archives of Neurology*, **34**, 308–9.

Perry, T. L., Wright, J. M., Hansen, S., Allan, B. A., Baird, P. A. & MacLeod, P. M. (1980). Failure of aminooxyacetic acid therapy in Huntington's disease. *Neurology*, **30**, 772–5.

Reed, L. J. (1981). Regulation of mammalian pyruvate dehydrogenase complex by a phosphorylation dephosphorylation cycle. In *Current Topics in Cellular Regulation*, vol. 18, ed. R. W. Estabrook & P. Srere, pp. 95–106. New York: Academic Press.

Reibling, A., Reyes, P. & Jameson, H. D. (1975). Dimethylaminoethanol ineffective in Huntington's chorea. *New England Journal of Medicine*, **293**, 274.

Reisine, T. D., Fields, J. Z., Stern, L. Z., Johnson, P. C., Bird, E. D. & Yamamura, H. I. (1977). Alterations in dopaminergic receptors in Huntington's disease. *Life Sciences*, **21**, 1123–8.

Sanberg, P. R. & Coyle, J. T. (1984). Scientific approaches to Huntington's disease. *CRC Critical Reviews in Clinical Neurobiology*, **1**, 1–44.

Sanberg, P. R., Lehmann, J. & Fibiger, H. C. (1978). Impaired learning and memory after kainic acid lesions of the striatum: A behavioural model of Huntington's disease. *Brain Research*, **149**, 546–51.

Scatton, B. & Lehmann, J. (1982). *N*-Methyl-D-aspartate type receptors mediate striatal ^{3}H-acetylcholine release evoked by excitatory amino acids. *Nature*, **297**, 422–4.
Scatton, B., Zivkovic, B., Dedek, J., Lloyd, K. G., Constantinidis, J., Tissot, R. & Bartholini, G. (1982). γ-Aminobutyric acid (GABA) receptor stimulation III. Effect of progabide (SL 76.002) on norepinephrine, dopamine and 5-hydroxytryptamine turnover in rat brain area. *The Journal of Pharmacology and Experimental Therapeutics*, **220**, 678–87.
Schwarcz, R. & Coyle, J. T. (1977a). Striatal lesions with kainic acid: Neurochemical characteristics. *Brain Research*, **127**, 235–49.
Schwarcz, R. & Coyle, J. T. (1977b). Neurochemical sequelae of kainate injections in corpus striatum and substantia nigra of the rat. *Life Sciences*, **20**, 431–6.
Schwarcz, R. & Meldrum, B. S. (1985). Excitatory amino acid antagonists provide a therapeutic approach to neurological disorders. *Lancet*, II, 140–3.
Schwarcz, R., Whetsell, W. O. & Mangano, R. M. (1983). Quinolinic acid; an endogenous metabolite that produces axon-sparing lesions in rat brain. *Science*, **219**, 316–8.
Shoulson, I. (1979). Huntington's disease: Overview of experimental therapeutics. In *Huntington's Disease, Advances in Neurology*, vol. 23, ed. T. N. Chase, N. S. Wexler & A. Barbeau, pp. 751–8. New York: Raven Press.
Shoulson, I, Goldblatt, D., Charlton, M. & Joynt, R. J. (1978). Huntington's disease: Treatment with muscimol, a GABA-mimetic drug. *Annals of Neurology*, **4**, 279–84.
Siesjo, B. K. (1978). *Brain Energy Metabolism*. Chichester: John Wiley & Sons.
Simon, R. P., Swan, J. H., Griffiths, T. & Meldrum, B. S. (1984). Blockade of *N*-methyl-D-aspartate receptors may protect against ischemic damage in the brain. *Science*, **226**, 850–2.
Simpson, J., Yates, C. M., Gordon, A. & St-Clair, D. M. (1984). Olfactory tubercle choline acetyltransferase activity in Alzheimer's-type dementia, Down's syndrome and Huntington's disease. *Journal of Neurology, Neurosurgery and Psychiatry*, **47**, 1138–9.
Sorbi, S., Bird, E. D. & Blass, J. P. (1982). Decreased pyruvate dehydrogenase complex activity in Huntington and Alzheimer brain. *Annals of Neurology*, **13**, 72–8.
Spokes, E. G. S. (1980). Neurochemical alterations in Huntington's chorea: A study of post-mortem brain tissue. *Brain*, **103**, 179–210.
Stahl, W. L. & Swanson, P. D. (1974). Biochemical abnormalities in Huntington's chorea brains. *Neurology*, **24**, 813–9.
Symington, G. R., Leonard, D. P., Shannon, P. J. & Vajda, F. J. E. (1978). Sodium valproate in Huntington's disease. *The American Journal of Psychiatry*, **135**, 352–4.
Tarsy, D., Leopold, N. & Sax, D. S. (1974). Physostigmine in choreiform movement disorders. *Neurology*, **24**, 28–33.
Tell, G., Böhlen, P., Schechter, P. J., Koch-Wester, J., Agid, Y., Bonnet, A. M., Coquillot, G., Chazot, G. & Fischer, C. (1981). Treatment of Huntington's disease with γ-acetylenic GABA, an irreversible inhibitor of GABA-transaminase: Increased CSF GABA and homocarnosine without clinical amelioration. *Neurology*, **31**, 207–11.

Tucek, S. & Cheng, S. M. (1974). Provenance of the acetyl group of acetyl choline and compartmentation of acetyl CO A and Krebs cycle intermediates in the brain *in vivo*. *Journal of Neurochemistry*, **22,** 893–914.

Walker, F. O., Young, A. B., Penney, J. B., Dovorini-Zis, K. & Shoulson, I. (1984). Benzodiazepine and GABA receptors in early Huntington's disease. *Neurology*, **34,** 1237–40.

Walker, J. E., Hoehn, M., Sears, E. & Lewis, J. (1973). Dimethylaminoethanol in Huntington's chorea. *Lancet*, I, 1512–13.

Wastek, G. J., Johnson, P. C., Stern, L. Z. & Yamamura, H. I. (1976a). Alterations in brain muscarinic cholinergic receptor binding and choline acetyltransferase activity in Huntington's disease. *Proceedings of the Western Pharmacological Society*, **19,** 170–1.

Wastek, G. J., Stern, L. Z., Johnson, P. C. & Yamamura, H. I. (1976b). Huntington's disease: Regional alteration in muscarinic cholinergic receptor binding in human brain. *Life Sciences*, **19,** 1033–40.

Wastek, G. J. & Yamamura, H. J. (1978). Biochemical characterization of the muscarinic cholinergic receptor in human brain: Alterations in Huntington's disease. *Molecular Pharmacology*, **14,** 768–80.

Weingartner, H., Caine, E. D. & Ebert, M. H. (1979). Encoding processes, learning and recall in Huntington's disease. In *Huntington's Chorea, Advances in Neurology*, vol. 23, ed. T. N. Chase, N. S. Wexler & A. Barbeau, pp. 215–26. New York: Raven Press.

Welch, M. J., Markham, C. H. & Jorden, D. J. (1976). Acetylcholine and choline in cerebrospinal fluid of patients with Parkinson's disease and Huntington's chorea. *Journal of Neurology, Neurosurgery and Psychiatry*, **390,** 367–74.

Wieloch, T. (1985). Hypoglycaemia-induced neuronal damage prevented by an *N*-methyl-D-aspartate antagonist. *Science*, **230,** 681–3.

Wong, P. T. H., McGeer, E. G., Rossor, M. & McGeer, P. L. (1982). Ornithine aminotransferase in Huntington's disease. *Brain Research*, **231,** 466–71.

Wu, J.-Y., Bird, E. D., Ceu, M. S. & Huang, W. M. (1979). Studies of neurotransmitter enzymes in Huntington's chorea. In *Huntington's Disease, Advances in Neurology*, vol. 23, ed. T. N. Chase, N. S. Wexler & A. Barbeau, pp. 527–36. New York: Raven Press.

Zaczek, R., Schwarcz, R. & Coyle, J. T. (1978). Long-term sequelae of striatal kainate lesion. *Brain Research*, **152,** 626–32.

Zaczek, R., Collins, J. & Coyle, J. T. (1981). *N*-methyl-D-aspartate: A convulsant with weak neurotoxic properties. *Neuroscience Letters*, **24,** 181–6.

2

GABA deficiency in Huntington's disease

Thomas L. Perry

2.1 Introduction

Huntington's disease (also originally and commonly called Huntington's chorea) is a severe progressive neurodegenerative disorder which is inherited in autosomal dominant fashion. Huntington's disease (HD) occurs in approximately one out of every 10 000 persons in white North American and European populations. Historical records describe the disease back at least to the early seventeenth century, and since its careful clinical description by George Huntington in 1872, it has been studied increasingly frequently.

2.2 GABA deficiency

The first biochemical abnormality involving a neurotransmitter to be found in autopsied brain in HD was the deficiency of γ-aminobutyric acid (GABA) in the basal ganglia (Perry *et al.*, 1973a,b). This was first described in 1972, on the occasion of the Centennial Symposium honouring George Huntington's pioneering studies. Soon thereafter, glutamic acid decarboxylase (GAD), the enzyme chiefly responsible for the synthesis of GABA, was reported to have reduced activity in the basal ganglia of autopsied brain in patients dying with HD (Bird *et al.*, 1983; Bird & Iversen, 1984).

Our discovery of the GABA deficiency in HD brain was a lucky one. We were not deliberately searching for a possible abnormality in this important inhibitory neurotransmitter, but were simply applying a technique we had developed earlier (Perry *et al.*, 1968; 1971a,b) for separating and quantitating a large number of amino acids and related amino compounds in specimens of autopsied or biopsied human brain. Figure 2.1 shows the degree of separation of amino compounds that can be obtained in brain with this method. When we began comparing the same regions of autopsied brain from patients dying with HD and patients dying without any neurological or psychiatric disorder, we were immediately struck by the great reduction in GABA content, especially in the globus pallidus and substantia nigra, in the HD patients.

Our original strategy of routinely measuring a wide variety of amino compounds in different regions of autopsied brain from patients dying with neurological or psychiatric diseases, and from appropriate control subjects, has paid off handsomely in a number of other disorders. In some of these, important biochemical abnormalities would have been missed had we measured only those compounds which we considered

Fig. 2.1. Tracing of a chromatogram of the free amino compounds in a deproteinized extract of a biopsy specimen of human temporal cortex equivalent to 0.1 g wet weight of brain. Abbreviations used are: Glycpea, glycerophosphoethanolamine; Tau, taurine; Pea, phosphoethanolamine; γ-Glu-Glu, γ-glutamyl-glutamic acid; Asp, aspartic acid; GSH, reduced glutathione; Thr, threonine; Ser, serine; Asn, asparagine; Glu, glutamic acid; Gln, glutamine; Pro, proline; GSSG, oxidized glutathione; Gly, glycine; Ala, alanine; Cit, citrulline; Aba, α-amino-n-butyric acid; Val, valine; Met, methionine; Cysta, cystathionine; Ile, isoleucine; Leu, leucine; Tyr, tyrosine; Phe, phenylalanine; GABA-Cysta, γ-aminobutyryl-cystathionine; GABA, γ-aminobutyric acid; Ea, ethanolamine; Orn, ornithine; Lys, lysine; His, histidine; HCarn, homocarnosine; GABA-Lys, γ-aminobutyryl-lysine; Put, putreanine; and Arg, arginine. (Taken from Perry (1978), by permission of Raven Press, New York.)

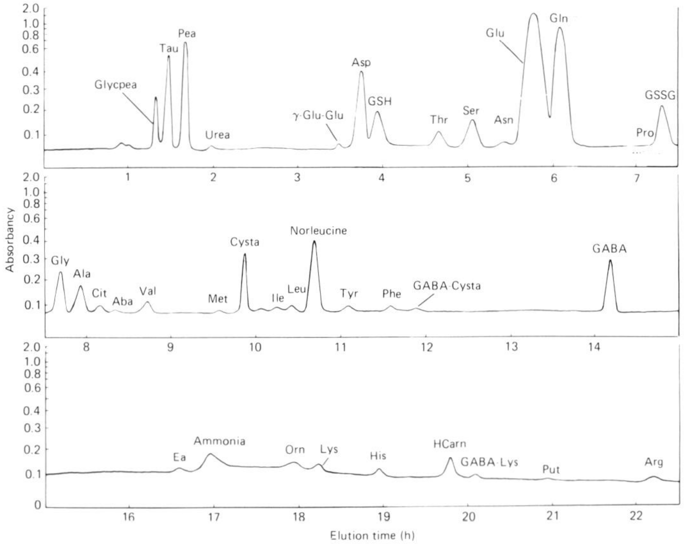

in advance to be relevant. Of course, valid comparisons cannot be made for all amino compounds in autopsied human brain, since the contents of many amino acids which are constituents of protein rise rapidly after death due to autolysis, while glutathione content drops rapidly after brain death. In general, valid comparisons can be made in studies of autopsied human brain between patients and controls for glycerophosphoethanolamine, taurine, phosphoethanolamine, glutamic acid, glutamine, cystathionine, GABA, and homocarnosine (Perry *et al.*, 1981a). Aspartic acid contents can be reliably compared if the death-to-freezing interval for brain specimens is less than four hours. GABA concentrations rise rapidly in brain after death, but have usually reached a stable maximum by one hour, a time interval before which few autopsies are ever done. Thus comparisons of GABA contents between similar regions of control and HD brain are reliable for almost all autopsies.

Table 2.1 shows the GABA contents of 10 different regions of autopsied brain for a large number of control subjects and HD patients. Reductions of GABA contents are marked in the caudate nucleus, putamen, globus pallidus, and substantia nigra, and are significantly but less markedly reduced in the occipital cortex and thalamus. However, in some regions of HD brain such as the frontal cortex, cerebellar cortex, and

Table 2.1. *GABA contents in various regions of autopsied human brain*

Subjects	Frontal cortex	Occipital cortex	Caudate nucleus	Putamen	Globus pallidus
Controls (neurologically normal)	1.67 ± 0.09 (26)	1.83 ± 0.11 (25)	2.90 ± 0.14 (32)	2.91 ± 0.20 (19)	7.32 ± 0.40 (16)
HD patients	1.64 ± 0.09 (20)	1.40 ± 0.08[b] (22)	1.37 ± 0.16[a] (23)	1.30 ± 0.15[a] (8)	2.75 ± 0.34[a] (9)

Subjects	Substantia nigra	Thalamus, medial–dorsal	Nucleus accumbens	Cerebellar cortex	Dentate nucleus
Controls (neurologically normal)	6.08 ± 0.25 (29)	2.05 ± 0.12 (35)	4.15 ± 0.29 (23)	1.65 ± 0.08 (26)	4.77 ± 0.23 (18)
HD patients	2.57 ± 0.18[a] (22)	1.72 ± 0.09[c] (30)	3.18 ± 0.39 (13)	1.52 ± 0.07 (20)	4.63 ± 0.35 (8)

Values (mean ± SEM) in μM/g wet weight, with number of patients in parentheses. [a]$P < 0.001$; [b]$P < 0.01$; [c]$P < 0.05$.

the dentate nucleus, there is no deficiency of GABA. Contents of homocarnosine, or γ-aminobutyryl-histidine, are diminished in HD in the same brain regions where GABA content is low (Perry *et al.*, 1973a; Urquhart *et al.*, 1975).

Although the deficiency of GAD activity in the basal ganglia in HD has been confirmed by several groups of investigators (Bird *et al.*, 1973; Bird & Iversen, 1974; Urquhart *et al.*, 1975; McGeer & McGeer, 1976; Spokes, 1980), this brain enzyme can be markedly affected by the manner of death, so that comparisons of GAD activity are not always meaningful. GAD activity in human brain is usually lower where death follows a prolonged period of anoxia or coma, than in cases where death occurs suddenly after normal or near-normal health (Perry & Perry, 1983). Surprisingly few attempts have been made to replicate our group's finding of a GABA deficiency in HD. To my knowledge, the only other reported efforts to measure GABA *itself* in HD are that of Bird & Iversen (1974), who used a fluorometric technique to demonstrate significantly reduced GABA contents in the caudate nucleus and putamen in autopsied brain, and the study of Kremzner *et al.* (1979) in which GABA was determined by an amino acid analyzer technique in instantly-frozen biopsies of frontal cortex from HD patients. The latter group found the mean GABA content in frontal cortex similar in HD patients and control subjects.

GABA aminotransferase (GABA-T), the first of the two sequential enzymes involved in the degradation of GABA, has normal activity in HD brain (Urquhart *et al.*, 1975), and thus the decreased GABA content cannot be ascribed to excessive activity of GABA-T. It is now generally assumed that the decreased GABA content and reduced GAD activity in the basal ganglia in HD are due to the loss of certain populations of GABAergic neurons, their progressive and premature death being programmed in a still-to-be-determined manner by the presence of the mutant HD gene, or by the absence of a double dose of the normal allele. It should be emphasized that not all neurons which utilize GABA as an inhibitory neurotransmitter are affected in HD. In the cerebellar cortex, where the neurotransmitter of one or more of the inhibitory interneurons is likely to be GABA, the content of this amino acid is normal in HD. And in the dentate nucleus, where the axons of the efferent GABAergic Purkinje neurons terminate, GABA content is always normal in HD. Similarly, GABA content is normal in the frontal cortex in HD, although decreased in the occipital cortex. GABA receptor sites have been reported decreased in number in the striatum in HD, perhaps due to local loss of other types of neurons, but no significant changes in binding affinity of GABA receptors were observed in any region of HD brain (Van Ness *et al.*, 1982). In another study (Enna *et al.*, 1976), GABA receptor binding was found normal in both cerebral cortex and caudate nucleus of HD patients.

2.3 Other neurochemical changes in HD

Additional neurochemical changes which have been established in autopsied brain of HD patients include a decrease in the striatum in activity of choline acetyltransferase (CAT), the enzyme which synthesizes acetylcholine (ACh), but CAT deficiency is not found in all HD patients (Bird & Iversen, 1974; McGeer & McGeer, 1976a). The significance of the loss of cholinergic neurons in HD is discussed in detail in Chapter 1 by Lloyd & Carter.

Substance P and cholecystokinin contents are reduced in the globus pallidus and substantia nigra in HD (Kanazawa *et al.*, 1977; Gale *et al.*, 1978; Emson *et al.*, 1980b), and there is also evidence for loss of methionine enkephalin in the striatopallidal and striatonigral neuronal pathways (Emson *et al.*, 1980a). Contents of the neuropeptide somatostatin surprisingly are increased in the striatum and globus pallidus in HD brain at autopsy (Aronin *et al.*, 1983), as well as in the nucleus accumbens, a brain region which is relatively spared pathologically in HD (Beal *et al.*, 1984). Contents of neurotensin and thyrotrophin-releasing hormone have also been reported significantly elevated in the caudate nucleus in postmortem HD brain (Nemeroff *et al.*, 1983). Thus, neurons which die off prematurely in the basal ganglia include GABAergic, cholinergic, and several peptidergic neuronal types.

Contents of dopamine, noradrenaline and serotonin have generally been found to be normal in the basal ganglia in HD, and there is no convincing evidence for a hyperactivity of dopaminergic nigrostriatal neurons (Melamud *et al.*, 1982). It is unlikely that neurons utilizing monoamine neurotransmitters are affected in HD. At this point, nothing is known about what kinds of neurons are lost in the cerebral cortex to account for the memory loss and dementia which is characteristic of HD. Neither is it clear just which symptoms and signs of HD are due to the loss of neuronal activity at inhibitory GABAergic synapses in the basal ganglia.

2.4 Cerebrospinal fluid GABA in HD

Since the GABA content is low in certain regions of autopsied brain from HD patients, and since it presumably is also low during life (as indicated by subnormal homocarnosine contents of the same brain regions), it was logical to look for reduced concentrations of GABA in cerebrospinal fluid (CSF) of living HD patients. Concentrations of GABA in human CSF are far lower than those of most amino acids, and they require techniques more sensitive than the average amino acid analyzer for accurate measurement.

HD patients, and even some healthy persons genetically at risk for HD, were originally reported to have GABA concentrations in their CSF well below those found in the CSF of normal subjects (Glaeser *et al.*, 1975; Manyam *et al.*, 1978, 1980). Our experience with a large group of HD patients, all with classical signs and symptoms, and with positive family histories, has been that GABA concentrations are normal in HD. We have used an ion exchange–fluorometric method, with post-column reaction of primary amines with *o*-phthalaldehyde (Perry *et al.*, 1982a). Our technique differs from that used by previous investigators in that only 10% as much sulfosalicylic acid is used for deproteinizing the CSF prior to column chromatography, and the sample is chromatographed on a cation exchange column with a much larger cross-sectional area. The result is that *on-column* hydrolysis of bound GABA compounds (such as homocarnosine) is much less likely to occur during chromatography, and formation of artefactual free GABA is prevented or greatly reduced. The details of technique in determination of GABA in CSF are crucial, and unless due care is taken, results will be meaningless.

Table 2.2 shows the mean GABA concentrations we have found in CSF from 36 neurologically normal adults who underwent lumbar puncture, and in 42 age-matched HD patients. The GABA levels in CSF did not differ significantly between the two groups. In addition, mean homocarnosine concentrations (determined with a standard amino acid

Table 2.2. *GABA Concentrations in CSF of control subjects and HD patients*

Subjects	Age (yr)	GABA (nM/l)
Neurologically normal controls (36)	44 ± 2.2	87 ± 7
HD patients (42)	45 ± 1.7	79 ± 8

Values shown are means ± SEM. Figures in parentheses indicate number of subjects examined. The mean GABA concentrations of the two groups do not differ statistically.

analyzer technique) were similar in CSF from the two groups of patients. GABA determination in CSF is clearly not useful for the diagnosis of suspected HD, nor is it of any value as a possible predictive test for persons genetically at risk. However, measurement of CSF GABA concentrations is useful in monitoring treatments of patients with drugs which inhibit the enzyme GABA-T and which can elevate brain GABA content.

2.5 Alterations in brain GABA content in other disorders

GABA deficiency in human brain is not confined to HD alone. Dialysis encephalopathy (dialysis dementia) is a progressive neurological syndrome, characterized by a unique language disorder, seizures, myoclonus, dyspraxia and dementia which commonly causes the deaths of patients treated for end-stage renal failure by repeated hemodialysis (Alfrey *et al.*, 1972). Aluminum toxicity is currently believed to be the most likely cause of dialysis fluid encephalopathy (Alfrey *et al.*, 1976; Berlyne, 1980; Sideman & Manor, 1982). Aluminum can cross into the brain from dialysis fluid from which this metal has not been carefully removed during preparation, as well as from aluminum absorbed in the gastrointestinal tract from the large amounts of phosphate-binding aluminum gels given most chronic renal failure patients. We have found (Sweeney *et al.*, 1985; Perry *et al.*, 1985d) that in dialysis encephalopathy patients at autopsy GABA contents are markedly decreased in frontal and occipital cortex, cerebellar cortex, dentate nucleus, medial dorsal thalamus, and caudate nucleus. Unlike the situation in HD, there is no deficiency of GABA in the putamen, globus pallidus, or substantia nigra of patients dying with dialysis encephalopathy.

GABA deficiency is present at autopsy in the cerebellar cortex in three of four biochemically and clinically different types of dominantly-inherited olivopontocerebellar atrophy (OPCA), and in the dentate nucleus in all four forms of OPCA (Perry *et al.*, 1981b; Perry, 1984). These reductions in GABA content presumably reflect marked neuronal loss of Purkinje cells and of one or more types of inhibitory interneuron in the cerebellar cortex. In the rare autosomal recessive disorder, Hallervorden–Spatz disease, GABA content is markedly decreased in the globus pallidus, the site of greatest neuropathological abnormality in this condition, and in the substantia nigra (Perry *et al.*, 1985c). Although not yet proven by neurochemical studies of human brain, it is also likely that local deficiencies of GABA may underlie tardive dyskinesia produced in psychiatric patients by chronic administration of neuroleptic drugs (Gunne *et al.*, 1984; Fibiger & Lloyd, 1984).

In two disorders, brain GABA content is elevated above normal levels. In Parkinson's disease, GABA content has been shown to be significantly higher than normal at autopsy in at least the putamen (Perry *et al.*, 1983). And in a recently-recognized genetically-determined disorder in which GABA-T enzyme activity is deficient (Jaeken *et al.*, 1984), GABA concentrations are greatly elevated in CSF, and are undoubtedly elevated in brain as well.

2.6 GABA replacement therapy in HD

The medical model which has been followed in most experimental therapies for HD has been that of Parkinson's disease. Since providing l-DOPA to sick and dying dopaminergic nigrostriatal neurons gives most Parkinson's disease patients significant relief of their symptoms for months or years, and generally improves their quality of life, it was logical for investigators to ask whether similar benefits could be achieved in HD. The efforts to correct presumed GABAergic neuronal dysfunction in HD patients have involved use either of GABAmimetic compounds, or of drugs which inhibit GABA-T and which would therefore be expected to elevate brain GABA content. Results of these therapies are summarized in Table 2.3.

Drugs that are agonists for GABA receptors in the brain have either failed to relieve the choreiform movements of HD patients, or in the case of muscimol, have increased dystonia. These GABAmimetic compounds have only been used for brief periods (usually less than six weeks) on HD patients, and primarily in efforts to diminish involuntary movements. Interested readers can consult the references listed in Table 2.3 for details.

Four drugs which inhibit GABA-T and which clearly elevate brain GABA content in experimental animals have been used in therapeutic trials on HD patients. These are isoniazid (INH), aminooxyacetic acid, γ-acetylenic GABA, and γ-vinyl GABA (Table 2.3). INH is itself not a GABA-T inhibitor, but is metabolized in the liver to form many breakdown products. One of the latter, hydrazine, has been shown to be the active agent in inhibiting GABA-T (Perry *et al.*, 1981c). Aminooxyacetic acid and γ-acetylenic GABA have both had unacceptable toxicities when tried on HD patients, while INH and γ-vinyl GABA have been better tolerated. Details can be found by consulting the references listed in Table 2.3.

That use of GABA-T inhibitors does indeed elevate brain GABA content in HD patients is supported by the substantial increases in CSF GABA concentrations found in patients given γ-acetylenic GABA (Tell

Table 2.3. *Neurotransmitter replacement therapies in HD*

Drug	Therapeutic effects	Comment	References
(a) *GABAmimetic compounds*			
GABA	Chorea unchanged	Fails cross blood–brain barrier	(Roberts & Kuriyama, 1968; Shoulson *et al.*, 1976)
Imidazoleacetic acid	Chorea unchanged	Fails cross blood–brain barrier	(Shoulson *et al.*, 1975)
Muscimol	Chorea rarely improved	Dystonia increased; other toxic side effects	(Shoulson *et al.*, 1978)
THIP (4,5,6,7-tetrahydro-isoxazolo-[5,4,-c]pyridin-3-ol)	Chorea unchanged	Causes unsteadiness of gait and somnolence	(Foster *et al.*, 1983)
SL 76002 (Progabide)	Mood elevation in early patients	No effects in patients with symptoms for > 5 years	(Bartholini *et al.*, 1979)
β-(p-chlorophenyl)-GABA (Baclofen)	No beneficial effects	*Not* a true GABA agonist	(Enna & Maggi, 1979)
(b) *GABA-T inhibitors*			
Isoniazid (hydrazine)	Mental improvement, minority of patients	Potentially hepatotoxic	(Perry *et al.*, 1979, 1982b; McLean, 1982; Stober *et al.*, 1983)
Aminooxyacetic acid	No beneficial effects	Unacceptable toxicities	(Perry *et al.*, 1980)
γ-acetylenic GABA	No beneficial effects	Unacceptable toxicities	(Tell *et al.*, 1981)
γ-vinyl GABA	No beneficial effects	No serious toxic effects	(Grove *et al.*, 1981; Scigliano *et al.*, 1984)
Sodium valproate	No beneficial effects	*Not* a GABA-T inhibitor	(Shoulson *et al.*, 1976)

et al., 1981), γ-vinyl GABA (Grove *et al.*, 1981), and INH (Perry *et al.*, 1982). We recently had the opportunity of studying the brain of a patient who committed suicide while on INH therapy for HD. GABA contents were higher in the basal ganglia than expected for HD, and they were supranormal in other brain areas (Perry *et al.*, 1985b). Amounts of hydrazine in this patient's brain at the time of his death were comparable to brain hydrazine contents of rats whose brain GABA had been elevated by daily injections of hydrazine (Perry *et al.*, 1981c).

As with the trials of GABAmimetic drugs, clinical trials with GABA-T inhibitors have usually been for brief periods only, and failure of HD patients to show clear *improvement* has generally been taken to indicate the uselessness of that particular form of therapy. In particular, the failure of choreiform movements to be relieved by drugs calculated to elevate brain GABA content has been interpreted by some investigators as indicating that GABA deficiency has little to do with the distressing symptoms of HD. It is hardly surprising that results of brief clinical trials of GABAmimetic agonists, and of GABA-T inhibitors, on HD patients should have been disappointing, when one remembers that many populations of neurons besides GABAergic ones are involved in this disorder, and that abnormal function probably affects many different types of synapses.

The only published reports of clinical improvement of HD patients treated with INH in high dosage (12–20 mg/kg/day) have been in patients treated for at least four months. A minority of those have had psychiatric improvement, with relief of depression, increased motivation, and an end to social withdrawal, but with little change in the movement disorder (Perry *et al.*, 1979, 1982b; Stober *et al.*, 1983).

What is of potentially greater importance is that a few HD patients supervised by our group (unpublished observations), ones maintained on INH plus supplemental pyridoxine steadily for long periods (three to five years), appear to have stopped deteriorating. Normally, HD follows a relentless downhill course without remissions, with a duration from first symptoms to death ranging from 10 to 25 years, and averaging 15 years. Shoulson (1981) devised a functional capacity rating scale for HD patients with 14 steps, ranging from a maximum of 13 for patients still retaining full abilities, down to zero for bed-ridden and terminal patients. In a large group of American HD patients receiving conventional drug treatments (neuroleptics and antidepressants), he observed a mean loss of 1.8 functional capacity units per year. In my view, it would be worthwhile to conduct a careful long-term (three to five years), double-blind clinical trial of either η-vinyl GABA or INH on a large group of early HD patients, repeatedly assessing their functional capacity on a scale like that of Shoulson (1981), to determine whether chronic elevation of brain GABA content slows down the neurological deterioration in HD. γ-Vinyl GABA might be the better choice of drug, since INH is often hepatotoxic in older patients. In the absence of any curative or preventive treatment for HD, a therapy which could give patients five additional years of reasonably good quality of life would be a distinct advance.

2.7 Possible effects of elevated brain GABA

It seems clear that increasing the total amounts of GABA in many brain regions (Perry *et al.*, 1985b) does not have beneficial effects in preventing the involuntary movements of HD. But GABA may well serve other functions in the brain besides acting as an important inhibitory neurotransmitter. Inhibition of GABA synthesis in rodent brain, with resulting lowered brain GABA content, leads to decreased protein synthesis (Sandoval *et al.*, 1976). Recently it has been shown that elevation of brain GABA content with GABA-T inhibitors in mice leads to increased activity of ornithine decarboxylase, the rate-limiting enzyme for production of putrescine and other polyamines (Lapinjoki *et al.*, 1983). The polyamines in turn play important roles in regulating synthesis of proteins, and synthesis and repair of RNA and DNA. It is believed that increasing brain GABA content may result in increased production by the anterior pituitary of growth hormone, and that the latter in turn causes increased ornithine decarboxylase activity. In this connection it is interesting that in the children with inherited deficiency of GABA-T who were investigated by Jaeken *et al.* (1984), there was unusually rapid physical growth, and fasting plasma growth hormone levels were increased.

We have measured polyamine concentrations in the CSF of a number of patients before and during treatment with high doses of INH. Putrescine and spermidine concentrations increase in CSF when GABA concentrations are elevated in CSF (and in brain) by the hydrazine produced from INH (unpublished observations) (Table 2.4). It is thus possible that GABA (and/or the polyamines) has an important trophic effect in brain. Progressive loss of GABAergic neurons in HD may not only result in involuntary movements secondary to lack of inhibition at key synapses in the basal ganglia, but might also cause further neuronal losses due to failures of protein synthesis. Thus it is conceivable that a general elevation of brain GABA content in various brain regions could delay or forestall further widespread neuronal losses which contribute to the mental depression, psychotic symptoms, and progressive dementia so characteristic of deteriorating HD patients.

2.8 What causes neuronal death in HD? Possible specific neurotoxins

How the mutant HD gene causes selective premature death of certain populations of GABA-utilizing and other neurons is still unknown. Numerous investigators have presented evidence that the HD gene codes for (i) a generalized membrane protein abnormality in all cells, including neurons, or (ii) that it produces a defective DNA repair mechanism which is particularly harmful to long-lived neurons. It is beyond the scope of this chapter to detail this evidence, but most of the claims have either been withdrawn by the original authors or effectively challenged by other investigators. Interested readers can find pertinent references in Perry *et al.* (1985a). In any case, the cell membrane abnormality and defective DNA repair hypotheses seem inadequate to explain why certain populations of neurons die prematurely in HD while others remain entirely undamaged.

Another hypothesis for premature neuronal loss in HD involves a specific neurotoxin, of either endogenous or exogenous origin, that is capable of binding to specific receptors on GABAergic and certain other neurons to cause their eventual destruction. The normal allele of the HD gene might code for an enzyme responsible for degrading the putative neurotoxin. Heterozygotes, or carriers of the HD gene, might produce insufficient enzyme for complete and regular degradation of the neurotoxin, and repeated presence of the latter in brain might cause progressive loss of susceptible neurons.

Intrastriatal injection of kainic acid, a powerful neurotoxic analogue

Table 2.4. *Concentrations of GABA, putrescine and spermidine in CSF before and during INH administration*

	GABA (pM/ml)	Putrescine (pM/ml)	Spermidine (pM/ml)
Before INH	65 ± 8 (19)	217 ± 26 (17)	101 ± 35 (6)
During INH	277 ± 23[a] (19)	354 ± 19[a] (17)	169 ± 37 (6)

Values given are means ± SEM. Numbers in parentheses indicate number of subjects. [a]$p < 0.001$.

of glutamate found in a Japanese seaweed, causes neuropathological and biochemical changes in rats closely resembling those found in human striatum in HD (Coyle & Schwarcz, 1976; McGeer & McGeer, 1976b; Coyle, 1983). In addition, quinolinic acid, an endogenous metabolite of tryptophan, has been shown to be a potent excitotoxin capable of producing neuronal lesions similar to those caused by kainic acid when injected intracerebrally in rats (Schwarcz *et al.*, 1983). However, we have been unable to detect increased amounts of quinolinic acid compared to controls in the brain, CSF, plasma or urine of HD patients (unpublished results). In addition, Foster *et al.* (1985) measured the enzyme which catalyzes the conversion of quinolinic acid to nicotinic acid mononucleotide, quinolinic acid phosphoribosyltransferase, in autopsied brain specimens from HD patients and controls and found no diminution of enzyme activity in caudate nucleus and putamen of HD patients. However, there are probably other as-yet-unidentified neurotoxins which might act like kainic and quinolinic acid.

In our laboratory, we have found (Perry *et al.*, 1985a) that repeated daily subcutaneous injections of large amounts of serum from drug-free HD patients into infant rats produces a significant reduction in mean striatal GABA content when the rats are sacrificed as adults. Infant rats injected with equal volumes of serum from control subjects have normal striatal GABA contents when killed as adults. This apparent loss of GABAergic striatal neurons is prevented if HD serum is first ultrafiltered through a membrane which retains compounds with a molecular weight greater than 10 000. These experiments suggest the possibility of a circulating neurotoxin in HD which is either a small molecule tightly bound to serum proteins, or less likely a molecule larger than 10 000 daltons.

We are currently pursuing these studies using newborn rat striatum grown in tissue culture and exposed to HD or control serum. These tissue culture experiments are showing more convincingly that serum from untreated HD patients, in contrast to serum from age- and sex-matched control subjects, contains one or more neurotoxins, probably small molecules, which reduce both GAD activity and GABA content in cultured rat striatal explants (unpublished results).

What effects this putative neurotoxin (or neurotoxins) has on neurons other than the GABAergic ones affected in HD remains to be explained. If a circulating neurotoxin can be confirmed as responsible for the premature neuronal losses in HD, and especially if it can be chemically identified, the way may open for either delaying or preventing the onset of symptoms in persons unfortunate enough to carry the HD gene.

2.9 Summary

(i) Reduced GABA content in the caudate nucleus, putamen, globus pallidus, substantia nigra, thalamus, and occipital cortex, and possibly in other brain regions not yet surveyed, is a biochemical abnormality regularly found in autopsied brain of HD patients. It is accompanied by reduced glutamic acid decarboxylase activity in the same brain regions, and the two findings reflect loss of GABAergic neurons. The GABA deficiency in brain is not reflected in the lumbar CSF of HD patients.

(ii) GABA deficiency is only one of a number of neurochemical abnormalities in HD, and it is clear that other types of neurons also die off prematurely.

(iii) Brain GABA content is reduced in some brain regions in several other neurological diseases besides HD. These include dialysis encephalopathy, dominantly inherited olivopontocerebellar atrophies, and Hallervorden–Spatz disease.

(iv) Short-term treatment of HD patients with GABAmimetic compounds, or with GABA aminotransferase inhibitors which increase GABA content throughout the brain, have not yielded clinical improvements nor relieved the choreiform movements. The latter presumably are due to more than mere lack of GABA at inhibitory synapses in the basal ganglia.

(v) Long-term treatment of a small number of HD patients with isoniazid in high dosage, plus supplemental pyridoxine, appears to slow or halt the normally inexorable neurological deterioration of HD. This observation has not been proven, but it merits further study, using either γ-vinyl GABA or isoniazid in an extended double-blind clinical trial of a sizeable group of HD patients. Elevating brain GABA with isoniazid increases putrescine concentrations in CSF, and GABA may possibly have trophic effects in brain acting through increased polyamine synthesis.

(vi) The serum of HD patients apparently contains one or more neurotoxins which reduce GABA content in rat striatum when animals are injected with large amounts of HD serum throughout infancy, and which reduce GABA content and glutamic acid decarboxylase in infant rat striatal explants grown in tissue culture. Confirmation of a causative neurotoxin in HD, and its chemical identification, might conceivably lead to a treatment for delaying or preventing onset of symptoms in carriers of the HD gene.

Research in the author's laboratory described in this chapter was supported by the Medical Research Council of Canada and by the Huntington Society of Canada. I appreciate much useful help from my colleagues Mrs Shirley Hansen and Dr James M. Wright, as well as from my former graduate student Dr Stephen J. Kish, and my present graduate student Voon Wee Yong.

References

Alfrey, A. C., LeGendre, G. R. & Kaehny, W. D. (1976). The dialysis encephalopathy syndrome: Possible aluminum intoxication. *The New England Journal of Medicine*, **294,** 184–8.

Alfrey, A. C., Mishell, J. M., Burks, J., Contiguglia, S. R., Rudolph, H., Lewin, E. & Holmes, J. H. (1972). Syndrome of dyspraxia and multifocal seizures associated with chronic hemodialysis. *Transactions of the American Society of Artificial Internal Organs*, **18,** 257–61.

Aronin, N., Cooper, P. E., Lorenz, L. J., Bird, E. D., Sagar, S. M., Leeman, S. E. & Martin, J. B. (1983). Somatostatin is increased in the basal ganglia in Huntington disease. *Annals of Neurology*, **13,** 519–26.

Bartholini, G., Scatton, B., Zivkovic, B. & Lloyd, K. G. (1979). On the mode of action of SL76000, a new GABA receptor agonist. In *GABA-Neurotransmitters: Pharmacochemical, Biochemical and Pharmacological Aspects*, ed. P. Krogsgaard-Larsen, J. Scheel-Krüger & H. Kofod, pp. 326–39. Copenhagen: Munksgaard.

Beal, M. F., Bird, E. D., Langlais, P. J. & Martin, J. B. (1984). Somatostatin is increased in the nucleus accumbens in Huntington's disease. *Neurology*, **34,** 663–6.

Berlyne, G. M. (1980). Aluminum toxicity in renal failure. *International Journal of Artificial Organs*, **3,** 80–1.

Bird, E. D. & Iversen, L. L. (1974). Huntington's chorea: Post-mortem measurement of glutamic acid decarboxylase, choline acetyltransferase and dopamine in basal ganglia. *Brain*, **97,** 457–72.

Bird, E. D., MacKay, A. V. P., Rayner, C. N. & Iversen, L. L. (1973). Reduced glutamic-acid-decarboxylase activity of post-mortem brain in Huntington's chorea. *Lancet*, I, 1090–2.

Coyle, J. T. (1983). Neurotoxic action of kainic acid. *Journal of Neurochemistry*, **41,** 1–11.

Coyle, J. T. & Schwarcz, R. (1976). Lesion of striatal neurons with kainic acid provides a model for Huntington's chorea. *Nature*, **263,** 244–6.

Emson, P. C., Arregui, A., Clement-Jones, V., Sandberg, B. E. B. & Rossor, M. (1980b). Regional distribution of methionine-enkephalin and substance P-like immunoreactivity in normal human brain and in Huntington's disease. *Brain Research*, **199,** 147–60.

Emson, P. C., Rehfeld, J. F., Langevin, H. & Rossor, M. (1980a). Reduction in cholecystokinin-like immunoreactivity in the basal ganglia in Huntington's disease. *Brain Research*, **198,** 497–500.

Enna, S. J., Bird, E. D., Bennett, J. P., Jr., Bylund, D. B., Yamamura, H. I., Iversen, L. L. & Snyder, S. H. (1976). Huntington's chorea: Changes in neurotransmitter receptors in the brain. *The New England Journal of Medicine*, **294,** 1305–9.

Enna, S. J. & Maggi, A. (1979). Biochemical pharmacology of GABAergic agonists. *Life Sciences*, **24,** 1727–38.

Fibiger, H. C. & Lloyd, K. G. (1984). Neurobiological substrates of tardive dyskinesia: The GABA hypothesis. *Trends in NeuroSciences*, **7,** 462–4.

Foster, N. L., Chase, T. N., Denaro, A., Hare, T. A. & Tamminga, C. A. (1983). THIP treatment of Huntington's disease. *Neurology*, **33,** 637–9.

Foster, A. C., Whetsell, W. O., Jr., Bird, E. D. & Schwarcz, R. (1985). Quinolinic acid phosphoribosyltransferase in human and rat brain: Activity in Huntington's disease and in quinolinate-lesioned rat striatum. *Brain Research*, **336,** 207–14.

Gale, J. S., Bird, E. D., Spokes, E. G., Iversen, L. L. & Jessell, T. (1978). Human brain substance P: Distribution in controls and Huntington's chorea. *Journal of Neurochemistry*, **30,** 633–4.

Glaeser, B. S., Vogel, W. H., Oleweiler, D. B. & Hare, T. A. (1975). GABA levels in cerebrospinal fluid of patients with Huntington's chorea: A preliminary report. *Biochemical Medicine*, **12,** 380–5.

Grove, J., Schechter, P. J., Tell, G., Koch-Weser, J., Sjoerdsma, A., Warter, J.-M., Marescaux, C. & Rumbach, L. (1981). Increased gamma-aminobutyric acid (GABA), homocarnosine and β-alanine in cerebrospinal fluid of patients treated with γ-vinyl GABA (4-amino-hex-5-enoic acid). *Life Sciences*, **28,** 2431–9.

Gunne, L.-M., Häggström, J.-E. & Sjöquist, B. (1984). Association with persistent neuroleptic-induced dyskinesia of regional changes in brain GABA synthesis. *Nature*, **309,** 347–9.

Jaeken, J., Casaer, P., deCock, P., Eeckels, R., Eggermont, E., Schechter, P. J. & Brucher, J.-M. (1984). Gamma-aminobutyric acid-transaminase deficiency: A newly recognized inborn error of neurotransmitter metabolism. *Neuropediatrics*, **15,** 165–9.

Kanazawa, I., Bird, E., O'Connell, R. & Powell, D. (1977). Evidence for a decrease in substance P content of substantia nigra in Huntington's chorea. *Brain Research*, **120,** 387–92.

Kremzner, L. T., Berl, S., Stellar, S. & Cote, L. J. (1979). Amino acids, peptides, and polyamines in cortical biopsies and venticular fluid in patients with Huntington's disease. In *Huntington's Disease, Advances in Neurology*, vol. 23, ed. T. N. Chase, N. S. Wexler & A. Barbeau, pp. 537–46. New York: Raven Press.

Lapinjoki, S. P., Pulkka, A. E., Laitinen, S. I. & Pajunen, A. E. I. (1983). Possible involvement of humoral regulation in the effects of elevated cerebral 4-aminobutyric acid levels on the polyamine metabolism in brain. *Journal of Neurochemistry*, **41,** 677–83.

Manyam, N. V. B., Hare, T. A., Katz, L. & Glaeser, B. S. (1978). Huntington's disease: Cerebrospinal fluid GABA levels in at-risk individuals. *Archives of Neurology*, **35,** 728–30.

Manyam, N. V. B., Katz, L., Hare, T. A., Gerber, J. C., III & Grossman, M. H. (1980). Levels of γ-aminobutyric acid in cerebrospinal fluid in various neurologic disorders. *Archives of Neurology*, **37,** 352–5.

McGeer, E. G. & McGeer, P. L. (1976b). Duplication of biochemical changes of Huntington's chorea by intrastriatal injections of glutamic and kainic acids. *Nature*, **263,** 517–9.

McGeer, P. L. & McGeer, E. G. (1976a). Enzymes associated with the metabolism of catecholamines, acetylcholine and GABA in human controls and patients with Parkinson's disease and Huntington's chorea. *Journal of Neurochemistry*, **26,** 65–76.

McLean, D. R. (1982). Failure of isoniazid therapy in Huntington disease. *Neurology*, **32,** 1189–91.

Melamed, E., Hefti, F. & Bird, E. D. (1982). Huntington chorea is not associated with hyperactivity of nigrostriatal dopaminergic neurons: Studies in postmortem tissues and in rats with kainic acid lesions. *Neurology*, **32,** 640–4.

Nemeroff, C. B., Youngblood, W. W., Manberg, P. J., Prange, A. J., Jr. & Kizer, J. S. (1983). Regional brain concentrations of neuropeptides in Huntington's chorea and schizophrenia. *Science*, **221,** 972–5.

Perry, E. K. & Perry, R. H. (1983). Human brain neurochemistry: Some postmortem problems. *Life Sciences*, **33,** 1733–43.

Perry, T. L. (1978). Taurine in dominantly inherited cerebellar atrophies and other human neurological disorders. In *Taurine and Neurological Disorders*, ed. A. Barbeau & R. J. Huxtable, pp. 441–51. New York: Raven Press.

Perry, T. L. (1984). Four biochemically different types of dominantly inherited olivopontocerebellar atrophy. In *The Olivopontocerebellar Atrophies, Advances in Neurology*, vol. 41, ed. R. C. Duvoisin & A. Plaitakis, pp. 205–16. New York: Raven Press.

Perry, T. L., Berry, K., Hansen, S., Diamond, S. & Mok, C. (1971a). Regional distribution of amino acids in human brain obtained at autopsy. *Journal of Neurochemistry*, **18,** 513–9.

Perry, T. L., Hansen, S., Berry, K., Mok, C. & Lesk, D. (1971b). Free amino acids and related compounds in biopsies of human brain. *Journal of Neurochemistry*, **18,** 521–8.

Perry, T. L., Hansen, S. & Gandham, S. S. (1981a). Postmortem changes of amino compounds in human and rat brain. *Journal of Neurochemistry*, **36,** 406–12.

Perry, T. L., Hansen, S. & Kloster, M. (1973a). Huntington's chorea: Deficiency of γ-aminobutyric acid in brain. *The New England Journal of Medicine*, **288,** 337–42.

Perry, T. L., Hansen, S., Lesk, D. & Kloster, M. (1973b). Amino acids in plasma, cerebrospinal fluid, and brain of patients with Huntington's chorea. In *Huntington's Chorea, 1872–1972, Advances in Neurology*, vol. 1, ed. A. Barbeau, T. N. Chase & G. W. Paulson, pp. 609–18. New York: Raven Press.

Perry, T. L., Hansen, S., Wall, R. A. & Gauthier, S. G. (1982a). Human CSF GABA concentrations: Revised downward for controls, but not decreased in Huntington's chorea. *Journal of Neurochemistry*, **38,** 766–73.

Perry, T. L., Javoy-Agid, F., Agid, Y. & Fibiger, H. C. (1983). Striatal GABAergic neuronal activity is not reduced in Parkinson's disease. *Journal of Neurochemistry*, **40,** 1120–3.

Perry, T. L., Kish, S. J., Hansen, S. & Currier, R. D. (1981b). Neurotransmitter amino acids in dominantly inherited cerebellar disorders. *Neurology*, **31,** 237–42.

Perry, T. L., Kish, S. J., Hansen, S., Wright, J. M., Wall, R. A., Dunn, W. L. & Bellward, G. D. (1981c). Elevation of brain GABA content by chronic low-dosage administration of hydrazine, a metabolite of isoniazid. *Journal of Neurochemistry*, **37,** 32–9.

Perry, T. L., Norman, M. G., Yong, V. W., Whiting, S., Chrichton, J. V., Hansen, S. & Kish, S. J. (1985c). Hallervorden–Spatz disease: Cysteine accumulation and cysteine dioxygenase deficiency in the globus pallidus. *Annals of Neurology*, **18,** 482–9.

Perry, T. L., Stedman, D. & Hansen, S. (1968). A versatile lithium buffer elution system for single column automatic amino acid chromatography. *Journal of Chromatography*, **38,** 460–6.

Perry, T. L., Wall, R. A. & Hansen, S. (1985b). Brain amino compounds in a Huntington's disease patient on isoniazid therapy. *Neurology*, **35,** 755–8.

Perry, T. L., Wright, J. M., Hansen, S., Allan, B. M., Baird, P. A. & MacLeod, P. M. (1980). Failure of aminooxyacetic acid therapy in Huntington disease. *Neurology*, **30,** 772–5.

Perry, T. L., Wright, J. M., Hansen, S., Baker-Thomas, S. M., Allan, B. M., Baird, P. A. & Diewold, P. A. (1982b). A double-blind clinical trial of isoniazid in Huntington disease. *Neurology*, **32,** 354–8.

Perry, T. L., Wright, J. M., Hansen, S. & MacLeod, P. M. (1979). Isoniazid therapy of Huntington disease. *Neurology*, **29,** 370–5.

Perry, T. L., Yong, V. W., Hansen, S., Foulks, J. G. & Kish, S. J. (1985a). Is a circulating neurotoxin involved in the pathogenesis of Huntington's chorea? *Journal of the Neurological Sciences*, **67,** 351–8.

Perry, T. L., Yong, V. W., Kish, S. J., Ito, M., Foulks, J. G., Godolphin, W. J. & Sweeney, V. P. (1985d). Neurochemical abnormalities in brains of renal failure patients treated by repeated hemodialysis. *Journal of Neurochemistry*, **45,** 1043–8.

Roberts, E. & Kuriyama, K. (1968). Biochemical-physiological correlations in studies of the γ-aminobutyric acid system. *Brain Research*, **8,** 1–35.

Sandoval, M.-E., Palacios, R. & Tapia, R. (1976). Studies on the relationship between GABA synthesis and protein synthesis in brain. *Journal of Neurochemistry*, **27,** 667–72.

Schwarcz, R., Whetsell, W. O., Jr. & Mangano, R. M. (1983). Quinolinic acid: An endogenous metabolite that produces axon-sparing lesions in rat brain. *Science*, **219,** 316–8.

Scigliano, G., Giovannini, P., Girotti, F., Grassi, M. P., Caraceni, T. & Schechter, P. J. (1984). Gamma-vinyl GABA treatment of Huntington's disease. *Neurology*, **34,** 94–6.

Shoulson, I. (1981). Huntington's disease: Functional capacities in patients treated with neuroleptic and antidepressant drugs. *Neurology*, **31,** 1333–5.

Shoulson, I., Chase, T. N., Roberts, E. & Van Balgooy, J. N. A. (1975). Huntington's disease: Treatment with imidazole-4-acetic acid. *The New England Journal of Medicine*, **293,** 504–5.

Shoulson, I., Goldblatt, D., Charlton, M. & Joynt, R. J. (1978). Huntington's disease: Treatment with muscimol, a GABA-mimetic drug. *Annals of Neurology*, **4,** 279–84.

Shoulson, I., Kartzinel, R. & Chase, T. N. (1976). Huntington's disease: Treatment with dipropylacetic acid and gamma-aminobutyric acid. *Neurology*, **26,** 61–3.

Sideman, S. & Manor, D. (1982). The dialysis dementia syndrome and aluminum intoxication. *Nephron*, **31,** 1–10.

Spokes, E. G. S. (1980). Neurochemical alterations in Huntington's chorea: A study of post-mortem brain tissue. *Brain*, **103,** 179–210.

Stober, T., Schimrigk, K., Holzer, G. & Ziegler, B. (1983). Quantitative evaluation of functional capacity during isoniazid therapy in Huntington's disease. *Journal of Neurology*, **229,** 237–45.

Sweeney, V. P., Perry, T. L., Price, J. D. E., Reeve, C. E., Godolphin, W. J. & Kish, S. J. (1985). Brain γ-aminobutyric acid deficiency in dialysis encephalopathy. *Neurology*, **35,** 180–4.

Tell, G., Böhlen, P., Schechter, P. J., Koch-Weser, J., Agid, Y., Bonnet, A. M., Coquillot, G., Chazot, G. & Fischer, C. (1981). Treatment of Huntington disease with γ-acetylenic GABA, an irreversible inhibitor of

GABA-transaminase: Increased CSF GABA and homocarnosine without clinical amelioration. *Neurology*, **31,** 207–11.

Urquhart, N., Perry, T. L., Hansen, S. & Kennedy, J. (1975). GABA content and glutamic acid decarboxylase activity in brain of Huntington's chorea patients and control subjects. *Journal of Neurochemistry*, **24,** 1071–5.

Van Ness, P. C., Watkins, A. E., Bergman, M. O., Tourtellotte, W. W. & Olsen, R. W. (1982). γ-Aminobutyric acid receptors in normal human brain and Huntington disease. *Neurology*, **32,** 63–8.

3

The role of central dopamine in movement disorders

Menek Goldstein and Emanuel Meller

3.1 Introduction

Histochemical and immunohistochemical studies reveal the existence of several different dopamine (DA)-containing neuronal pathways in the CNS. The mesencephalic DA cell groups have been extensively studied and subdivided into three groups: A-8, A-9, A-10 (Bjorklund & Lindvall, 1984). The A-8 group represents the caudally located supralemniscal cells, the A-9, the cells in the substantia nigra, and the A-10, the cells in the ventral tegmental area. DA-containing cell bodies give rise to descending and ascending projections, and the latter innervate three principal sets of targets: neostriatum, limbic cortex, and other limbic structures. The degeneration of the nigrostriatal DA neuronal pathway is associated with the extrapyramidal dysfunctions in Parkinson's disease (Hornykiewicz, 1972). However, the role of other DA neuronal systems in various movement disorders is not yet well established. We have recently obtained evidence that a central DA dysfunction might be involved in self biting (SB) behavior (Goldstein *et al.*, 1986). The findings that the levels of DA and its metabolites are reduced in postmortem brain of Lesch–Nyhan patients (Lloyd *et al.*, 1981), and that some DA agonists induce SB behavior in monkeys with supersensitive DA receptors, suggest abnormal dopaminergic function in this disorder. Animal models are useful in investigating the pathological and biochemical abnormalities of specific disorders. Monkeys with unilateral lesions in the ventromedial tegmental (VMT) area of the brain stem exhibit neurochemical and neurological deficits which are similar to those observed in Parkinson's disease (Poirier & Sourkes, 1965). We have evaluated the antiParkinsonian activities of various DA agonists in such lesioned monkeys (Goldstein *et al.*, 1973). During the course of these studies we observed that in a group of monkeys with unilateral VMT lesions of the brain stem the administration of specific DA agonists elicited SB behavior similar to that observed in Lesch–Nyhan patients. Thus, we have used monkeys with unilateral VMT lesions of the brain stem as a model for two different disorders. One group of monkeys with unilateral VMT lesions of the brain stem which developed hypokinesia and tremor of the extremities contralateral to the lesion side were used as a model for Parkinson's disease, while another group, which upon administration of specific DA agonists developed SB behavior, were used as a model for Lesch–Nyhan syndrome. In this presentation we will describe our studies in these two animal models and we will discuss mechanisms which might be responsible for the antiParkinsonian activities of some DA agonists.

3.2 Monkeys with unilateral surgical VMT lesions of the brain stem as a model for Parkinson's disease

The surgically induced tremor in monkeys with unilateral VMT lesions of the brain stem has a frequency (4–6 Hz) similar to that in Parkinson's patients (Goldstein *et al.*, 1973). We have shown that l-DOPA relieves tremor and induces abnormal involuntary movements (AIMs) in these monkeys, and these effects are similar to those observed in Parkinson's patients undergoing treatment with l-DOPA (Goldstein *et al.*, 1973). Thus, stimulation of supersensitive post-synaptic DA receptors by l-DOPA ameliorates the Parkinsonian-tremor and concomitantly produces AIMs.

Our studies have shown that not only l-DOPA, but several other DA agonists, relieve tremor and evoke AIMs in monkeys with unilateral VMT lesions of the brain stem (Table 3.1). We examined whether the relief of tremor and the occurrence of AIMs are related to stimulation of D_1, D_2 or both DA receptors. DA formed from administered l-DOPA stimulates both D_1 and D_2 DA receptors and effectively relieves tremor as well as produces AIMs (Table 3.1). Pergolide predominantly stimulates D_2 DA receptors (Goldstein *et al.*, 1980) and relieves tremor more effectively and for a longer time period than other tested ergot derivatives. The selective D_2 DA agonist and the partial ergoline derivative LY 141865 also effectively relieves tremor and produces AIMs, whereas the selective D_1 DA agonist SKF 38393 only slightly diminishes surgically induced tremor in monkeys. However, SKF 38393 poorly penetrates the blood brain barrier and it might therefore be ineffective as an antitremor agent. Based on our studies in monkeys with unilateral VMT lesions of the brain stem, we conclude that relief of tremor and occurrence of AIMs are related to stimulation of D_2 DA receptors, but simultaneous stimulation of D_1 and D_2 DA receptors may potentiate these effects. It is also evident from Table 3.1 that several partial DA agonists, such as the indolyl-3-butylamine derivative EMD 23 448 (Seyfried *et al.*, 1982) or the troponyl-piperazine derivative AY 27-110 (Ahmed & Bagli, 1982), also effectively relieve tremor and evoke AIMs in monkeys with unilateral VMT lesions of the brain stem. However, the AIMs elicited after administration of partial DA agonists are usually less severe than after administration of full DA agonists.

The therapeutic effectiveness of several different DA agonists in Parkinsonian patients is now under investigation. Since the tested DA agonists are usually less therapeutically effective than l-DOPA, most clinical trials evaluate the effects of the DA agonist in combination with l-DOPA. It is therefore of importance to consider the mechanisms which may be responsible for the therapeutic action of l-DOPA in combination with specific DA agonists (see next section).

3.3 Possible molecular mechanisms underlying the action of partial DA agonists

We and others have shown that the central DA agonist activity of bromocriptine and of other partial DA agonists is decreased when the synaptic levels of DA are reduced by treatment of animals with the l-DOPA synthesis inhibitor α-methyl-*p*-tyrosine (α-MPT) (Goldstein *et al.*, 1978; Gershanik *et al.*, 1983). On the other hand, the central DA agonists activity of full DA agonists such as apomorphine is not affected by treatment with α-MPT. To explain these observations we

Table 3.1. *The effects of DA agonists on tremor and on the occurrence of AIMs in monkeys with unilateral VMT lesion of the brain stem*

Drug (mg/kg, i.m.)	Response	
	Antitremor	Propensity to develop AIMs
L-DOPA (100)	very effective	high
Pergolide (0.2)	very effective	high
Quinpirole (LY 141865) (0.5)	very effective	low
Bromocriptine (5.0)	effective	low
EMD 23 448 (1.0)	effective	low
AY 27-110 (3.0)	effective	low
SKF 38393-A (3.0)	slightly effective	?

The experimental details were reported previously (Goldstein *et al.*, 1973).

have suggested the following hypothesis (Goldstein *et al.*, 1985). Bromocriptine, unlike classical DA agonists, does not induce a conformational change at the DA receptor leading to the conversion of the receptor from a low to a high affinity state for agonists (Sibley & Creese, 1983). However, the DA agonist activity of bromocriptine is enhanced in the presence of synaptic DA, since the latter induces a conformational change of the receptor and leads to the formation of a ternary complex which mediates DA agonist effects (Sibley *et al.*, 1982). Although bromocriptine does not differentiate between the high and low affinity states of the receptor, it might replace DA from the ternary complex and, by virtue of its higher affinity, enhance the duration of the agonist activity (Goldstein *et al.*, 1985). This hypothesis predicts that bromocriptine and other DA agonists with low intrinsic efficacy will be therapeutically more effective when combined with low doses of l-DOPA (Goldstein *et al.*, 1986).

3.4 Receptor reserve at pre-synaptic DA receptors

It is now well established that several new DA agonists such as (+)3-PPP and EMD 23 448 exert high activity at pre-synaptic and supersensitive post-synaptic, but not at normosensitive post-synaptic DA receptors (Goldstein *et al.*, 1984; Clark *et al.*, 1985). It has been postulated that the intrinsic activity of these DA agonists may be a function of the degree of previous agonist occupancy at the receptor, leading to variable conformational changes in the receptor (Clark *et al.*, 1985). Many studies have shown that in some receptor systems (those with a receptor reserve), partial agonists require a larger fractional receptor occupancy to produce a specific level of response than do full agonists (Ruffolo, 1982). Thus, full agonists are often able to produce a maximal response even when they occupy only a small fraction of the total number of receptors, whereas partial agonists require the occupancy of all the receptors to elicit a maximal response. The existence of such a receptor reserve could explain the selectivity of some partial DA agonists for pre-synaptic DA receptors (autoreceptors) and for supersensitive post-synaptic DA receptors. Indeed, we have recently shown that a large receptor reserve exists at the striatal DA autoreceptor. Furthermore, selective autoreceptor agonists such as EMD 23 448 and (+)3-PPP, although they demonstrate full intrinsic (tissue) *activity*, are actually partial agonists (Meller *et al.*, 1986; Meller *et al.*, unpublished data). The selectivity of these DA autoreceptors could be explained by a differential receptor reserve at pre- vs post-synaptic DA receptors. It is also possible that the increase in receptor density which accompanies the development of supersensitive DA receptors creates a substantial population of 'spare' receptors, which might explain the selectivity of some DA agonists for these receptors.

3.5 Monkeys with surgical unilateral VMT lesions of the brain stem as a model for Lesch–Nyhan syndrome

We have observed that in a group of monkeys with unilateral VMT lesions of the brain stem the administration of DA agonists elicits SB behavior of the forelimb digits contralateral to the lesion and spasticity of the contralateral hindlimb (Goldstein *et al.*, 1986). Preliminary studies suggest that the location and extent of the surgical VMT lesion of the brain stem which produces tremor and hypokinesia differs from that which produces DA agonist-induced SB behavior. The unilateral VMT lesion which produces the DA agonist-induced SB behavior seems to be confined to the dorsal area of the lateral part of the ventromedial area (A. Deutch and M. Goldstein, unpublished data). Thus, the neuropathological defect in monkeys with VMT lesions of the brain stem which mimics Parkinson's disease differs from that which elicits SB behavior upon DA agonist administration.

The administration of mixed D_1/D_2 DA agonists such as l-DOPA (in combination with the peripheral dopa decarboxylase inhibitor MK-486), apomorphine or Abeorphine 201–678 (Markstein *et al.*, 1984) results in the occurrence of SB behavior (Table 3.2). The SB behavior occurs within a few minutes after the administration of the DA agonist and it is manifested as biting, predominantly of the forelimb digits contralateral to the lesion. The mixed D_1/D_2 agonist Abeorphine 201–678

Table 3.2. *Effect of DA agonists on SB behavior in monkeys with a specific surgical unilateral lesion in the ventromedial tegmental area of the brain stem*

DA agonist (mg/kg, i.m.)	Occurrence of SB behavior
L-DOPA (100) + MK 486 (10)	(++)
Apomorphine (0.5)	(++)
Abeorphine 201–678 (0.1)	(++)
Quinpirole (LY 141865) (0.2)	–
SKF 38393-A (2.5)	–
Quinpirole (0.2) + SKF 38393 (2.5) SKF 38393 (2.5)	(+)

(++) Persistent SB behavior for at least 20 min.
(+) Intermittent SB behavior for 20 min.

produces SB behavior at a lower dose and for a longer duration than apomorphine or l-DOPA. Pergolide, which predominantly exerts D_2 DA agonist activity, and the selective D_2 DA agonist quinpirole (LY 171555), do not produce SB behavior. The selective D_1 DA agonist SKF 38393-A, by itself, does not produce SB behavior, but in combination with the D_2 agonist quinpirole, it elicits SB behavior for a short period of time. As previously pointed out, SKF 38393-A poorly penetrates the blood brain barrier, and therefore it might by itself be ineffective at low doses, while the combined administration of D_1 and D_2 DA agonists might produce a potentiating effect. The results obtained with DA antagonists also indicate that SB behavior is mediated by D_1 or by D_1 and D_2 DA receptors. Thus, the selective D_1 DA antagonist SCH 23390 or the mixed D_1/D_2 antagonist fluphenazine prevent the DA agonist-induced SB behavior, while the selective D_2 antagonist (±)sulpiride does not (Table 3.3) (Goldstein *et al.*, 1986).

3.6 Discussion

Recent studies suggest that partial DA agonists which selectively stimulate pre-synaptic and suspersensitive post-synaptic DA receptors might have therapeutic potential in treatment of Parkinson's disease and some mental disorders which are associated with abnormal central dopaminergic functions. Clinical studies indicate that although administration of DA agonists in combination with l-DOPA results in reduction of disability in Parkinsonian patients with advanced disease, it also produces adverse side effects. It will be of interest to determine whether a low dose of l-DOPA in combination with a partial DA agonist is therapeutically more advantageous than when combined with a full DA agonist. One might expect that treatment with partial DA agonists in combination with low doses of l-DOPA will produce a therapeutic effect

Table 3.3. *Effects of DA antagonists on blockade of SB behavior elicited by administration of the DA agonist Abeorphine 201–678*

DA antagonist (mg/kg, i.m.)	Effect on SB behavior induced by Abeorphine 201–678[a]
None	SB behavior for a period of 3–5 h
(±) sulpiride (100)	SB behavior for a period of 3–5 h
SCH 23390 (0.3)	Complete blockade
Fluphenazine (1.5)	Complete blockade

[a] The DA agonist Abeorphine 201–678 (0.1 mg/kg) was given 10–20 min after administration of the DA antagonists.

with a lower incidence of undesired side effects. The sudden freezing episodes, 'on–off' effects, which occur during treatment with higher doses of l-DOPA might be less pronounced during treatment with partial DA agonists in combination with low doses of l-DOPA.

Our preliminary studies indicate that the neuroanatomical lesion which produces tremor and other Parkinsonian-like symptoms in monkeys with unilateral VMT lesions differs from the lesion which produces SB behavior. It is noteworthy that Parkinsonian patients treated with l-DOPA or various DA agonists apparently do not display SB behavior. These observations also imply that the dopaminergic dysfunction in Parkinson's disease differs from the dopaminergic dysfunction associated with SB behavior in Lesch–Nyhan syndrome. At present, we can only speculate on the relationship between the major biochemical defects in Lesch–Nyhan syndrome, namely the deficiency in hypoxanthine–guanine phosphoribosyltransferase (HPRT) (salvage enzyme) (Wilson *et al.*, 1983), and dopaminergic dysfunction in this disorder. The defective HPRT enzyme in Lesch–Nyhan brain could lead to reduced production of striatal GTP which is a precursor for pteridines (Kapatos *et al.*, 1982). Since pteridine is the cofactor for the catecholamine-synthesizing enzyme tyrosine hydroxylase (TH), a reduction in its levels will result in decreased TH activity leading to decreased DA synthesis. Thus, decreased synthesis of DA might result from low levels of striatal pteridine, and this might be responsible for the low levels of central DA in postmortem Lesch–Nyhan brain. The prolonged deficiency of DA at the synapse might produce supersensitivity at DA receptors. Furthermore, GTP is involved in the regulation of the activity state of DA receptors and reduced GTP levels could also result, via a compensatory feedback mechanism, in the development of supersensitive DA receptors. The role of GTP in disorders with abnormal dopaminergic function is still not well understood and its involvement in CNS functions might be of greater importance than presently credited.

These studies were supported in part by grants NINCDS 06801–19 and MH 35976–6.

References

Ahmed, F. R. & Bagli, J. (1982). Troponoid V[1]. Crystallographic studies on AY 27–110 – a dopamine agonist of the troponylpiperazine series[2]. *Canadian Journal of Chemistry*, **60**, 2687–91.

Bjorklund, A. & Lindvall, O. (1964). Dopamine-containing systems in the CNS. In *Classical Transmitters in the CNS, Handbook of Chemical Neuroanatomy*, vol. 2, pt. 1, ed. A. Bjorklund & T. Hokfelt, pp. 55–122. Holland: Elsevier.

Clark, D., Hjorth, S. & Carlsson, A. (1985). Dopamine-receptor agonists: Mechanisms underlying autoreceptor selectivity. *Journal of Neural Transmission*, **62,** 1–52

Gershanik, O., Heikkila, R. H. & Devoisin, R. C. (1983). Effect of dopamine depletion on rotational behavior to dopamine agonists. *Brain Research*, **261,** 358–60.

Goldstein, M., Battista, A. F., Ohmoto, T., Anagnoste, B. & Fuxe, K. (1973). Tremor and involuntary movements in monkeys: effect of L-dopa and of a dopamine receptor stimulating agent. *Science*, **179,** 816.

Goldstein, M., Kuga, S., Kusano, N., Meller, E., Dancis, J. & Schwarcz, R. (1986). *Brain Research*, **367,** 114–20.

Goldstein, M., Lew, J. Y. & Nakamura, S. (1978). Dopaminephilic properties of ergot alkaloids. *Federal Proceedings*, **37,** 2202–5.

Goldstein, M., Lieberman, A. & Battista, A. F. (1984). The therapeutic potential of centrally acting dopamine agonists. *Trends in Pharmacological Sciences*, **5,** 227–30.

Goldstein, M., Lieberman, A., Lew, J. Y., Asano, T., Rosenfeld, M. & Makman, M. H. (1980). Interaction of pergolide with central dopaminergic receptors. *Proceedings of the National Academy of Sciences, USA*, **77,** 3725–8.

Goldstein, M., Lieberman, A. & Meller, E. (1985). A possible molecular mechanism for the antiparkinsonian action of bromocriptine in combination with levodopa. *Trends in Pharmacological Sciences*, **6,** 436–7.

Hornykiewicz, O. (1972). Dopamine and extrapyramidal motor function and dysfunction. In *Neurotransmitters, Association for Research in Nervous and Mental Disease, Research Publications*, vol. 50, pp. 390–415. New York: Raven Press.

Kapatos, G., Katoh, S. & Kaufman, S. (1982). Biosynthesis of biopterin by rat brain. *Journal of Neurochemistry*, **39,** 1152–62.

Lloyd, K. G., Hornykiewicz, O., Davidson, L., Shannak, K., Farley, I., Goldstein, M., Shibuya, M., Kelly, W. N. & Fox, I. H. (1981). Biochemical evidence of dysfunction of brain neurotransmitters in the Lesch–Nyhan syndrome. *The New England Journal of Medicine*, **305,** 1106–11.

Markstein, R., Jaton, J. L., Vigouret, J. M., Giger, R., Closse, A., Briner, U. & Enz, A. (1984). Pharmacological properties of 201–678 a new dopamine agonist. *Clinical Neuropharmacology,* **7,** 800–1.

Meller, E., Helmer-Matyjek, E., Bohmaker, K., Adler, C. H., Friedhoff, A. J. & Goldstein, M. (1986). Receptor reserve at striatal dopamine autoreceptors: Implications for selectivity of dopamine agonists. *European Journal of Pharmacology,* **123,** 311–4.

Poirier, L. J. and Sourkes, T. L. (1965). Influence of the substantia nigra on the catecholamine content of the striatum. *Brain*, **88,** 181–92.

Ruffolo, R. (1982). Important concepts of receptor theory. *Journal of Autonomic Pharmacology,* **2,** 277–95.

Seyfried, C., Fuxe, K., Wolf, H.-P & Agnati, L. F. (1982). Neurochemical and functional studies with EMD 23 448, a novel dopamine agonist. *Acta Pharmaceutica Suecica*, **2,** 243–7.

Sibley, D. R. & Creese, I. (1983). Interaction of ergot alkaloids with anterior pituitary D-2 dopamine receptors. *Molecular Pharmacology*, **23,** 585–93.

Sibley, D. R., De Lean, A. & Creese, I. (1982). Anterior pituitary dopamine receptors. *Journal of Biological Chemistry*, **257,** 6351–61.

Wilson, J. M., Young, A. B. & Kelley, W. N. (1983). Hypoxanthine-guanine phosphoribosyltransferase deficiency: The molecular basis of the clinical syndromes. *The New England Journal of Medicine*, **309,** 900–10.

4

Tardive dyskinesia – a historical review

Caroline M. Tanner and Harold L. Klawans

4.1 Introduction

'Tardive dyskinesia' is the term used to describe the syndrome of abnormal involuntary movements produced by chronic treatment with neuroleptic agents. The predominant involuntary movement in tardive dyskinesia (TD) is chorea, although dystonia, tics, myoclonus and the subjective sensation of akathisia have all been described as part of the TD syndrome (Fahn, 1983). This chapter will review the historical development of clinical and preclinical understanding of tardive dyskinesia.

4.2 Early clinical descriptions

The successful treatment of schizophrenia with chlorpromazine was reported in 1952 (Delay & Deniker, 1952). Reserpine (1954) and the butyrophenone, haloperidol (1959) were soon recognized to have similar therapeutic properties. These 'major tranquilizers' or 'neuroleptics' were distinguished from the minor tranquilizers by five points (Delay & Deniker, 1968): '(i) The production of a peculiar psychomotor apathy. (ii) Value in the treatment of agitation and excitement. (iii) Progressive amelioration of acute and chronic psychotic states. (iv) Production of diencephalic and extrapyramidal syndromes. (v) A site of action which is primarily at subcortical levels.' It was at first believed that the acute movement disorders (dystonia and parkinsonism) produced by neuroleptics related directly to their antipsychotic efficacy. The introduction of thioridazine, a potent antipsychotic which produces relatively few motor disturbances, disproved this claim (Cole & Clyde, 1961). The neuroleptics gained rapid and widespread use – between the years 1955 and 1965 chlorpromazine alone was estimated to have been given to over 50 million patients (Jarvik, 1970).

Shortly after the introduction of neuroleptics, several acute and subacute movement disorders, including parkinsonism (Steck, 1954) and akathisia, were recognized as side effects of neuroleptic administration. These were known to abate with anticholinergic therapy and to resolve after cessation of the neuroleptic (Delay & Deniker, 1968). A persistent movement disorder with different clinical characteristics was described five years later (Schonecker, 1957). Three middle aged women with lipsmacking which had developed after weeks or months of chlorpromazine treatment and which did not improve with anticholinergic drugs were reported, along with an adolescent with a typical acute dystonia which did respond to anticholinergic drugs. These movements persisted for up to 11 weeks after drug withdrawal. A more extensive description of the TD syndrome was published two years later (Sigwald *et al.*, 1959). In this report, four non-psychotic middle aged women were reported to develop involuntary movements of the mouth and trunk which persisted for months after neuroleptic therapy was discontinued. The authors believed the movements to result from chronic neuroleptic treatment, and postulated that the movements would gradually abate during a long drug-free period.

The report of Sigwald and colleagues was soon followed by an epidemiologic survey of 155 women chronically treated with perphenazine (Uhrbrand & Faurbye, 1960). Although the investigators did not clearly distinguish all cases of acute dystonia and Parkinsonism from chronic movement abnormalities, they reported 29 patients with a particular movement abnormality of oral and trunk musculature which sometimes persisted for months after neuroleptic discontinuation. A special susceptibility of the elderly, and of those with pre-existing brain injury was proposed for the first time in their report. Subsequently, numerous clinical descriptions and several additional epidemiologic studies verified the existence of this iatrogenic disorder (Crane, 1968).

Nonetheless, interest in and concern about TD was not great during the fifties and sixties. Many authors considered TD to be a rare phenomenon. In a review of the published reports of irreversible dyskinesia after neuroleptic use, Kline concluded that the majority of those reported had pre-existing brain damage. He summarized: 'Since there are less than two dozen reported cases in non-brain-damaged patients among 100 million estimated users the finding is interesting but not of great clinical significance' (Kline, 1968). Others, citing descriptions of abnormal movements in early descriptions of schizophrenia by Kraepelin, ignored the reports of irreversible movements in nonpsychotic patients and argued that the movements called 'tardive dyskinesia' in neuroleptic treated patients were not the result of drug therapy, but rather were manifestations of the disease itself. Interest in pathogenetic mechanisms was minimal, and generally limited to postulates of underlying brain damage. Increased doses of neuroleptic drugs had been observed to ameliorate the movements of TD, and neuroleptic withdrawal or increase were the sole recommended therapies (Delay & Deniker, 1968).

Crane played a critical, and, at times, lonely role in establishing TD as a disease entity. In 1968, he reviewed over 500 cases included in the 21 papers published since 1959 and proposed this definition of TD: '(i) involuntary movements; (ii) late occurrence in the course of treatment and often after discontinuation of drug administration; (iii) persistence of disabling manifestations for months or years in a high percentage of cases; and (iv) poor response to any type of therapy' (Crane, 1968). Crane went on to explore the range of clinical presentation of TD, and possible risk factors for its development. In addition to the classic buccal masticatory syndrome, he recognized choreic movements of other body parts, sometimes leading to their own complications, such as dysarthria, shortness of breath and dysphagia with weight loss. He recognized that 'movements of the lips and tongue are . . . often socially objectionable, and thus a source of considerable embarrassment to the patient and his family', qualifying the commonly held belief, based on reviews of institutionalized populations, that patients are unaware of their symptoms. Crane assessed the role of age, sex, type of drug, dose of drug, psychiatric and other diagnoses, and concurrent therapies in TD. Crane found that older patients, women, and those with pre-existing brain damage appeared to be most prone to develop TD, but he was unable to establish a relationship between diagnosis, type or dose of neuroleptic, or concurrent therapies and TD.

During the early seventies, recognition of TD as a serious iatrogenic problem became widespread. In 1973, the American College of Neuropharmacology – Food and Drug Administration Task Force published a general warning to all physicians, stating that: 'Tardive dyskinesia is sufficiently prevalent to warrant an educational campaign advising the medical profession of its occurrence' (Schiele *et al.*, 1973). In this report, signs of TD were represented as choreic only, and largely limited to the mouth. Women and older persons were identified as at increased risk, but the occurrence of TD in non-psychotic outpatients was also described. Physicians were encouraged to use the lowest possible dose of neuroleptic, to avoid use of antipsychotic drugs for non-psychotic conditions when possible, and to give psychiatric patients periodic drug-free trials, under supervision, when possible.

In the same year, Crane again challenged those who questioned the importance or existence of TD by reviewing those cases reported since 1967, as well as the literature describing the prevalence of movement abnormalities in untreated psychiatric patients (Crane, 1973). These latter included his own studies in Turkey, where neuroleptics were rarely used, and led him to the conclusion that 'the high incidence of tardive dsykinesias in drug-treated populations and the relative rarity of such abnormalities in similar untreated populations provide compelling evidence to indicate that tardive dyskinesia is related to the use of phenothiazines or similar agents'. In this report, Crane also carefully distinguished TD from other neuroleptic-induced movements disorders, observing that both TD and drug-induced Parkinsonism ('pseudoparkinsonism') could occur together. The relationship of changes in neuroleptic therapy, with increased TD as neuroleptics were decreased and the apparent 'resolution' of TD after increased neuroleptic doses was also described. Finally, a review of the two postmortem studies, as well as the one surgical observation, led to the postulate that the area of dysfunction was in the upper brainstem. This was coupled with a review of early pharmacologic postulates, attempting to identify an anatomic and pharmacologic basis for TD, once again focusing on the scientific description of this iatrogenic disease.

4.3 Pharmacologic hypotheses

The next important development in TD research resulted from a revolutionary breakthrough in the treatment of a chronic neurologic illness, Parkinson's disease, with the precursor of the neurotransmitter dopamine (Hornekiewicz, 1966). L-DOPA was dramatically effective in decreasing the akinesia, tremor, rigidity and postural reflex deficits of Parkinson's disease, but was soon noted to cause choreic lipsmacking, tongue-protrusion, and sometimes more generalized chorea, which phenomenologically resembled the movements of TD (Cotzias *et al.*, 1969). At about the same time, neuroleptic drugs were recognized to block central nervous system dopamine receptors (van Rossum, 1966), and their ability to produce a Parkinsonian syndrome was attributed to this property.

The clinical similarities of TD and l-DOPA-induced dyskinesias led to the hypothesis of a common pharmacologic pathophysiology for all choreic disorders (Klawans *et al.*, 1970). Chorea was proposed to represent a relative overactivity of striatal dopamine activity, resulting from chronic dopamine receptor blockade in TD ('denervation hypersensitivity'), and from the combined result of a partially denervated striatum and exogenous 1-DOPA therapy in Parkinson's disease (Klawans, 1973). In this way chorea was the pharmacologic opposite of Parkinsonism, which resulted from decreased striatal dopamine activity, whether as the result of receptor blockade in neuroleptic-induced Parkinsonism, or actual loss of substantia nigra dopaminergic neurons in Parkinson's disease. This pharmacologic observation explained the decrease in TD movements after an increase in neuroleptic dose (with consequent increased blockade of striatal dopamine receptors) as well as the exacerbation of movements with drug discontinuation (and consequent decreased blockade of the same receptors). Additionally, since Parkinsonism was known to respond to central antimuscarinic drugs, a reciprocal antagonism between dopamine and acetylcholine in the striatum was proposed. TD would be postulated to worsen after anticholinergic treatment, and improve during enhanced cholinergic activity. Such a relationship was subsequently demonstrated in TD patients who were acutely treated with such agents (Klawans & Rubovits, 1974).

This proposal of a pharmacologic pathophysiology for TD led to a variety of clinical and preclinical investigations, whose common goal was treatment or prevention of this iatrogenic disorder.

4.4 Animal studies

Animal models for TD have largely used either non-human primates or rodents and guinea pigs. Ideally, an animal model should mimic the human disorder, thereby providing a setting in which to address questions of prevention and therapy.

The primate models of TD have been proposed to best approximate the human condition. In initial studies, when neuroleptics were chronically administered to non-human primates, acute dystonic reactions and mouthing movements which resolved with cessation of neuroleptic therapy were observed, but persistent dyskinesias were not (Paulson, 1973). The failure of these studies to produce a disorder similar to persistent dyskinesias, plus the expense and small numbers of animals available for any one study, precluded the application of this model to questions of treatment or prevention. More recently, a few investigators have produced dyskinesias which persist for weeks after neuroleptic discontinuation in certain monkeys (Domino & Kovacic, 1983). Although this model may be the closest to the human condition, the small numbers of affected animals and reversibility of the condition limit further applications.

The acute production of quantifiable stereotypic behaviors in rodents and guinea pigs after administration of a dopaminergic agent was well accepted by the mid-sixties (Randrup & Munkvad, 1967). These acute stereotypies were shown to directly reflect striatal dopamine activity, by the local application of dopaminergic agents and neuroleptics to these and other brain areas (Ernst & Smelik, 1966, Fog *et al.*, 1967) and were consequently proposed as a model of TD (Rubovits & Klawans, 1972). This model was subsequently criticized, however, since the signs of TD develop after chronic, not acute, drug therapy. In 1972, Klawans and Rubovits described the production of the same stereotypic behavioral response to apomorphine, a dopamine receptor agonist, in guinea pigs who had been chronically treated with chlorpromazine, then withdrawn before apomorphine challenge. The same dose of apomorphine was too low to produce stereotypic behavior in control animals not exposed to neuroleptics. They proposed that this hypersensitive behavioral response to dopaminergic agents after chronic neuroleptic therapy, which more closely resembled the clinical and pharmacologic conditions felt to underlie TD, was preferable to acute stereotypic behaviors as an animal model. In subsequent studies, numbers of striatal dopamine receptors were found to be increased after chronic neuroleptic administration in this model, and TD was proposed to reflect striatal denervation hypersensitivity (Hitri *et al.*, 1978).

More recently, this model has been used to address a variety of questions of potential clinical relevance. A hypersensitive behavioral response to a dopaminergic agent after chronic treatment with and subsequent withdrawal of a neuroleptic agent (termed 'behavioral hypersensitivity' or BH) has been shown to result from doses of most neuroleptics, including chlorpromazine, haloperidol, trifluoperazine, and prochlorperazine, but not from doses of the 'atypical' neuroleptics thioridazine (Klawans *et al.*, 1980) and clozapine (Kobayashi, 1977), given in equal antipsychotic doses. BH is increased in direct relationship to dose and duration of the neuroleptic (Klawans *et al.*, 1981). Attempts to use this model to develop preventive or therapeutic regimens have resulted in observations that concurrent therapy with neuroleptics and antimuscarinic drugs (Carvey *et al.*, 1986), apomorphine (Christiansen & Moller-Nielson, 1980), and amantadine prevent the development of BH (Borison *et al.*, 1980). Friedhoff and colleagues found that low doses of l-DOPA could reverse established BH (Friedhoff *et al.*, 1978).

Others have criticized the use of the above rodent model, since it differs from the human condition in its distribution (occurring in 100% of animals), its time course (occurring in three weeks and resolving in six weeks), and in its failure to produce spontaneous movements, but rather to produce BH only after neuroleptic withdrawal and dopaminergic challenge. In an attempt to produce spontaneous dyskinesias in a model without the attendant economic restraints of primates, two groups (Clow *et al.*, 1980; Iversen *et al.*, 1980) have treated rats for up to 12 months. Although both observed spontaneous mouth movements after chronic therapy, in each case these resolved with removal of neuroleptic, thus suggesting a closer resemblance to neuroleptic-induced Parkinsonism than to TD.

4.5 Recent clinical studies

From the middle seventies to the present day, TD research has focused on an epidemiologic approach to identification of risk factors, the search for an underlying pathology, and the development of effective prevention or treatment protocols.

In order to describe a disease epidemiologically, accurate clinical criteria for its diagnosis must be determined. Thus, during the seventies a variety of rating scales was developed to facilitate the assessment of movement disorder in neuroleptic-treated patients (Fann *et al.*, 1980). Unfortunately, many of these scales included movements such as tremor which are not part of TD, and to some extent contributed to confusion in the clinical differentiation of TD from other movements disorders in the same population. An example of this is the description of a late-onset neuroleptic-induced disorder, named the 'rabbit syndrome' (Villeneuve *et al.*, 1973), which was characterised by rhythmic involuntary movements of the masticatory musculature, at five cycles per second, which were diminished after anticholinergic therapy. Little consideration is needed to determine that 'rabbit syndrome' applies to drug-induced Parkinsonian tremor of the jaw and oral musculature, but its proposal as a separate late consequence of neuroleptic therapy is typical of the diagnostic confusion which occurred.

Variations in the clinical course of TD were also described in the seventies. Although persistent TD had been recognized from the earliest descriptions of TD, the possibility that dyskinesias might reverse was not well recognized. The concept of 'withdrawal dyskinesias' (Jacobson *et al.*, 1974) led to questions concerning the early reversibility of TD. Others identified the potential mortality of TD (Mehta *et al.*, 1978; Casey *et al.*, 1978).

Many epidemiologic studies, especially prevalence studies in institutionalized psychiatric populations, attempted to clarify the role of such factors as dose, duration and type of neuroleptic to the development of TD. By 1979, Tepper and Haas identified 44 studies and attempted to apply these data to evaluate at least some of these questions (Tepper

& Haas, 1979). They estimated 2.2 million Americans had received neuroleptic prescriptions in 1978, of whom at least 27% were potential chronic users. Using the prevalence range of 24% to 56% from the studies reviewed, they concluded that at least 33%, or 198 000 patients will develop TD. They concluded that increasing age and female sex are risk factors for TD, but could not demonstrate effects of dose, duration, type of neuroleptic or other diagnoses in the development of TD.

Attempts to define an underlying pathologic or anatomic abnormality were another active area of enquiry during this period, although largely unsuccessful. Early researchers evaluated pneumoencephalogram and electroencephalogram (Jeste *et al.*, 1979) reports without clearly demonstrating differences. Later, a particular EEG pattern was described in TD, but this has not been replicated (Wegner *et al.*, 1979). Studies of CAT scans have similarly been unable to demonstrate a specific pathology (Jeste *et al.*, 1980). Postmortem evaluations of routine and pharmacologic measures have similarly been unable to distinguish clearly TD patients from neuroleptic-treated controls (Jellinger, 1977).

Although treatment with tetrabenazine was reported to be useful in TD in 1961 (Brandrup, 1961), therapeutic trials in TD followed the development of a pharmacologic hypothesis of this disorder. By the early seventies, dopamine depleting agents were reported by many researchers to benefit TD (McCallum, 1979; Villeneuve & Bosormenyi, 1970). Others attempted to increase central cholinergic activity (Klawans *et al.*, 1975; Davis *et al.*, 1976), or GABAergic systems (Korsgaard, 1976), but with less success. The literature of the seventies and early eighties abounds with anecdotal reports of therapeutic successes in TD which are not replicated in larger series (Tanner, 1983), while the treatment of choice remains that of presynaptic dopamine depleting agents, both for their efficacy and their lack of risk for continuing the pathogenesis of the disorder (Fahn, 1983).

By the early 1980s, the experience of the last decade of research was summarized by the American Psychiatric Association Task Force (Baldessarini *et al.*, 1980). This report concludes that clinically recognizable TD occurs in 10–20% of patients receiving chronic neuroleptics for more than one year, perhaps somewhat more in the elderly and in women. One fourth to one half of patients who are withdrawn from neuroleptics may undergo remission or improvement after one year. Recommendations for management included the use of neuroleptics only when clearly indicated, with constant reassessment of the continuing need for such therapy. When neuroleptic agents are necessary to control the psychiatric illness, the committee comments: 'since tardive dyskinesia seems not to be a uniformly relentless and progressive disorder, it may be prudent to continue neuroleptic therapy temporarily if the psychiatric indications are sufficiently compelling'. Finally, the search for a specific neuroleptic agent, with antipsychotic activity but no motor side effects, is encouraged.

The five years since 1980 have seen the redefinition of clinical subcategories of TD (Fahn, 1983). 'Tardive dyskinesia' is used to designate the choreic disorder, while tardive dystonia, a term first used in 1973 (Keegan & Rajput, 1973), is once again applied to neuroleptic-induced movements which are predominantly dystonic (Burke *et al.*, 1982). Most recently, a syndrome of persistent motor restlessness occurring independently of chorea ('tardive akathisia') has been described (Fahn, 1983). The advances in clinical pharmacotherapy which have occurred in the treatment of disorders with the same clinical signs but different etiologies have been applied to neuroleptic-induced movements. Thus, although dopamine depleting agents are used in all cases, anticholinergic drugs may benefit tardive dystonia but aggravate chorea. Tardive akathisia may respond to narcotic analgesics, which are of no benefit in other neuroleptic-induced syndromes.

References

Appenzeller, O. & Biehl, J. P. (1967). Mouthing in the elderly. *Neurology*, **17,** 290.

Baldessarini, R. J., Cole, J. O., Davis, J. M., Simpson, G., Tarsy, D., Gardos, G. & Preskorn, S. H. (1980). Tardive Dyskinesia: Summary of a Task Force Report of the American Psychiatric Association. *American Journal of Psychiatry*, **137,** 1163–72.

Borison, R. L. & Diamond, B. I. (1980). Anticholinergics promote neuroleptic-induced tardive dyskinesia. In *Long-term Effects of Neuroleptics, Advances in Biochemical Psychopharmacology*, vol. 24, ed. F. Cattabeni, G. Racgni, P. F. Spano & E. Casta, pp. 359–62. New York: Raven Press.

Boszormenyi, Z. (1970). Treatment of drug-induced dyskinesia. *Lancet*, I, 353–4.

Brandrup, E. (1961). Tetrabenacine treatment in persisting dyskinesia caused by psychopharmaca. *American Journal of Psychiatry*, **118,** 551–2.

Burke, R. E., Fahn, S., Jankovic, J., Marsden, C. D., Lang, A. E., Gollomp, S. & Ilson, J. (1982). Tardive dystonia: Late-onset and persistent dystonia caused by antipsychotic drugs. *Neurology*, **32,** 1335–46.

Carvey, P. M., Kao, L. C., Tanner, C. M., Goetz, C. G. & Klawans, H. L. (1986). The effect of antimuscarinic agents on haloperidol-induced behavioral hypersensitivity. *European Journal of Pharmacology*, **120,** 193–9.

Casey, D. E. & Rabins, P. (1978). Tardive dyskinesias as a life-threatening illness. *American Journal of Psychiatry*, **135,** 486–8.

Christensen, A. V. & Moller-Neilsen, I. (1980). On the supersensitivity of DA receptors after single and repeated administration of neuroleptics. In *Tardive*

Dyskinesia, ed. W. E. Fann, R. C. Smith, J. M. Davis & E. F. Domino, pp. 35–50. New York: Medical & Scientific Books.

Clow, A. T., Jenner, P. & Marsden, C. D. (1980). Changes in cerebral dopamine function induced by a year's administration of trifluoperazine or thioridazine and their subsequent withdrawal. In *Long-term Effects of Neuroleptics, Advances in Biochemical Psychopharmacology*, vol. 24, ed. F. Cattabeni, G. Racgni, P. F. Spano & E. Costa, pp. 335–40. New York: Raven Press.

Cole, J. O. & Clyde, D. J. (1961). Extrapyramidal side effects and clinical response to the phenothiazines. *Revue can. Biol.*, **20,** 565–74.

Cotzias, C. G., Papavasiliou, P. S. & Gellene, R. (1969). Modification of parkinsonism – chronic treatment with L-dopa. *The New England Journal of Medicine*, **280,** 338–44.

Crane, G. E. (1968). Tardive dyskinesias in patients treated with major neuroleptics. A review of the literature. *American Journal of Psychiatry*, **124** (Feb. Suppl.), 40–8.

Crane, G. E. (1973). Persistent dyskinesia. *British Journal of Psychiatry*, **122,** 395–405.

Davis, K. L., Hollister, L. E., Barchas, J. D. & Berger, P. A. (1976). Choline in tardive dyskinesia and Huntington's disease. *Life Science*, **19,** 1507–16.

Delay, J. & Deniker, P. (1952). Trente-huit cas de psychoses traitées par la cure prolongée et continué de 4560 RP. Le Congrès des Al. et Neurol. de Langue Fr. In *Compte rendu du Congrès*. Paris: Masson et Cie.

Delay, J. & Deniker, P. (1968). Drug-induced extrapyramidal syndromes. In *Handbook of Clinical Neurology*, vol. 6, ed. P. J. Vinken & G. W. Bruyn, pp. 248–66. Amsterdam, North Holland: Elsevier.

Domino, E. F. & Kovacic, B. (1983). Monkey models of tardive dyskinesia. *Modern Problems in Pharmacopsychiatry*, **21,** 21–2.

Ernst, A. M. & Smelik, P. G. (1966). Site of action of dopamine and apomorphine on compulsive gnawing behavior in rats. *Experientia (Basel)*, **22,** 837.

Fahn, S. (1983). Treatment of tardive dyskinesia with dopamine depleting agents. *Clinical Neuropharmacology*, **6,** 151–8.

Fann, W. E., Smith, R. C., Davis, J. M. & Domino, E. F. (ed.) (1980). Tardive dyskinesia scales in current use. In *Tardive Dyskinesia: Research & Treatment*, pp. 243–67. New York: SP Medical & Scientific Books.

Fog, R. L., Randrup, A. & Pakkenberg, H. (1968). Neuroleptic action of quaternary chlorpromazine and related drugs injected into various brain areas in rats. *Psychopharmacologia (Berlin)*, **12,** 428.

Friedhoff, A. J., Rosengarten, H. & Bonnet, K. (1978). Receptor cell sensitivity modification as a model for pathogenesis and treatment of tardive dyskinesia. *Psychopharmacology Bulletin*, **14,** 77–9.

Hitri, A., Weiner, W. J., Borison, R. L., Diamond, B. I., Nausieda, P. A. & Klawans, H. L. (1978). Dopamine receptor binding in an animal model of tardive dyskinesia. *Annals of Neurology*, **3,** 134–40.

Hornykiewicz, O. (1966). Dopamine (3-hydroxytyramine) and brain function. *Pharmacology Review*, **18,** 925–64.

Iversen, S. D., Howels, R. B. & Hughes, R. P. (1980). The behavioral consequences of long-term treatment with neuroleptic drugs. In *Long-term Effects of Neuroleptics, Advances in Biochemical Psychopharmacology*, vol. 24, ed. F. Cattabeni, G. Racgni, P. F. Spano & E. Costa, pp. 305–14. New York: Raven Press.

Jacobson, G., Baldessarini, R. J. & Manschreck, T. (1974). Tardive and withdrawal dyskinesia associated with haloperidol. *American Journal of Psychiatry*, **131**, 910–3.
Jarvik, M. E. (1958). Are there any psychotherapeutic or psychotomimetic drugs? In *Psychopharmacology: Pharmacologic Effects on Behavior*, ed. H. H. Pennes, pp. 203–21. New York: Paul B. Hoeber, Inc.
Jellinger, K. (1977). Neuropathologic findings after neuroleptic longterm therapy. In *Neurotoxicology*, ed. L. Roizin, H. Shiraki & N. Grecevic, pp. 25–42. New York: Raven Press.
Jeste, D. V., Potkin, S. G., Sinha, S., Feder, S. & Wyatt, R. J. (1979). Tardive dyskinesia: reversible and persistent. *Archives of General Psychiatry*, **36**, 585–90.
Jeste, D. V., Wagner, R. L., Weinberger, D. R., Reith, K. G. & Wyatt, R. J. (1980). Evaluation of CT Scans in tardive dyskinesia. *American Journal of Psychiatry*, **137**, 247–8.
Jones, M. Hunter, R. (1969). Abnormal movements in patients with chronic psychiatric illness. In *Psychotropic Drugs and Dysfunctions of the Basal Ganglia*, ed. G. E. Crane & R. Gardner, Jr, pp. 53–8. Washington D.C.: Public Health Service Publication, 1938.
Keegan, D. L. (1973). Drug induced dystonia tarda: treatment with L-Dopa. *Diseases of the Nervous System*, **38**, 167–9.
Klawans, H. L. (1973). *The Pharmacology of Extrapyramidal Movement Disorders*. Basel: S. Karger.
Klawans, H. L., Carvey, P., Nausieda, P. A., Goetz, C. G. & Weiner, W. J. (1980). Effect of dose and type of neuroleptic in an animal model of tardive dyskinesia. *Neurology*, **30**, 384.
Klawans, H. L. Jr, Ilahi, M. M. & Shenker, D. (1970). Theoretical implications of the use of L-dopa in parkinsonism. *Acta Neurologica Scandinavica*, **46**, 409.
Klawans, H. L., Nausieda, P. A., Goetz, C. G., Carvey, P. & Weiner, W. J. (1981). Effect of duration of neuroleptic therapy in an animal model of tardive dyskinesia. *Neurology* **31**, 103.
Klawans, H. L. & Rubovits, R. (1972). An experimental model of tardive dyskinesia. *Journal of Neural Transmission*, **33**, 235–46.
Klawans, H. L. & Rubovits, R. (1974). The effect of cholinergic and anticholinergic agents on tardive dyskinesias. *Journal of Neurology, Neurosurgery and Psychiatry*, **37**, 941–7.
Klawans, H. L., Topel, J. L. & Bergen, D. (1975). Deanol in the treatment of levodopa-induced dyskinesias. *Neurology*, **25**, 290–3.
Kline, N. S. (1968). On the rarity of 'irreversible' oral dyskinesias following phenothiazines. *American Journal of Psychiatry* **124** *(Feb. Suppl.) 8*, 48–54.
Korsgaard, S. (1976). Baclofen (Lioresal) in the treatment of neuroleptic-induced tardive dyskinesia. *Acta Psychiatrica Scandinavica*, **54**, 17–24.
McCallum, W. A. G. (1970). Tetrabenazine for extrapyramidal movement disorders. *British Medical Journal*, I, 760.
Mehta, D., Mallya, A. & Volavka, J. (1978). Mortality of patients with tardive dyskinesia. *American Journal of Psychiatry*, **135**, 371–2.
Randrup, A. & Munkvad, I. (1967). Stereotyped activities produced by amphetamine in several animal species and man. *Psychopharmacology*, **11**, 300.
Rubovits, R. & Klawans, H. L. (1972). Implications of amphetamine-induced stereotyped behavior as a model for tardive dyskinesias. *Archives of General Psychiatry*, **27**, 502–7.

Rubovits, R., Patel, B. C. & Klawans, H. L. (1973). Effect of prolonged chlorpromazine pretreatment on the threshold of amphetamine-induced stereotypy: a model for tardive dyskinesias. *Advances in Neurology*, **1,** 671–5.

Schiele, B. C., Gallant, D., Simpson, G., Gardner, E. A. & Cole, J. O. (1973). Tardive dyskinesia: A persistent neurological syndrome associated with antipsychotic drug use. *Annals of Internal Medicine*, **79,** 99–100.

Schonecker, V. M. (1957) Ein eigentumliches Syndrom in oralen Bereich bei Megphen applikation. *Nervenarzt*, **28,** 35–43.

Sigwald, J., Bouttier, D., Raymondeaud, C. & Piot, C. (1959). Quatre cas de dyskinesie facio-buccal-linguo-masticatrice à l'evolution prolongée secondaire a un traitement par les neuroleptiques. *Revue Neurologique*, **100,** 750–5.

Steck, H. (1954). Le syndrome extra-pyramidal et di-encephalique au cours des traitements au Largactil et au Serpasil. *Ann. med.-psychol.*, **112,** 737–43.

Tanner, C. (1983). Treatment of tardive dyskinesia; other therapies. *Clinical Neuropharmacology*, **2,** 159–67

Tepper, S. J. & Haas, J. F. Prevalence of tardive dyskinesia. *Journal of Clinical Psychiatry*, **40,** 508–16.

van Rossum, J. M. (1966). The significance of dopamine receptor blockade for the action of neuroleptic drugs. In *Neuro-Psychopharmacology*, ed. H. Brill, J. O. Cole, P. Deniker, H. Hippius & P. Bradley, p. 166. Proceedings of the 5th International Congress of the Collegium Internationale Neuropsychopharmacologicum, Washington, DC, March, 1966. International Congress Series no. 129.

Villeneuve, A. (1972). Rabbit syndrome – a peculiar extrapyramidal reaction. *Canadian Psychiatric Association Journal*, **17,** 69–72.

Wegner, J. T., Struve, F. A. & Kanton, J. S. (1979). Relationship between the B mitten EEG pattern and tardive dyskinesia. *Archives of General Psychiatry*, **36,** 599–603.

Yarden, P. E. & Di Scipio, W. J. (1971). Abnormal movements and prognosis in schizophrenia. *American Journal of Psychiatry*, **128,** 317–23.

5

Gilles de la Tourette syndrome

Jack W. Schweitzer and Arnold J. Friedhoff

5.1 Introduction

One hundred years ago, George Gilles de la Tourette (1885) identified a cluster of verbal behaviors and motor tics which he characterized as a syndrome. His original description is still used as the basis for the diagnosis of a disorder that has since come to be known as Tourette's syndrome (TS) in the United States. Patients with this disorder have frequent motor tics and coprolalia, echolalia or echopraxia (Goetz & Klawans, 1982).

Because of the nature of the symptoms, there has been considerable controversy in the past as to whether TS is primarily a psychiatric or neurologic disorder. Whereas Gilles de la Tourette believed that the disorder was primarily neurological, psychiatric approaches to therapy prevailed during the first half of the twentieth century. Current consensus is that the disease is, fundamentally, neurologic in origin but that it is rare for a patient to be free of secondary or associated psychiatric symptoms (Montgomery *et al.*, 1982).

There has been a suspicion that at least some forms of the disorder may be genetically transmitted because of the occurrence of the illness in several generations of some families; however, TS typically appears in isolated cases without family history of the illness. The study of genetic aspects of TS is complicated by the fact that its symptoms may not be fully expressed in all cases. Obsessive compulsive symptoms, for example, have been found in high frequency in relatives of TS patients (Montgomery *et al.*, 1982). For the moment no definitive mode of genetic transmission has been established although interesting work is in progress (Kidd *et al.*, 1980; Comings, 1984).

Over the last decade, therapeutic success, to a greater or lesser degree, has been attained with drugs acting on the dopaminergic system.

Recently, cholinergic and serotonergic drugs have, in experimental settings, provided transient relief and therefore these pathways have also been implicated in TS. Involvement of the noradrenergic system in TS may also be of significance because of the reported beneficial effects of the α_2-agonist, clonidine.

In this review we will discuss possible mechanisms in TS as well as mechanisms that may be involved in the action of drugs used for treatment of TS.

5.2 The dopaminergic system

At a time when dopamine was considered to be simply a metabolic intermediate in the tyrosine-to-norepinephrine biosynthetic pathway, neuroleptics were found effective in TS (Bockner, 1959; Mesnikoff, 1959; Caprini & Melotti, 1961; Seignot, 1961). Their early use stemmed from the view then that TS was, primarily, a psychiatric disorder (reviewed by Shapiro & Shapiro, 1982).

Neuroleptics remain the drugs of choice in TS. From a compilation of neuroleptic drug activity in relation to the dopaminergic system, Stahl & Berger (1982a) found a direct relationship between the rank order of neuroleptic potency in TS and in schizophrenia. The same order has been found for potency toward blockade of rat striatal dopamine D_2 receptors. Further evidence for the involvement of the dopaminergic system in TS comes from clinical trials with other classes of dopaminergic drugs. Thus, α-methyl-*p*-tyrosine (Sweet *et al.*, 1974) which blocks dopamine synthesis, and tetrabenazine (Jankovic *et al.*, 1984) which prevents intraneuronal storage of dopamine, are also ameliorative. Interestingly, apomorphine, a dopamine agonist, is somewhat effective at low doses (Feinberg & Carroll, 1979). Its positive effects are attributed to its ability to stimulate dopamine autoreceptors which, in turn, start a chain of events leading to a reduction in the release of dopamine (Cutler *et al.*, 1982). At higher doses, dopamine agonists, as might be expected, tend to exacerbate symptoms of TS (Pollack *et al.*, 1977).

In addition to the D_2 receptor a dopamine D_1 receptor is also present. The D_1 receptor activates a system that stimulates the production of c-AMP. Unlike the D_2 receptor, the affinity of neuroleptics for the D_1 receptor does not correlate with their therapeutic effects (Table 5.1). In a seminal report, Stoof & Kebabian (1981) demonstrated that the simultaneous blockade of D_2 receptors and specific stimulation of D_1

receptors by the new drug, SKF 38393, greatly augmented the production of c-AMP. On the other hand, stimulation of the D_2 receptor with the specific D_2 agonist, LY 141865 reduced the accumulation of c-AMP to a level below the basal value.

Rosengarten *et al.* (1983), in our laboratories, set out to determine whether a specific behaviour might emerge under conditions where stereotypic D_2-mediated behaviors such as biting, chewing, licking and rearing (Tarsy & Baldessarini, 1972; Costall & Naylor, 1973) could be specifically blocked. Using a low dose of spiroperidol (40 μg/kg), a neuroleptic that is about 7000 times more potent against the D_2 than the D_1 receptor (Hyttel, 1978), followed one hour later (at the peak of spiroperidol's potency) by either apomorphine (0.3 mg/kg) or SKF 38393 (5 mg/kg) a new behavior emerged. Best described as repetitive jaw movements, it consisted of rapid bursts of jaw activity, occasional tongue thrusting and rapid movement of the cheeks. This is the first recognized D_1-mediated behavior. Similar effects were seen when spiroperidol was replaced by another D_2 antagonist and neuroleptic, sulpiride. The same pattern but at a lower rate appeared when rats were treated with the specific D_1 agonist, SKF 38393. More recently, the Schering Corp. has made available the first specific D_1 antagonist, SCH 23390 (Iorio *et al.*, 1983). Its effects in mental disorders are presently unknown. The oral behaviors we have described are completely blocked with this antagonist (Rosengarten, Schweitzer & Friedhoff, 1986). A summary of the actions of newer drugs on the D_1 and D_2 systems is given in Table 5.2.

Table 5.1. *Rank order of neuroleptic efficacy in Tourette syndrome and in inhibition of dopamine stimulatable adenylate cyclase*

Drug	TS efficacy	Inhibition of adenylate cyclase
Haloperidol	1	4
Droperidol	1	8
Pimozide	1	7
Fluphenazine	2	1
Perphenazine	3	2
Chlorpromazine	4	3
Trifluoperazine	5	3
Thioridazine	6	5
Clozapine	7	6

TS efficacies were adapted from Stahl & Berger (1982a) and the rank order for inhibition of adenylate cyclase was derived from data reported by Hyttel (1978).

As a consequence of the introduction of these specific drugs differential effects of D_1 and D_2 receptors are at present being newly evaluated (Casey *et al.*, 1985). It has been found, for example, that stereotypic behaviors, formerly considered to be inducible only by D_2 stimulation, appear to be inducible by D_1 stimulation as well, under appropriate conditions. Stoof *et al.* (1985) have found that both a D_1 and a D_2 receptor regulate the electrical activity of growth hormone producing cells of the pond snail, *Lymnaea stagnalis*.

Another curious relationship between the two synaptic receptor systems occurs with the destruction of the nigrostriatal dopaminergic system. Prior to the intracranial administration of 6-hydroxydopamine, post-synaptic D_1 and D_2 receptors are capable of being stimulated or inhibited by agonists and antagonists specific to the individual receptors, as measured by behavioral changes. After such treatment, however, the two receptors no longer respond only to their 'own' agonist; however, antagonist specificity is retained (Arnt, 1985). This may occur because of the induction of supersensitivity as a consequence of the massive denervation caused by 6-hydroxydopamine. The supersensitive D_1 neurons might be expected to respond to D_2 agonists at lower dose inasmuch as some crossover specificity normally exists between D_1 and D_2 agonists.

In a book that is remarkable for the author's sensitivity to the subject, Sacks (1974) gives his insights on the ravages of Parkinson's disease and of the reversals shortly after the immediately striking effects obtained with l-DOPA. In an effort to reduce the bizarre behavior and thinking that most of the patients underwent while on l-DOPA, Sacks initiated the coadministration of carefully measured amounts of phenothiazine or butyrophenone neuroleptics. Both good effects and side effects were reduced or exacerbated idiosyncratically with such combinations. His findings and those of others provide evidence to indicate that changes

Table 5.2. *Effects of specific D_1 and D_2 receptor agonists and antagonists*

Treatment of rat or striatal tissue	Action	Behavior[a]	c-AMP level
SKF 38393	D_1 agonist	Repetitive jaw movements	Increased[b]
Sulpiride	D_2 antagonist	Repetitive jaw movements	Increased[b]
LY 141865	D_2 agonist	Stereotypy only	Decreased[b]
SCH 23390	D_1 antagonist	None	Decreased[c]

[a]From Rosengarten *et al.* (1983). [b]From Stoof & Kebabian (1981). [c]From Onali *et al.* (1984).

produced by the destruction of the nigrostriatal dopaminergic system may involve more than a permanent information loss between the dopaminergic–cholinergic synaptic link.

The reason for common acceptance of this singular relationship can be understood from the way in which most neuroleptic drugs have been developed. Potential neuroleptics, often structurally related to the earliest ones discovered, are identified as such by their ability to produce catalepsy and ability to block a conditioned avoidance response. Catalepsy is one behavioral response to D_2 blockade. It is not surprising, therefore, that neuroleptic potency against D_2 receptors, as measured, for example, by radioligand binding techniques, should parallel neuroleptic potency in schizophrenia and, as well, blockade of the D_2-mediated behaviors such as the cluster of behaviors commonly referred to as stereotypic movements. If, under normal circumstances, the D_2 system predominates, in that D_2 behaviors are more easily elicited by D_2 stimulation than are D_1 behaviors initiated by D_1 stimulation, and, if some of the same behaviors are inducible by both receptors, as discussed earlier, then neuroleptic intervention will be perceived, in the main, as blocking all dopaminergic behaviors and functions. Perhaps the reason for Sacks' inability to control the side effects of l-DOPA therapy in parkinsonism by means of neuroleptic blockade was that, largely, only D_2 functions were blocked and D_1 functions (side effects) were now being seen or actually augmented because of the selective blockade.

In Table 5.1 several neuroleptics are ranked for their efficacy against TS and for their inhibition of dopamine stimulatable adenylate cyclase. There is good agreement when the phenothiazines are taken alone ($r = 0.86$, $n = 5$, where r is correlation coefficient, n number of neuroleptics tested) but not when all of the neuroleptics are considered ($r = 0.3$, $n = 9$). It will only be determined if D_1 receptors play a role in the mediation of some TS symptoms when specific D_1 agonists and antagonists have been developed.

It should also be noted that the two most effective neuroleptics, haloperidol and pimozide, at the doses used in TS, are relatively specific D_2 antagonists, probably having little spillover to D_1 receptors. Many of the phenothiazines, in contrast, although they tend to be primarily D_2 blockers, have a relatively high affinity for D_1 receptors when compared with haloperidol or pimozide.

Another approach to the treatment of TS has been to reduce the activity of the dopaminergic system by persistent exposure to agonist. We have shown previously (Friedhoff *et al.*, 1977) that the return of supersensitive dopamine receptors to the control level was faster when rats were treated with l-DOPA. We call such treatment receptor sensitivity modification (RSM) (Friedhoff & Miller, 1983). This approach has been somewhat successful in schizophrenia (Schweitzer *et al.*, 1984) and has been applied in TS (Friedhoff, 1982). Transient amelioration was observed following some initial worsening in patients who were unable to tolerate the side effects of haloperidol treatment. In this pilot study, recurrence occurred in all six cases within four months to two years. Several patients have been successfully retreated.

5.3 The serotonergic system

Serotonin is capable of blocking glutamate excitation of dopamine neurons (Aghajanian & Bunney, 1974) and therefore, would be expected to reduce dopamine release (Hutson *et al.*, 1981). Fostering antidopaminergic activity should be beneficial in TS and, indeed, transient amelioration of tics has been reported with tryptophan administration (Yaryura-Tobias, 1979). In contrast, Barabas *et al.* (1984) have found a tenuous association between serotonergic agonist activity and TS in that a subgroup of TS patients, mostly young boys, also suffered from migraine headaches. Serotonin agonists can bring on such attacks and methylsergide, a serotonin antagonist, is an effective treatment (Goodman & Gilman, 1965).

No consistent evidence has emerged for alterations in serotonin metabolism in TS. Leckman *et al.* (1984), for example, found tryptophan, but not serotonin, to be lower in whole blood of TS patients. 5-hydroxyindoleacetic acid, the principal metabolite of serotonin has also been measured in CSF of TS patients and controls. Butler *et al.* (1979) measured lumbar CSF 5-HIAA in nine TS children and 39 non-TS neurological patients. Additionally, TS patients, but not the controls, were given probenecid to allow for a greater accumulation of the 5-HT metabolite in CSF. Control values for this part of the study were obtained from estimates on adults in other studies. Results showed a trend toward lower levels of 5-HIAA in TS patients and some of the TS children also showed impaired post-probenecid accumulation of the metabolite. In a similar study, Cohen *et al.* (1979) failed to observe a lower baseline of 5-HIAA in TS but agreed that accumulated 5-HIAA was lower after probenecid. These results, although clouded by problems associated with the use of probenecid (Koslow *et al*, 1982), are compatible with the proposal that serotonin may be underutilized in TS.

5.4 The GABAergic system

Certain behaviors seen in TS are reminiscent of seizure-like responses. As described by Cohen *et al.* (1982) the TS patient has '. . .

a crescendo of bodily tension ... which he resists. The ... act becomes irresistible and the patient eventually collapses, allowing for breakthrough of the motor discharge.' Roberts (1980) believes that seizures may occur when excitatory activity within the neuronal tissue exceeds the ability of that tissue to modulate the activity. The origins of such a state may reside in an increase in nerve membrane excitability, blockade of inhibitory transmitter function or a decrease in the amount of available inhibitory transmitter. Such considerations, derived from observations of behaviors in Huntington's chorea where GABAergic and dopaminergic deficits are found (Lloyd *et al.*, 1980; Barbeau *et al.*, 1973) have prompted inquiries into the possible role of GABA (γ-aminobutyric acid) in TS.

Attempts at treating TS with GABAergic drugs – agonists as well as antagonists and antianxiety agents have not been successful (Shapiro & Shapiro, 1981; Shapiro *et al.*, 1981). In an examination of body fluid levels of GABA in TS, Van Woert *et al.* (1982) found CSF and blood levels to be lower, but the decreases were not statistically significant. Thus, at the present time, biochemical and clinical observations have not been in support of the largely intuitive association of GABA with TS.

5.5 The noradrenergic system

Clonidine, a potent α_2-adrenergic agonist, has been reported to be effective in treatment of TS (Cohen *et al.*, 1979a,b). Shapiro *et al.* (1983) have reported some beneficial effects of clonidine but failed to achieve as high a success rate as that of Cohen's group. They have suggested that this might result from the higher doses used in their study. This conclusion was based on an observation by Cederbaum & Aghajanian (1977) that, at low doses clonidine, through its autoreceptor action, would decrease the release of norepinephrine, whereas at high doses the drug would itself activate noradrenergic post-synaptic receptors. Thus if this biphasic action of clonidine on TS symptoms is correct, any therapeutic effect of clonidine would presumably be through its decrease of norepinephrine release at relatively low doses. Borison *et al.* (1982) have reported that higher doses of clonidine actually exacerbate TS symptoms. Leckman *et al.* (1982) have reported that the maximum benefit from clonidine often took place after months of treatment. This suggests that a change in α_2-receptor number due to agonist-induced down-regulation may be important. Interestingly, however, they found that effective responses to long term treatment were reasonably predictable from positive physiological responses such as sedation, release of growth hormone, hypotension and a decline in plasma MHPG, the major metabolite of norepinephrine (NE), with acute treatment.

In contrast to the evidence for the participation of the noradrenergic system in the action of clonidine in TS, a consistent pattern of metabolic alterations in noradrenergic activity in TS has not emerged. As summarized in Table 5.3, urinary MHPG is reported variously as decreased or not changed with respect to control values. In addition, dopamine-β-hydroxylase (DBH), the enzyme responsible for the conversion of dopamine to NE, monoamine oxidase (MAO) and catechol-*O*-methyltransferase (COMT), catabolic enzymes, remained unaltered in activity; however, Leckman *et al.* (1983) have reported that both clonidine and the neuroleptic, haloperidol, were capable of elevating plasma homovanillic acid (HVA), the principal metabolite of dopamine.

Other evidence points to a possible indirect relationship between the noradrenergic system and TS. The serotonergic system has been implicated in the mediation of responses by the dopaminergic system following challenges to the noradrenergic system. Thus, Bunney *et al.* (1982) found that α_2 antagonism (by piperoxane) reversed dopamine agonist-induced depression of dopaminergic activity in the intact animal but not after the serotonergic system was destroyed by means of 5,7-dihydroxytryptophan administration. In a previous study by this group (Svensson *et al.*, 1975) it was shown that clonidine was capable of inhibiting raphe noradrenergic neurotransmission which, in turn, suppressed serotonergic activity in that area of the brain. Unexpectedly, Leckman *et al.* (1984) found that whole blood serotonin was elevated following chronic clonidine treatment in TS. The changes, however, did not correspond to

Table 5.3. *Norepinephrine metabolism in Tourette syndrome*

Substance	Change *vis-à-vis* controls	Reference
Plasma NE	↔	Lake *et al.* (1977); Eldridge *et al.* (1977)
CSF MHPG	↔	Butler *et al.* (1979)
Urinary MHPG	↓	Sweeney *et al.* (1978)
Urinary MHPG	↓	Ang *et al.* (1982)
Urinary MHPG	↔	Cohen *et al.* (1979a)
Plasma DBH	↔	Lake *et al.* (1977); Eldridge *et al.* (1977)
Platelet MAO	↔	Lake *et al.* (1977)
Erythrocyte COMT	↔	Lake *et al.* (1977)
Fibroblast COMT	↔	Giller *et al.* (1980)
Fibroblast MAO	↑	Giller *et al.* (1980)

therapeutic outcome which led them to conclude that elevated serotonin is not directly related to the ameliorative effects of clonidine in TS.

5.6 The cholinergic system

Physostigmine (Sweet *et al.*, 1976), a cholinesterase inhibitor, and the acetylcholine precursors, lecithin (Polinsky *et al.*, 1980) and choline (Stahl & Berger, 1981; Barbeau, 1980) give transient relief of tics in TS. All three approaches are known to elevate acetylcholine levels in the CNS (Haubrich *et al.*, 1976; Cohen & Wurtman, 1976; Hanin *et al.*, 1979; Rosenberg & Davis, 1982). Conversely, anticholinergics such as benztropine (Sweet *et al.*, 1976) and atropine (Stahl & Berger, 1981) tend to exacerbate the frequency of tics. As treatments, however, acetylcholine precursors and cholinomimetics are short-acting and the ingestion of choline itself can induce nausea (Barbeau, 1978). These drugs therefore have served largely to reveal cholinergic involvement in TS.

Post-synaptic D_2 receptors are known to be located on cholinergic interneurons in the striatum. Blockade of these receptors disinhibits these neurons leading to a release of acetylcholine. Since hyperdopaminergia can exacerbate TS, so should drugs that are capable of blocking cholinergic (muscarinic) receptors. It may not, therefore, be by accident that the order of potency of neuroleptic drugs for efficacy in TS is inversely related to their abilities to block muscarinic receptors (Stahl & Berger, 1982a,b). The outstanding efficacy of haloperidol in TS, therefore, may not be due solely to its potency toward blockade of D_2 receptors but also because of its relatively weak ability to bind to muscarinic receptors. In contrast, the neuroleptics thioridazine and clozapine are reported to be less effective in TS, despite their abilities toward blockade of D_2 receptors, perhaps because they happen to be potent muscarinic receptor antagonists as well.

5.7 Animal models of Tourette syndrome

In contrast to models of fairly well-defined illnesses, such as Huntington's chorea, Parkinson's disease or phenylketonuria, where a specific biochemical abnormality has been recognized and, therefore, ramifications of the induced effect should be strongly related to the human disorder, no such defect has been identified in TS; however, in TS, many have assumed that a state of hyperdopaminergia exists because of the success with dopamine receptor blocking neuroleptic medication. Thus most of the proposed models have attempted to induce a hyperdopaminergic state. Some of these models are listed in Table

5.4. We have pointed out that the fact that dopamine antagonists such as haloperidol have therapeutic effects does not, in itself, warrant concluding that the primary condition results from hyperdopaminergia (Friedhoff, 1983; Friedhoff & Miller, 1983). Dopamine may be a mediator in a compensatory system designed to protect the CNS against perturbations of many different etiologies. From the fact that drugs that are effective in the treatment of schizophrenia and other psychoses also act in TS, it seems probable that antidopaminergic drugs are not interacting with the specific TS etiological factor, but rather are activating a dopamine dependent CNS restitutive system.

Iversen & Alpert (1982) have suggested that the caudate–putamen, which receives input from cortical regions involved with association and movement may be a site of dysfunction in TS. Another potential model is self-evident from a report by Pulst *et al.* (1983) in which is described the effects of carbon monoxide on an otherwise normal, healthy man. There developed several of the symptoms of TS, including coprolalia, echolalia, palalia and fits of shouting. Tics of the head and neck were also seen. Carbon monoxide poisoning has been studied in the primate (Ginsberg *et al.*, 1974) but there has been no attempt to develop a TS model in primate or rat.

Features of TS appear in encephalitis lethargica (Sacks, 1974) and it has been suggested (Devinsky, 1984) that, for this reason and with knowledge of the CNS location of vocalization lesions, damage to the periductal gray and midbrain tegmentum brain areas may be present in TS. Models with such lesions have not as yet been explored.

5.8 Conclusions

TS is a disorder that can have devastating consequences for its victims and their families. Frequently mistaken for a behavior disorder, patients have been subjected to inappropriate psychotherapy which has little effect on the tics, or worse, to punishment for bad behavior and cursing. The discovery that the tics were responsive to medication led to a reorientation about the disorder by knowledgeable

Table 5.4. *Animal models of Tourette syndrome associated with alterations in dopaminergic activity*

Treatment	Reference
l-DOPA	Friedhoff (1982)
6-hydroxydopamine	Shaywitz *et al.* (1982)
Iminodipropionitrile	Diamond *et al.* (1982)
Tail pinch	Knott & Hutson (1982)

physicians; however, the disorder being relatively uncommon, many physicians to this day have little familiarity with it or its treatment.

The disorder is of great scientific interest (for reviews of recent clinical findings see Friedhoff & Chase, 1982; Cohen & Leckman, 1984) because the pathology involves episodic release of control of both motor and higher speech centers. Although there may be associated pathology such as obsessions, compulsions, learning disabilities or attention deficit disorder, there is no impairment of intellectual function. Additionally, voluntary movement is not impaired and tics tend to be quiescent during vigorous activity. Many TS patients are excellent athletes, some even champions.

Thus the clinical symptomatology is not compatible with any known localized CNS lesions. It is more likely that there is an episodic collapse of a central inhibitory system that regulates highly integrated speech and motor phenomena. Which transmitter systems, if any, play a primary etiological role, and which are involved in compensatory roles, remains an enigma.

Some insight may be gained from the fact that the disorder is much more common in boys and in families of Mediterranean origin. The former is compatible with either a genetic factor or a hormonal role, whereas from the latter it would seem that there is a genetic factor. The suspicion that at least vulnerability may be inherited makes it worthwhile to initiate a search for an abnormal gene in patients with the disorder. The new genetic technology involving cutting of the human genome into several hundred fragments with restriction enzymes and searching for restriction fragment length polymorphisms (RFLP) that may be a marker for the disorder, hold promise, although the approach is tedious.

Other approaches may be dependent on our developing further insight into the basic regulation of tic motor and speech systems.

The authors are appreciative of helpful discussions with Helen Rosengarten, MD and Emanuel Meller, PhD regarding interactions of D_1 and D_2 dopamine receptors. This review was supported, in part, by a Research Scientist Award MH 14024 to A.J.F. and by Program Project Grant MH 08618, both from the National Institute of Mental Health.

References

Aghajanian, G. K. & Bunney, B. S. (1974). Dopaminergic and non-dopaminergic neurons of the substantia nigra: differential responses to putative transmitters. In *Proceedings of the 9th International Congress of the Collegium Internationale Neuropsychopharmacologicum*, ed. J. R. Bossier, H. Hippus & P. Pichot, pp. 444–52. Amsterdam: Excerpta Medica.

Ang, L., Borison, R., Dysken, M. & Davis, J. M. (1982). Reduced excretion of MHPG in Tourette Syndrome. In *Gilles de la Tourette Syndrome, Advances in Neurology*, vol. 35, ed. A. J. Friedhoff & T. N. Chase. New York: Raven Press.

Arnt, J. (1985). Independent dopamine D-1 and D-2 receptor function after denervation and after prolonged reserpine treatment. 4th World Cong. Biol. Psychiatry, Phila., Sept.

Barabas, G., Matthews, W. S. & Ferrari, M. (1984). Tourette syndrome and migraine. *Arch. Neurol.*, **41,** 871–2.

Barbeau, A. (1978). Emerging treatments: replacement therapy with choline or lecithin in neurological diseases. *Can. J. Neurol. Sci.*, **5,** 157–61.

Barbeau, A. (1980). Cholinergic Treatment in Tourette Syndrome. *New Engl. J. Med.*, **302,** 1310–1.

Barbeau, A., Chase, T. N. & Paulson, G. W. (1973) (ed.). *Huntington's Chorea: 1872–1972, Advances in Neurology*, vol. 1, pp. 1–801. New York: Raven Press.

Bockner, S. (1959). Gilles de la Tourette's disease. *J. Ment. Sci.*, **105,** 1078.

Borison, R. L., Ang, L., Chang, S., Dysken, M., Comaty, J. E. & Davis, J. M. (1982). New pharmacological approaches in the treatment of Tourette syndrome. In *Gilles de la Tourette Syndrome, Advances in Neurology*, vol. 35, ed. A. J. Friedhoff & T. N. Chase, pp. 377–82. New York: Raven Press.

Bunney, B. S. & De Riemer, S. (1982). Effect of clonidine on dopaminergic neuron activity in the substantia nigra; possible indirect mediation by noradrenergic regulation of the serotonergic raphe system. In *Gilles de la Tourette Syndrome, Advances in Neurology*, vol. 35, ed. A. J. Friedhoff & T. N. Chase, pp. 99–104. New York: Raven Press.

Butler, I. J., Koslow, S. H., Siefert, W. E., Jr., Caprioli, R. M. & Singer, H. S. (1979). Biogenic amine metabolism in Tourette syndrome. *Ann. Neurol.*, **6,** 37–9.

Casey, D. E., Chase, T. N., Christensen, A. V. & Gerlach, J. (ed.) (1985). *Dyskinesia: Research and Treatment*, pp. 2–223. New York: Springer Verlag.

Caprini, G. & Melotti, V. (1961). Un grave sindrome ticcose guerita con haloperidol. *Riv. Sper. Freniatr.*, **85,** 191–6.

Cederbaum, J. M. & Aghajanian, G. K. (1977). Catecholamine receptors on locus ceruleus neurons: pharmacological characterization. *Eur. J. Pharmacol.*, **44,** 375–85.

Cohen, D. J., Detlor, J., Shaywitz, B. A. & Leckman, J. F. (1982). Interaction of biological and psychological factors in the natural history of TS: A paradigm for childhood neuropsychiatric disorders. In *Gilles de la Tourette Syndrome, Advances in Neurology*, vol. 35, ed. A. J. Friedhoff & T. N. Chase, pp. 31–40. New York: Raven Press.

Cohen, D. J. & Leckman, J. F. (1984). (Special section on Tourette Syndrome). *J. Am. Acad. Child Psychiatry*, **23,** 123–81.

Cohen, D. J., Shaywitz, B. A., Young, J. G., Carbonaria, C. M., Nathanson, J. A., Lieberman, D., Bowers, M. B., Jr. & Mass, J. W. (1979a). Central biogenic amine metabolism in children with the syndrome of chronic multiple tics of Gilles de la Tourette: norepinephrine, serotonin and dopamine. *J. Am. Acad. Child Psychiatry*, **18,** 320–41.

Cohen, E. L. & Wurtman, R. J. (1976). Brain acetylcholine: control by dietary choline. *Science*, **191,** 561–2.

Cohen, D. J., Young, J. G., Nathanson, J. A. & Shaywitz, B. A. (1979b). Clonidine in Tourette's syndrome. *Lancet*, II, 551–3.

Comings, D. E. (1984). Detection of major gene for Gilles de la Tourette's syndrome. *Am. J. Hum. Genet.*, **36,** 586–600.
Costall, B. & Naylor, R. J. (1973). Neuroleptic and non-neuroleptic catalepsy. *Arzneim. Forsch.*, **23,** 674–83.
Cutler, N. R., Jeste, D. V., Karoum, F. & Wyatt, R. J. (1982). Low dose apomorphine reduces serum homovanillic acid concentration in schizophrenic patients. *Life Sci.*, **30,** 753–6.
Devinsky, O. (1983). Neurochemistry of Gilles de la Tourette's syndrome – possible midbrain involvement. *Arch. Neurol.*, **40,** 508–14.
Diamond, B. I., Reyes, M. G. & Borison, R. (1982). A new animal model for Tourette syndrome. In *Gilles de la Tourette Syndrome, Advances in Neurology*, vol. 35, ed. A. J. Friedhoff & T. N. Chase, pp. 221–5. New York: Raven Press.
Eldridge, R., Sweet, R., Lake, C. R., Ziegler, M. & Shapiro, A. K. (1977). Gilles de la Tourette's syndrome: Clinical, genetic, psychologic and biochemical aspects in 21 selected families. *Neurology*, **27,** 115–24.
Feinberg, M. & Carroll, B. J. (1979). Effects of dopamine agonists and antagonists in Tourette's disease. *Arch. Gen. Psychiatry*, **36,** 979–85.
Friedhoff, A. J. (1982). Receptor maturation in pathogenesis and treatment of Tourette syndrome. In *Gilles de la Tourette Syndrome, Advances in Neurology*, vol. 35, ed. A. J. Friedhoff & T. N. Chase, pp. 133–40. New York: Raven Press.
Friedhoff, A. J. (1983). A strategy for developing novel drugs for the treatment of schizophrenia. *Schizophr. Bull.*, **9,** 556–62.
Friedhoff, A. J., Bonnet, K. A. & Rosengarten, H. (1977). Reversal of two manifestations of dopamine receptor supersensitivity by administration of L-dopa. *Res. Commun. Chem. Pathol. Pharmacol.*, **16,** 411–23.
Friedhoff, A. J. & Chase, T. N. (ed.) (1982). *Gilles de la Tourette Syndrome, Advances in Neurology*, vol. 35, pp. 1–454. New York: Raven Press.
Friedhoff, A. J. & Miller, J. C. (1983). Clinical implications of receptor sensitivity modification. *Ann. Rev. Neurosci.*, **6,** 121–48.
Giller, E. L., Young, J. G., Breakefield, X. O., Carbonari, C., Braverman, M. & Cohen, D. J. (1980). Monamine oxidase and catechol-O-methyl transferase activities in cultured fibroblasts and blood cells from children with autism and the Gilles de la Tourette syndrome. *Psychiatry Res.*, **2,** 187–97.
Gilles de la Tourette, G. (1885). Etude sur une affection nerveuse characterisée par d'incoordination motrice accompagnée d'écholalie et de coprolalie. *Arch. Neurol. (Paris)*, **9,** 19–42; 185–200.
Ginsberg, M. D., Meyers, R. E. & McDonagh, B. F. (1974). Experimental carbon monoxide poisoning encephalopathy in the primate: II. Clinical aspects, neuropathology and physiologic correlation. *Arch. Neurol.*, **30,** 209–16.
Goetz, C. G. & Klawans, H. L. (1982). Gilles de la Tourette on Tourette syndrome. In *Gilles de la Tourette Syndrome, Advances in Neurology*, vol. 35, ed. A. J. Friedhoff & T. N. Chase, pp. 1–16. New York: Raven Press.
Goodman, L. S. & Gilman, A. (1965). *The Pharmacological Basis of Therapeutics*, pp. 1–652. Macmillan Co: New York.
Hanin, I., Merikangas, J. R., Merikangas, K. R. & Kopp, U. (1979). Red cell choline and Gilles de la Tourette syndrome. *New Engl. J. Med.*, **301,** 661–2.
Haubrich, D. R., Wedeking, P. W. & Wang, P. F. L. (1974). Increase in tissue concentration of acetylcholine in guinea pigs in vivo induced by administration of choline. *Life Sci.*, **14,** 921–7.

Hutson, P. H., Knott, P. J. & Curzon, G. (1981). Voltammetric and Behavioral effects of fenfluramine. In *Central Neurotransmitter Turnover*, ed. C. J. Pycock & P. V. Taberner, pp. 155–61. London: Croom Helm.
Hyttel, J. (1978). Effects of neuroleptics on ^{3}H-haloperidol and ^{3}H-cis(Z)-flupenthixol binding and on adenylate cyclase activity in vitro. *Life Sci.*, **23**, 551–6.
Iorio, L. C., Barnett, A., Leitz, F. H., Houser, V. P. & Korduba, C. A. (1983). SCH 23390, a potential benzazepine antipsychotic with unique interactions on dopaminergic systems. *J. Pharmacol. Exp. Ther.*, **226**, 462–8.
Iversen, S. & Alpert, J. E. (1982). Functional organization of the dopaminergic system in normal and abnormal behavior. In *Gilles de la Tourette Syndrome, Advances in Neurology*, vol. 35, ed. A. J. Friedhoff & T. N. Chase, pp. 69–76. New York: Raven Press.
Jankovic, J., Glaze, D. G. & Frost, J. D., Jr. (1984). Effect of tetrabenazine on tics and sleep of Gilles de la Tourette's syndrome. *Neurology*, **34**, 688–92.
Kidd, K. K., Prusoff, B. A. & Cohen, D. J. (1980). Familial pattern of Gilles de la Tourette syndrome. *Arch. Gen. Psychiatry*, **37**, 1336–9.
Knott, P. J. & Hutson, P. H. (1982). Stress-induced stereotypy in the rat: neuropharmacological similarities to Tourette syndrome. In *Gilles de la Tourette syndrome, Advances in Neurology*, vol. 35, ed. A. J. Friedhoff & T. N. Chase, pp. 233–8. New York: Raven Press.
Koslow, S. H. & Cross, C. K. (1982). Cerebrospinal fluid monoamine metabolites in Tourette syndrome and their neuroendocrine implications. In *Gilles de la Tourette Syndrome, Advances in Neurology*, vol. 35, ed. A. J. Friedhoff & T. N. Chase, pp. 185–97. New York: Raven Press.
Lake, C. R., Ziegler, M. G., Eldridge, R. & Murphy, D. L. (1977). Catecholamine metabolism in Gilles de la Tourette's syndrome. *Am. J. Psychiatry*, **134**, 257–60.
Leckman, J. F., Anderson, G. M., Cohen, D. J., Ort, S., Harderik, D. F., Hoder, E. L. & Syawitz, B. A. (1984). Whole blood serotonin and tryptophan levels in Tourette's disorder: effects of acute and chronic clonidine treatment. *Life Sci.*, **35**, 2497–503.
Leckman, J. F., Cohen, D. J., Detlor, J., Young, J. G., Harcherik, D. & Shaywitz, B. A. (1982). Clonidine in the treatment of Tourette syndrome: a review of data. In *Gilles de la Tourette Syndrome, Advances in Neurology*, ed. A. J. Friedhoff & T. N. Chase, pp. 391–401. New York: Raven Press.
Leckman, J. F., Cohen, D. J., Gertner, J. M., Ort, S. & Harcherik, D. F. (1984). Growth hormone response to clonidine in children ages 4–17; Tourette's syndrome vs. children with short stature. *J. Am. Acad. Child Psychiatry*, **23**, 174–81.
Leckman, J. F, Detlor, J., Harcherik, D. F., Young, J. G., Anderson, G. M., Shaywitz, B. A. & Cohen, D. J. (1983). Acute and chronic clonidine treatment in Tourette's syndrome: a preliminary report on clinical response and effect on plasma and urinary catecholamine metabolites, growth hormone and blood pressure. *J. Am. Acad. Child Psychiatry*, **22**, 433–40.
Lloyd, K. G., Beaumont, K. & Ziegler, M. (1980). Assessment of GABA receptors in different CNS diseases by means of radioligand assays. In *Psychopharmacology and Biochemistry of Neurotransmitter receptors*, ed. H. I. Yamamura, R. Wolson & E. Usdin, pp. 551–68. New York: Elsevier.
Mereu, G., Collu, M., Ongini, E., Biggio, G. & Gessa, G. L. (1985). SCH 23390, a selective dopamine D_1 antagonist, activates dopamine neurons but fails to prevent their inhibition by apomorphine. *Eur. J. Pharmacol.*, **111**, 393–6.

Mesnikoff, A. M. (1959). Three cases of Gilles de la Tourette's syndrome treated with psychotherapy and chlorpromazine. *Arch. Neurol. Psychiatry*, **81,** 710.
Montgomery, M. A., Clayton, P. M. & Friedhoff, A. J. (1982). Psychiatric illness in Tourette syndrome patients and first-degree relatives. In *Gilles de la Tourette Syndrome, Advances in Neurology*, vol. 35, ed. A. J. Friedhoff & T. N. Chase, pp. 335–9. New York: Raven Press.
Onali, P., Olianas, M. C. & Gessa, G. L. (1984). Selective blockade of dopamine D-1 receptors by SCH 23390 discloses striatal D-2 receptors mediating the inhibition of adenylate in rats. *Eur. J. Pharmacol.*, **99,** 127–8.
Polinsky, R. J., Ebert, M. H., Caine, E. D., Ludlow, C. & Bassich, C. J. (1980). Cholinergic treatment in the Tourette syndrome. *New Engl. J. Med.*, **302,** 1310.
Pollack, M. A., Cohen, N. L. & Friedhoff, A. J. (1977). Gilles de la Tourette syndrome: Familial occurrence and precipitation by methylphenidate therapy. *Arch. Neurol.*, **34,** 630–2.
Pulst, S. M., Walshe, T. M. & Romero, J. A. (1983). Carbon monoxide poisoning with features of Gilles de la Tourette's syndrome. *Arch. Neurol.*, **40,** 443–4.
Roberts, E. (1980). GABA receptor-related phenomena in seizures. In *Psychopharmacology and Biochemistry of Neurotransmitter Receptors*, ed. H. I. Yamamura, R. W. Olsen & E. Usdin, pp. 569–91. New York: Elsevier.
Rosenberg, G. S. & Davis, K. L. (1982). Precursors of acetylcholine: considerations underlying their use in Tourette syndrome. In *Gilles de la Tourette Syndrome, Advances in Neurology*, vol. 35, ed. A. J. Friedhoff & T. N. Chase, pp. 407–12. New York: Raven Press.
Rosengarten, H., Schweitzer, J. W. & Friedhoff, A. J. (1983). Induction of oral dyskinesias in naive rats by D_1 stimulation. *Life Sci.*, **33,** 2479–82.
Rosengarten, H., Schweitzer, J. W. & Friedhoff, A. J. (1985). Exposure to haloperidol in utero decreases the striatal D_2:D_1 ratio and permanently enhances a spontaneous oral behavior in rats. *4th Capo Boi Conf. on Neurosci. Villasimius, Sardinia*, June.
Rosengarten, H., Schweitzer, J. W. & Friedhoff, A. J. (1986). Tardive dyskinesia-like oral movements in rats: modulation by dopamine D_2 receptor activity. In *Fidea Research Series*, in press.
Sacks, O. W. (1974). *Awakenings*, p. 44. Garden City: Doubleday & Co. Inc.
Schweitzer, J. W., Bonnet, K. A. & Friedhoff, A. J. (1984). Receptor adaptation to psychotropic drugs. In *Handbook of Neurochemistry*, vol. 6, ed. A. Lajtha, pp. 639–60. New York: Plenum.
Seignot, M. J. N. (1961). Un cas de maladie des tics de Gilles de la Tourette gueri par le R-1625. *Ann. Med. Psychol.*, **119,** 578–9.
Shapiro, A. K. & Shapiro, E. (1981). The treatment and etiology of tics and Tourette syndrome. *Compr. Psychiatry*, **22,** 193–205.
Shapiro, A. K. & Shapiro, E. (1982). Tourette syndrome: history and present status. In *Gilles de la Tourette Syndrome, Advances in Neurology*, vol. 35, ed. A. J. Friedhoff & T. N. Chase, pp. 17–23. New York: Raven Press.
Shapiro, A. K., Shapiro, E. & Eisenkraft, G. J. (1983). Treatment of Gilles de la Tourette's syndrome with clonidine and neuroleptics. *Arch. Gen. Psychiatry*, **40,** 1235–40.
Shapiro, A. K., Shapiro, E. & Sweet, R. D. (1981). Treatment of tics and Tourette syndrome. In *Disorders of Movement*, ed. A. Barbeau, pp. 105–32. Lancaster, England: MTP Press Ltd.

Shaywitz, B. A., Wolf, A., Shaywitz, S. E., Loomis, R. & Cohen, D. J. (1982). Animal models of neuropsychiatric disorders and their relevance for Tourette syndrome. In *Gilles de la Tourette Syndrome, Advances in Neurology*, vol. 35, ed. A. J. Friedhoff & T. N. Chase, pp. 199–202. New York: Raven Press.

Stahl, S. M. & Berger, P. A. (1980). Physostigmine in Gilles de la Tourette's syndrome. *New Engl. J. Med.*, **302,** 298.

Stahl, S. M. & Berger, P. A. (1981). Physostigmine in Tourette syndrome: evidence for cholinergic underactivity. *Am. J. Psychiatry*, **138,** 240–2.

Stahl, S. M. & Berger, P. A. (1982a). Cholinergic and dopaminergic mechanisms in Tourette syndrome. In *Gilles de la Tourette Syndrome, Advances in Neurology*, vol. 35, ed. A. J. Friedhoff & T. N. Chase, pp. 141–50. New York: Raven Press.

Stahl, S. M. & Berger, P. A. (1982b). Neuroleptic effects in Tourette syndrome predict dopamine excess and acetylcholine deficiency. *Biol. Psychiatry*, **17,** 1047–53.

Stoof, J. C., De Vlieger, T. A. & Lodder, J. C. (1985). Opposing roles for D_1 and D_2 dopamine receptors in regulating the excitability of growth hormone-producing cells in the snail Lymnaea stagnalis. *Eur. J. Pharmacol.*, **106,** 431–5.

Stoof, J. C. & Kebabian, J. W. (1981). Opposing roles for the D_1 and D_2 dopamine receptors in efflux of c-AMP from rat neostriatum. *Nature*, **294,** 366–8.

Svensson, T. H., Bunney, B. S. & Aghajanian, G. K. (1975). Inhibition of both noradrenergic and serotonergic neurons in brain by the alpha adrenergic agonist clonidine. *Brain Res.*, **92,** 291–6.

Sweeney, D., Pickar, D., Redmond, D. E., Jr. & Maas, J. (1978). Noradrenergic and dopaminergic mechanisms in Gille de la Tourette syndrome. *Lancet*, I, 872.

Sweet, R. D., Bruun, R. D., Shapiro, A. K. & Shapiro, E. (1976). The pharmacology of Gilles de la Tourette's syndrome. In *Clinical Neuropharmacology*, vol. 1, ed. H. L. Klawans, pp. 81–106. New York: Raven Press.

Tarsy, D. & Baldessarini, R. J. (1974). Behavioral supersensitivity to apomorphine following chronic treatment with drugs which interfere with the synaptic function of catecholomines. *Neuropharmacology*, **13,** 927–40.

Van Woert, M. H., Rosenbaum, D. & Enna, S. J. (1982). Overview of pharmacological approaches to therapy for Tourette syndrome. In *Gilles de la Tourette Syndrome, Advances in Neurology*, vol. 35, ed. A. J. Friedhoff & T. N. Chase, pp. 369–75. New York: Raven Press.

Yaryura-Tobias, J. A. (1979). Gilles de la Tourette syndrome. Interactions with other neuropsychiatric disorders. *Acta Psychiatr. Scand.*, **59,** 9–16.

6

Aluminum and Alzheimer's disease

D. R. Crapper McLachlan

6.1 Introduction

Alzheimer's disease is a common, fatal metabolic disorder of the brain. Neither the etiology nor the pathogenesis of this degenerative disease of older people is understood.

The morphological changes which characterize the disorder include brain atrophy, loss of large neurons, senile (neuritic) plaques, neurofibrillary degeneration composed of paired helical filaments (PHFs) and granulovacuolar degeneration. Each of these morphological changes may occur in other degenerative diseases but the primary pathogenic events which initiate Alzheimer's disease release this unique combination of tissue responses.

Three major hypotheses have been advanced to account for this disease: an infectious agent, a cytopathic immunological response and an error in gene expression.

An incomplete conventional virus has been sought. Several authors have reported neurofibrillary degeneration composed of PHFs to be a delayed sequellae of virus infections (Hallervorden, 1933; Hadfield *et al.*, 1974; Mandybur *et al.*, 1977). Definitive experimental support for this hypothesis is wanting: viral DNA sequences have so far not been detected for vaccinia, herpes simplex I and II, hepatitis B, adenovirus 2 and SV40 (Middleton *et al.*, 1980; Taylor *et al.*, 1984; Pogo & Elizan, 1985).

An unconventional virus akin to the agent of scrapie and Jacob–Creutzfeldt has been postulated by numerous workers. Recent intensive investigations into the nature of the scrapie agent and the associated amyloid of the infectious neuritic plaque do not support this hypothesis. Alzheimer's disease has never been transmitted to laboratory animals and there is no epidemiological evidence for transmission in human populations. Furthermore, spongioform degeneration does not occur in Alzheimer's disease and PHFs never occur in the unconventional transmissible encephalopathies (Bruce, 1984; Somerville, 1985). Powers *et al.* (1981) reported that of eight intracellular antibodies tested, Alzheimer amyloid reacts only with neurofilament, and Glenner *et al.* (1984) reported that the amino acid composition of Alzheimer amyloid does not resemble that of scrapie amyloid. Recently, a gene has been identified whose expression is increased in the brain of scrapie affected animals and in the region of senile plaques of Alzheimer's disease (Wietgrefe *et al.*, 1985). A probable interpretation of these important findings is that both scrapie and the primary events which initiate Alzheimer's disease induce the expression of common genes. While exploitation of the unconventional virus hypothesis may provide useful markers for studying Alzheimer's disease, there is no firm support for a transmissible component to the illness at this time.

A cytotoxic immunological mechanism lacks experimental support, particularly in view of the increasing evidence that the proteins responsible for the amyloid of the Alzheimer plaque appear to arise from within the brain (Glenner, 1979; Powers *et al.*, 1981) rather than from circulating tissue destructive antibodies. The presence of circulating antibodies in senile plaques probably represents a post mortem artifact secondary to loss of the blood brain barrier after death (Torack & Lynch, 1981; Mann *et al.*, 1982).

6.2 Alzheimer's disease and altered gene expression: an hypothesis

This hypothesis views Alzheimer's disease to be the result of a disorder in gene expression, possibly triggered by environmental factors. The primary pathogenic events which initiate the illness probably result in reduced transcription of genetic information. The consequences of altered gene transcription is a reduction in protein synthesis and loss of cell homeostasis.

Fundamental to the regulation of gene expression is the controlled access of the enzyme RNA polymerase to genetic messages coded within DNA. Access to DNA is controlled by a number of DNA associated proteins which regulate the folding of DNA. Physical states of DNA range from dense compaction of completely repressed genes, through various stages of partial compaction to readily accessible and repeatedly expressed genetic information. Application of two independent techniques, sonication followed by differential centrifugation and enzymatic digestion with micrococcal nuclease, revealed an unique change in chromatin structure associated with Alzheimer's disease occurring in both neuron and glia enriched fractions (Crapper *et al.*, 1979; Lewis *et al.*, 1981; Crapper McLachlan *et al.*, 1984). Strong circumstantial evidence now indicates that a change in the physical accessibility of DNA to RNA polymerase in Alzheimer's disease may explain reduced RNA synthesis resulting in reduced protein synthesis (Crapper McLachlan & Lewis, 1985). Reduced protein synthesis may contribute to an impairment of cell homeostasis through a number of mechanisms including impairment in the regulation of energy metabolism, intracellular calcium content (McLachlan & Farnell, 1985), neurofilament metabolism or the failure to inactive potentially toxic substances such as aluminum (Crapper *et al.*, 1976) and excitatory toxic amino acids (De Boni & McLachlan, 1985). Our studies lead to the hypothesis that Alzheimer's disease results from a disorder in a 'master' gene which is responsible for the control of a large number of other genes, possibly through an action upon chromatin structure. This model parallels the idea of global regulators, 'regulons', of global regulatory networks, a concept which has been useful in elucidating regulation of bacterial homeostasis (Gottesman, 1984). Applied to Alzheimer's disease, this concept suggests that the 'master' gene regulates a defined set of genes crucial to neuronal homeostasis, particularly the barriers to aluminum.

There is other evidence in support of a genetic contribution to Alzheimer's disease: no animal, other than man, exhibits the histopathological features of the disease suggesting that the hominid genome is a necessary prerequisite for expression of the illness. Trisomy of chromosome 21, Down syndrome, is a major risk factor for pre-senile Alzheimer's disease (Jervis, 1948, Malamud *et al.*, 1972, Dalton *et al.*, 1974, Dalton & Crapper McLachlan, 1984). Greater than 95% of people with Down syndrome who are over the age of 40 exhibit the histopathological and, eventually, the clinical manifestations of pre-senile Alzheimer's disease. Finally, familial Alzheimer's disease with dominant inheritance, although rare, is well documented (Nee *et al.*, 1983) and evidence for susceptible loci on chromosomes 6 and 14 has been advanced (Weitkamp *et al.*, 1983). Furthermore, studies based upon consecutive series of patients with 'sporadic' Alzheimer's disease have suggested a pattern of expression compatible with autosomal dominance with extremely low penetrance or multifactorial inheritance (Heston & Mastri, 1977; Heyman *et al.*, 1983).

The exact role of environmental factors in the disease is uncertain but the extremely high frequency of the histopathological manifestations of the disease in the elderly, virtually 100% after age 70 years (Matsuyama & Nakamura, 1978) with clinical disability in 10% of individuals over the age of 65 (Katzman, 1976), suggests that a mutation is unlikely. Head injury has been implicated as a risk factor (Heyman *et al.*, 1984; Mortimer *et al.*, 1985). However, strong circumstantial evidence indicates that the neurotoxic element, aluminum, may play a role in the pathogenesis of Alzheimer's disease, particularly the neurofibrillary component of the illness (Crapper *et al.*, 1976; Yase, 1980) and, possibly, in gene expression.

6.3 Aluminum tolerance gene hypothesis

Although aluminum is the third most common element in the earth's crust and composes 8% by weight, there is no known biological function for this element. The brain tissues of six common species of mammal have low, closely similar concentrations ranging between 1.1 μg and 1.9 μg Al/g dry weight (Crapper *et al.*, 1976). The small crystal ionic radius and high charge (0.05 nm and valence 3) endow aluminum with prolonged ligand dissociation times, perhaps preventing the incorporation of this element into biological systems which require rapid, energy efficient, dissociation kinetics. Despite high bioavailability, the low cellular concentrations of aluminum implicate a genetically determined mechanism for exclusion which may operate broadly in biological systems. Indeed, chromosome locations for the genes controlling aluminum tolerance in wheat, rye and triticale have been localized to loci on chromosomes 2, 3, 4, 6 and 7 (Aniol Gustafson, 1984). Unfortunately, no information is available on the genetic loci important in the exclusion or turnover of aluminum in the mammalian brain. Nevertheless, the wide range of sensitivity to the neurotoxic effects of aluminum in mammals indicate genetic determinants for exclusion, detoxification and turnover. Once inside the blood brain barrier, rats and mice have considerably higher aluminum tolerance than cats and rabbits (King *et al.*, 1975). One explanation for the presence of aluminum in human degenerative brain disease is that the primary etiological events responsible for the initiation of the disease, among other disturbances, alters the aluminum tolerance gene permitting aluminum to accumulate in the central nervous system.

6.4 Aluminum in Alzheimer's disease

Following the initial reports that elevated concentrations approaching those found to be lethal in certain laboratory animals occur in Alzheimer's disease (Crapper *et al.*, 1973, 1976), a controversy arose concerning the universal reproducibility of these findings. The advent of improved technology, particularly instruments capable of performing elemental analysis in small tissue samples or intracellular loci has left little doubt that increased concentrations of aluminum occur in this disease. Table 6.1 lists those authors who have reported aluminum to be elevated in cerebral tissues associated with Alzheimer histopathology. Examination of the table indicates that four different techniques have been employed in at least ten independent laboratories. Table 6.1 also includes those authors who failed to find aluminum to be significantly elevated in Alzheimer's disease. Possible explanations for the failure to detect aluminum elevation in association with Alzheimer's histopathology have been presented elsewhere (Crapper *et al.*, 1980; Krishnan *et al.*, 1987).

The tissue sites which have so far been identified as loci of aluminum accumulation in Alzheimer's disease are given in Table 6.1. The principal loci are the nucleus, the neurofibrillary tangle, ferritin and the amyloid

Table 6.1. *Aluminum in neurodegenerative disease*

Author	Year	Technique	Site
(a) *Aluminum elevated in Alzheimer's disease*			
1 Crapper *et al.*	1973, 1976	AA	Total tissue
2 Duckett & Galle	1976	XMA	Neuritic plaque cores
3 Trapp *et al.*	1978	AA	Total tissue
4 Crapper *et al.*	1980	AA	Nucleus
5 Perl & Brody	1980	XMA	Nucleus
6 Perl *et al.*	1982	XMA	Tangle bearing neuron
7 Perry *et al.*	1985	XMA	Amyloid of neuritic plaque core
8 Masters *et al.*	1985	AA	Tangle & plaque cores
9 Yoshimasu *et al.*	1985	INA	Total tissue
10 Joshi *et al.*	1985	AA	Ferritin
(b) *Aluminum elevated in Alzheimer tangle bearing neurons*			
1 Liss *et al.*	1979	AA	Adjacent to hamartoma
2 Yase	1980	INA	Guam & Kii ALS/PD
3 Garruto *et al.*	1984	XMA	Guam ALS/PD
4 Yoshimasu *et al.*	1985	INA	Guam ALS/PD
(c) *Aluminum not found elevated in Alzheimer's disease*			
1 McDermott *et al.*	1977	AA	Total tissue
2 Markesbery *et al.*	1981	INA	Total tissue

Abbreviations for analytical techniques: AA: Atomic absorption spectrophotometry, INA: Instrumental neutron activation, XMA: X-ray microanalysis and wavelength dispersive spectrometry.

Other abbreviation: ALS/PD: Amyotrophic lateral sclerosis and Parkinsonian dementia syndrome of Guam.

core of senile plaques. The known neurotoxic manifestations of aluminum and the consequences of aluminum accumulation in these compartments are reviewed below.

6.5 Neurotoxic effects of aluminum

Four important neurotoxic responses induced in laboratory animals following intracerebral or systemic application of aluminum are: (i) disorders in learning–memory performance; (ii) changes in the cytoskeleton of certain types of neurons known as neurofibrillary degeneration; (iii) changes in nuclear function and (iv) altered electrical properties of neurons.

6.5.1 *Aluminum and behavior*

Changes in short-term memory during the early stage of the encephalopathy occur in cats trained to perform a delayed response task in the Wisconsin test apparatus. In fully trained animals, intracerebral injection of 6 μM to 9 μM of aluminum produced no changes in memory performance for eight to ten days but at the end of this asymptomatic period both delayed matching to sample and the rate of acquisition of a conditioned avoidance task became progressively impaired (Crapper & Dalton, 1973). The behavioral deficits are selective in the early stages of the encephalopathy because no changes in performance of visual discrimination tasks were noted and the speed of motor response was not altered. Intracerebral injection of 5 μM of aluminum in adult rabbits induced deficits in both acquisition of an active avoidance task ten days post-aluminum and in retention of the task three days later (Petit *et al.*, 1980). Infant rabbits injected intracerebral with 3.7 μM of aluminum also demonstrated impaired learning in a water maze (Rabe *et al.*, 1982). Furthermore, repeated subcutaneous injections of aluminum in mature rabbits affects classical conditioning (Yokel, 1983). Rabbits receiving accumulated doses of 4 mM or 8 mM over four weeks demonstrated a decrease in acquisition and increased latency to onset of the conditioned nictitating membrane response. Animals receiving a total of 2 mM, 1 mM or 0.5 mM aluminum did not exhibit altered responses. Thus, several laboratories have reported changes in learning and memory performance as an early sign of the aluminum encephalopathy in susceptible species.

At brain aluminum concentrations five-fold higher than cats, rats demonstrate a deficit in active avoidance response acquisition immediately following intracranial injection. However, rats do not readily develop a progressive encephalopathy, neurofibrillary degeneration or a chronic memory deficit (King *et al.*, 1975). A study, employing oral administration of aluminum in rats, reported that increased brain concentrations were associated with increased general activity, decreased ability to maintain roto-rod activity and increased sensitivity to flicker (Bowdler *et al.*, 1979). These authors did not observe impairment of acquisition of a shock avoidance task, but brain aluminum levels did not exceed twice the control levels. Furthermore, King *et al.* (1975) found interstrain variability in response to aluminum between hooded and Wistar rats as did Commissari *et al.* (1982) between Fisher and Sprague–Dawley rats in various behavioral tasks.

The behavioral effects of aluminum ingestion on elderly human behavior have also been studied. High serum concentrations of aluminum were found to be associated with decreased visuo-motor coordination, poor long-term memory and increased sensitivity to flicker fusion, (Bowdler *et al.*, 1979).

The major brain disorders in man in which aluminum has been implicated, Alzheimer's disease (Crapper *et al.*, 1973, 1976), dialysis dementia (Alfrey *et al.*, 1976), and the Parkinson-dementia-amyotrophic lateral sclerosis complex of Guam (Yase, 1980; Perl *et al.*, 1982) are dementing illnesses associated with changes in learning–memory performance.

In addition to changes in the performance of learning–memory tasks, other neurological signs develop in the experimental aluminum encephalopathy in cats which resemble, in part, the evolution of signs frequently encountered in protracted Alzheimer's disease. Following the appearance of impaired performance at the delayed response task, cats may develop disorders of limb movement, closely resembling the motor dyspraxias frequently seen in advanced Alzheimer's disease. Furthermore, in the latter stages of the encephalopathy cats develop a general increase in muscle tone, myoclonic jerks and seizures. Both of these changes may accompany the advanced stages of Alzheimer's disease. While the clinical course of the untreated experimental encephalopathy is only three to four weeks in duration and the animals usually die in status epilepticus (Crapper & Dalton, 1973a,b), the clinical course of Alzheimer's disease extends over many years and pneumonia, not status epilepticus, is usually the terminal event (Crapper McLachlan *et al.*, 1983). Nevertheless, the similarity in the clinical course between the two conditions is compatible with the hypothesis that aluminum may play an active role in the pathogenesis of the disease.

6.5.2 *Aluminum and the cytoskeleton*

An important manifestation of aluminum neurotoxicity is the induction of neurofibrillary degeneration. The soluble salts of aluminum, applied either intracerebrally or systemically, induce in several classes of neurons, including the large pyramidal shaped neurons of the neo- and pyriform cortex and anterior horn cells of the spinal cord, a marked accumulation of bundles of 10 nm single filaments which have immunochemical epitopes identical to those of neurofilaments. The neurofilaments of the aluminum induced tangles have epitopes indicative of hyperphosphorylation (Tronocoso *et al.*, 1985). A recent hypothesis postulates that the accumulation of neurofilaments in the soma and proximal processes in the aluminum encephalopathy is related to a failure of anterograde movement of the neurofilaments into axons (Bizzi *et al.*, 1984), possibly because hyperphosphorylation has altered the mechanisms responsible for the transport of neurofilaments (Sternberger *et al.*, 1985).

The neurofibrillary tangles of Alzheimer's disease differ morphologically from the aluminum induced tangle in laboratory animals. The Alzheimer tangle is composed of paired 10 nm filaments wound in a helix, (PHFs). The chemical composition of the PHFs is uncertain at present. There are two principal concepts concerning PHFs: in the most widely held model, PHFs are considered to be composed of modified cytoskeletal proteins. A large number of immunohistochemical studies from several laboratories indicate that PHFs share epitopes with the 150 kD and 200 kD moieties of neurofilaments (Rasool *et al.*, 1984; Perry *et al.*, 1985). The neurofilaments are also hyperphosphorylated, although the epitopes may differ from those induced by aluminum (Sternberger *et al.*, 1985). Epitopes for microtubule associated proteins, (MAP 2 proteins) and vimentin (Yen *et al.*, 1983) have also been detected in association with the Alzheimer tangle. A unique antigenic site in Alzheimer tangles gives origin to the 'PHF' antibody which reacts immunologically with Alzheimer's tangles, Pick bodies (Rasool *et al.*, 1985) and the tangles of supranuclear palsy (Dickson *et al.*, 1985) but does not recognize normal brain proteins (Ihara *et al.*, 1983). Selkoe (1985) has recently reported that both purified plaques and tangles exposed to 89% formic acid release a protein of approximately 5–7 kD molecular weight which reacts with PHF antibody. Thus neurofibrillary degeneration and amyloid share epitopes in common and are possibly of similar origin.

PHFs have never been reported following aluminum application in appropriate laboratory models, although aluminum is present in the human tangle (Perl *et al.*, 1982: Garruto *et al.*, 1984).

Another group of workers have presented evidence that PHFs arise from an unique protein not known to occur in normal brain tissue. Masters *et al.* (1985a,b) reported that the amino acid sequences of purified cerebral amyloid and purified neurofibrillary tangles are identical and postulate that cerebral amyloid may be of neuronal origin. The monomeric form of these proteins appears to be about 3.5 kD and also reacts with the antibody raised to PHFs by Selkoe. The dimeric form of the protein may be identical to the protein which Selkoe's group has eluted from amyloid. The amino acid sequence of the 3.5 kD protein reported by Masters *et al.* (1985) is unrelated to any known protein except amyloid. Resolution of the controversy concerning the chemical composition of PHFs must await further investigations.

In addition to the unique protein of amyloid and tangles, Masters *et al.* (1985b) report that the insoluble residue, remaining after formic acid extraction of protein from PHFs and amyloid cores, contains aluminum silicate. These authors speculate that the aluminum silicates could form a linear crystal with cationic exchange sites capable of ordering molecules in a linear array. Perry *et al.* (1985, personal communication) have also reported aluminum silicate in the amyloid cores of senile plaques from Alzheimer's disease and Down syndrome but at present neither report has presented evidence which indicates the exact physical state of the aluminum silicate. There are two aluminum silicate crystal arrays which are of particular biological interest: montmorillonite and imogolite clays. The surface chemistry of these clays is of interest because the crystal lattice offers cationic exchange sites capable of cleaving peptide bonds and organizing biological molecules (Weiss, 1981). These hypotheses demand that the PHFs and amyloid cores be closely examined for an aluminum silicate skeleton which contributes both to the unique structure and the highly insoluble nature of the PHFs. Determination of the exact physical state of aluminum in the Alzheimer tangle and plaque will aid in determining whether aluminum on these structures is merely a coincidence or an active cofactor in the assembly of PHFs.

In summary, aluminum may influence PHF formation through two mechanisms: one which results in the cytoplasmic accumulation of neurofilaments, as in the aluminum encephalopathy, and the other by crystal formation with silicon which contributes to the regular organization of peptide moieties into the unique PHF structure.

6.5.3 *Toxic effects of aluminum upon nuclear mechanisms*

The nucleus is a major intracellular site of aluminum accumulation in brains of experimental animals, normal human control and in Alzheimer's disease (Crapper *et al.*, 1980; Perl & Brody, 1980). In control human cerebral cortex, approximately 95% of total tissue aluminum can be accounted for in the nuclear compartment. In aluminum sensitive animals approximately 80% of the total tissue aluminum content in the encephalopathy occurs in the nucleus whereas only 20% to 30% of the total occurs in the nucleus of aluminum resistant animals such as the rat. One potential intranuclear effect of aluminum, demonstrated *in vitro*, is an interaction with DNA (Karlik *et al.*, 1980). Observations from this laboratory indicate that aluminum alters the binding of linker histones to DNA when isolated human brain nuclei are exposed to increasing concentrations of sodium chloride (Lukiw *et al.*, 1987). At aluminum concentrations approaching those found in Alzheimer's disease (30 aluminum atoms per dinucleosome, Crapper *et al.*, 1980) the elution pattern closely resembles that reported in Alzheimer's disease (Crapper McLachlan *et al.*, 1984: Table 4). Remarkably, this effect of aluminum upon histone elution from chromatin was not observed in either rabbit or rat brain nuclei. Linker histones exhibit considerable species variation and these observations support the hypothesis that aluminum may have toxic effects which are unique to human brain as a consequence of the complement of species specific linker histones and other DNA associated proteins. Furthermore, aluminum may contribute to the reduction in general transcription through a change in chromatin condensation. It is noteworthy that the aluminum content of intermediate euchromatin, expressed per gram of DNA, was a predictor for the percentage of heterochromatin prepared from Alzheimer neocortex (Crapper *et al.*, 1980).

A number of *in vivo* nuclear effects have been reported in the experimentally induced encephalopathy. Alterations in corticosterone binding to nuclei of the rabbit hippocampus, presumed to be a consequence of chromatin bound aluminum were reported by Sanderson *et al.* (1982). At aluminum concentrations of 3.3 $\mu g/ml$, cultured human lymphocytes demonstrated a significant reduction in sister chromatid exchanges (De Boni *et al.*, 1980). Direct experimental evidence indicating that aluminum alters gene expression in the experimental encephalopathy has been obtained by employing northern hybridization techniques in a quantitative dot–blot system to measure messenger RNA yield of calmodulin. These experiments reveal that twenty-four hours after the intracranial injection of aluminum lactate, rabbits exhibit a 40% decrease in calmodulin messenger RNA yield which persists for at least the next seven days (VanBerkum *et al.*, 1986). Total messenger RNA was not reduced. This is evidence in favor of a direct effect of aluminum upon the gene expression of a principal calcium receptor protein critical for the calcium regulation of several cellular functions. Thus, several intranuclear toxic effects upon nuclear function have been reported for the mammalian brain.

6.5.4 *Aluminum and ferritin*

Joshi *et al.* (1985) have reported that ferritin exists in human brain and that ferritin extracted from Alzheimer affected brain contains 10 times more aluminum than age and sex matched controls. Aluminum bound to ferritin alters the binding properties of this important iron storage molecule and it has been postulated by these workers that unbound iron(II) salts might contribute to free radical formation and membrane damage through peroxidation of lipid membranes. *In vitro* experiments of Gutteridge *et al.* (1985) indicate that aluminum greatly accelerates peroxidation of membrane lipids stimulated by iron salts.

6.5.5 *Aluminum and the electrical properties of neurons*

Changes in the electrophysiological properties of neurons in the aluminum encephalopathy involve both neurotransmitter effects and changes in membrane electrical effects. The electrical properties appear to change through a mechanism which disconnects excitatory post-synaptic potentials from the spike generator regions of neurons inducing electrical silence (Crapper & Tomko, 1975; Farnell *et al.*, 1982, 1985) and may occur in neurons other than those which are affected by neurofibrillary degeneration. Neurotransmitter effects as well as a number of neurochemical disturbances which affect excitability have been reviewed elsewhere (Crapper McLachlan *et al.*, 1985).

6.6 Aluminum concentration and neurotoxicity

Although a large number of neurotoxic effects of aluminum are now known, one of the most important issues is whether the aluminum concentration at a particular site in a human disease is in sufficient concentration to exert a toxic effect. While atomic absorption spectroscopy is quantitative and sensitive (10^{-11} g/1% absorption), the technique destroys tissue and requires a relatively large amount of tissue, 10–20 mg dry weight. Electronmicroscopic techniques employing x-ray emission are very sensitive, capable of detecting as little as 10^{-18} g of aluminum within a 1 μm diameter locus, however, the techniques have not yet been developed for reliable quantitative measurement. In the neocortex of Alzheimer's disease, only about 1–3% of large pyramidal shaped neurons are affected by neurofibrillary degeneration. If a defect in aluminum exclusion were to occur in only those cells which are either potentially susceptible to or actually undergoing neurofibrillary degeneration, very high local concentrations would be expected within a very small population of cells. Since neurons with neurofibrillary degeneration are not uniformly distributed in the neocortex and account for a minor percentage of the total cell population, large scale sampling procedures employed in atomic absorption spectroscopy or neutron activation would be expected to reveal only small changes in overall bulk tissue aluminum concentration. By these techniques the average aluminum content of control human brains in the age range between 50 and 65 years, completely free of neurofibrillary degeneration by light microscopic criteria, have an average aluminum content of 1.9 μg/g dry weight (±0.7 S.D.) as measured in our laboratory (Crapper *et al.*, 1976) and 1.53 μg/g as measured by McDermott *et al.*, (1977). While the mean overall value for 585 samples from ten Alzheimer affected brains was 3.8 μg Al/g dry weight, approximately 30% of the neocortical areas sampled had aluminum concentrations greater than the mean value of control brain plus three standard deviations of the mean, or 4 μg/g. In experimental animals the concentration of aluminum found to be toxic, as assessed by histopathology and electrophysiological means and measured in total tissue by atomic absorption spectrophotometry, is in the range of 4–8 μg/g, (Crapper & Tomko, 1975). Thus a third of the areas sampled in neocortex from Alzheimer's disease exhibit concentrations in the range which are associated with toxicity in rabbits and cats. Imaging techniques indicate high local concentration in neurons undergoing neurofibrillary degeneration but are not sufficiently sensitive enough to detect aluminum with normal cells. Thus information concerning whether aluminum does or does not accumulate prior to PHF formation in susceptible neurons is not yet available.

Intranuclear concentrations of aluminum, based on bulk isolation of nuclei of both neurons and glia also indicate an approximate increase of 200% in Alzheimer's disease: control = 716 μg Al/g DNA in the nucleus, Alzheimer = 1487 μg Al/g DNA. Cats, dying with an aluminum encephalopathy, reveal about a 366% increase in intranuclear aluminum following a dose which is lethal to 100% of animals: control = 705 μg Al/g DNA, aluminum treated = 2582 μg Al/g DNA (Crapper *et al.*, 1980).

6.7 Conclusions and future directions

The neurotoxic properties of aluminum are well documented. Studies of brains of patients undergoing renal dialysis indicate that the healthy human brain is capable of detoxifying large amounts of aluminum. Indeed, the aluminum sensitive laboratory animals such as cats and rabbits are apparently considerably more sensitive than normal humans to this agent. However, the circumstantial evidence implicating aluminum in the primary neurodegenerative diseases, such as Alzheimer's disease, are based on the presence of aluminum in the affected tissues and the similarities in the pathogenesis of the human and experimental models. The lack of understanding of the cellular mechanisms which control the barriers and turnover of aluminum in nervous tissue is a major difficulty in evaluating the role of aluminum in the pathogenesis of Alzheimer's disease. It has not yet been possible to determine when in the course of cellular events leading to neurodegeneration aluminum enters nervous tissue. Perhaps the strongest evidence upon which to evaluate the contribution of aluminum in human neurodegenerative disease will come from an examination of the disorders in gene expression which occur in Alzheimer's disease and in the human experimental aluminum encephalopathies. Application of the powerful tools of recombinant DNA to both the human and the experimental encephalopathies has only just begun. Until definitive evidence to the contrary has been obtained, aluminum must continue to be considered a potential contributor to the pathogenesis of certain human neurodegenerative diseases.

This work was supported by the Ontario Mental Health Foundation.

References

Alfry, A. C., Le Gendre, G. R. & Kaehny, W. D. (1976). The dialysis encephalopathy syndrome: possible aluminum intoxication. *New Engl. J. Med.*, **294,** 184–8.

Aniol, A. & Gustafson, J. P. (1984). Chromosome location of genes controlling aluminum tolerance in wheat, rye and triticale. *Can. J. Genet. Cytol.*, **26,** 701–5.

Bizzi, A., Crane, R. C. & Autilio-Gambitti, L. (1984). Aluminum effects of slow oxonal transport. A novel impairment of neurofilament transport. *J. Neurosci.*, **4,** 722–31.

Bowdler, N. C., Beasley, D. S. & Fritze, C. (1979). Behavioral effects of aluminum ingestion on animal and human subjects. *Pharmacol. Biochem. Behav.*, **10,** 505–12.

Bruce, M. (1984). Scrapie and Alzheimer's disease. *Psychol. Med.*, **14,** 497–500.

Commisaris, R. L., Cordon, J. S. Sprague, S., Keiser, I., Mayor, G. & Rich, R. (1982). Behavioral changes in rats after chronic aluminum and parathyroid hormone changes in rats after chronic aluminum and parathyroid hormone administration. *Neurobehav. Toxicol. Teratol.*, **4,** 403–10.

Crapper, D. R. & Dalton, A. J. (1973a). Alterations and short-term retention, conditioned avoidance response acquisition and motivation following aluminum induced neurofibrillary degeneration. *Physiol & Behav.*, **10,** 925–33.

Crapper, D. R. & Dalton, A. J. (1973b). Aluminum induced neurofibrillary degeneration, brain electrical activity and alterations in acquisition and retention. *Physiol. & Behav.*, **10,** 935–45.
Crapper, D. R., Krishnan, S. S. & Dalton, A. J. (1973). Brain aluminum distribution in Alzheimer's disease and experimental neurofibrillary degeneration. *Science*, **180,** 511–3.
Crapper, D. R., Krishnan, S. S. & Quittkat, S. (1976). Aluminum, neurofibrillary degeneration and Alzheimer's disease. *Brain*, **99,** 67–80.
Crapper, D. R., Quittkat, S. & De Boni, U. (1979). Altered chromatin conformation in Alzheimer's disease. *Brain*, **102,** 483–95.
Crapper, D. R. & Tomko, G. S. (1975). Neuronal correlates of an encephalopathy induced by aluminum neurofibrillary degeneration. *Brain Res.*, **97,** 253–64.
Crapper McLachlan, D. R., Dalton, A. J., Galin, H., Schlotterer, G. & Daicar, E. (1984). Alzheimer's disease: Clinical course and cognitive disturbances *Acta Neurologia Scand.*, **69** *(Supp. 99)*, 83–90.
Crapper McLachlan, D. R. & De Boni, U., (1980). Aluminum in human brain disease – an overview. *Neurotoxicol.*, **1,** 3–16.
Crapper McLachlan, D. R., Kruck, T. & Van Berkum, M. (1985). Aluminum and neurodegenerative disease: therapeutic implications. *Am. J. Kidney Diseases*, **6,** 322–9.
Crapper McLachlan, D. R., Lewis, P. N., Lukiw, W. J., Senia, A., Bergeron, C. & De Boni, U. (1984). Chromatin structure in dementia. *Ann. Neurol.*, **15,** 329–34.
Crapper McLachlan, D. R. & Lewis, P. N. (1985). Alzheimer's disease: errors in gene expression. *Can. J. Neurol. Sci.*, **12,** 1–5.
Dalton, A. J., Crapper, D. R. & Schlotterer, G. R. (1974). Alzheimer's disease in Down's syndrome: visual retention deficits. *Cortex*, **10,** 366–77.
Dalton, A. J. & McLachlan Crapper, D. R. (1984). Incidence of memory deterioration in aging persons with Down's syndrome. In *Perspectives and Progress in Mental Retardation*, ed. J. M. Berg., pp. 55–62. Baltimore: University Park Press.
De Boni, U. & McLachlan Crapper, D. R. (1985). Controlled induction of paired helical filaments of the Alzheimer's type in cultured human neurons, by glutamate and aspartate. *J. Neuro. Sci.*, **68,** 105–18.
De Boni, U., Seger, M. & Crapper McLachlan, D. R. (1980). Functional consequences of chromatin bound aluminum in cultured human cells. *Neurotoxicol.*, **1,** 65–82.
Dickson, P. W., Kress, Y., Crowe, A. & Yen, S. (1985). Monoclonal antibodies to Alzheimer's neurofibrillary tangles. *Am. J. Pathol.*, **120,** 292–303.
Duckett, S. & Galle, P. (1976). Mise en evidence de l'aluminum dans les plaques de la maladie d'Alzheimer: étudie à la microsonde de Castaing. *C.R. Acad. Sci. Paris*, **282:** 393–5.
Farnell, B. J., Crapper McLachlan, D. R., Bainbridge, K., De Boni, U., Wong. L. & Wood, P. L. (1985). Calcium metabolism in aluminum encephalopathy. *Exp. Neurol.*, **88,** 68–83.
Farnell, B. J., De Boni, U. & Crapper McLachlan, D. R. (1982). Aluminum neurotoxicity in the absence of neurofibrillary degeneration in CAI hippocampal pyramidal neurons in vitro. *Exp. Neurol.*, **78,** 241–58.
Garruto, R. M., Fukaton, R., Yongihara, R., Gajdusek, D. C., Hook, G. & Fiore, C. (1984). Imaging of calcium and aluminum in neurofibrillary tangle-hearing neurons in parkinsonism-dementia of brain. *Proc. Nat. Acad. Sci. USA*, **81,** 1875–9.

Glenner, G. C. (1979). Congophilic microangiopathy in the pathogenesis of Alzheimer's syndrome (presenile dementia). *Med. Hypotheses*, **5,** 1231–6.
Glenner, G. C. & Wong, W. C. (1984). Alzheimer's disease and Down's syndrome: sharing of a unique cerebrovascular amyloid fibril protein. *Biochem. Biophys. Res. Commun.*, **122,** 1131–5.
Gutteridge, J., Quinlan, G., Clark, I. & Halliwell, B. (1985). Aluminum salts accelerate peroxidation of membrane lipids stimulated by ion salts. *Biochim. Biophys. Acta.*, **835,** 441–7.
Hadfield, M. G., Martinez, A. H. & Gilmartin, R. C. (1974). Progressive multifocal leukoencephalopathy with paramyxovirus-like structures, Hirano bodies and neurofibrillary tangles. *Acta Neuropathol. (Berlin)*, **27,** 277–88.
Hallervorden, J. (1933). Zur Pathogenesis des Post Encephalitischen Parkinsonismus. *Klin. Wochenschr.*, **12,** 692–5.
Heston, L. & Mastvi, A. (1977). The genetics of Alzheimer's disease. *Arch. Gen. Psychiatry*, 976–81.
Heyman, A., Wilkinson, W. E., Hurwitz, B. J., Schmechel, D., Sigmon, A., Weinberg, T., Helms, M. & Swift, M. (1983). Alzheimer's disease: genetic aspects and associated, clinical disorders. *Ann. Neurol.*, **14,** 507–15.
Heyman, A., Wilkinson, W. E., Stafford, J. A., Helms, M. J., Sigmon, A. H. & Weinberg, T. (1984). Alzheimer's disease: a study of epidemiologic aspects. *Ann. Neurol.*, **15,** 335–341.
Ihara, Y., Abraham, C. & Selkoe D. J. (1983). Antibodies to paired helical filaments in Alzheimer's disease do not recognize normal brain proteins. *Nature (Lond.)*, **304,** 727–30.
Jervis, G. A. (1948). Early senile dementia in mongoloid idiocy. *Am. J. Psychiatry*, **105,** 102–6.
Joshi, J. G., Fleming, J. & Zimmerman, A. (1985). Ferritin and aluminum binding. Thirteenth World Congress of Neurology, Hamburg, Abstract 05.07.03.
Karlik, S. J., Eichorn, G. L., Lewis, P. N. & Crapper McLachlan, D. R. (1980). Interaction of aluminum species with DNA. *Biochemistry*, **19,** 5991–8.
Katzman, R. (1976). The prevalence and malignancy of Alzheimer's disease. *Arch. Neurol.*, **33,** 217–8.
King, G. A., De Boni, U. & Crapper, D. R. (1975). Effect of aluminum upon conditioned avoidance response acquisition in the absence of neurofibrillary degeneration. *Pharmacol. Biochem. Behavior.*, **3,** 1003–9.
Krishnan, S. S., Harrison, J. E. & Crapper McLachlan, D. R. (1987). Origin and resolution of the aluminum controversy concerning Alzheimer neurofibrillary degeneration. *Biochemical Trace Element Research.* (In press.)
Lewis, P. N., Lukiw, W. J., De Boni, U. & Crapper McLachlan, D. R. (1981). Changes in chromatin structure associated with Alzheimer's disease. *J. Neurochem.*, **37,** 1193–202.
Liss, L., Ebner, K. & Couri, D. (1979). Neurofibrillary tangles induced by a sclerosing angioma. *Hum. Pathol.* **10,** 104–8.
Lukiw, W. J., Kruck, T. P. A. & Crapper McLachlan, D. R. (1987). Alterations in human linker histones – DNA binding in the presence of aluminum salts in vitro and in Alzheimer's Disease. *Neurotoxicol.*, **8,** 291–302.
Malamud, N. (1972). Neuropathology of organic brain syndrome associated with aging. In *Aging and the Brain*, 3rd edn, ed. C. M. Gaitz, pp. 63–87. New York: Plenum Press.

Mandybur, T. I., Naypaul, A. S., Pappus, Z. & Niklowitz, W. S. (1977). Alzheimer neurofibrillary changes in subacute sclerosing parencephalitis. *Ann. Neurol.*, **1**, 103–7.
Mann, D. M. A., Davies, J. S., Hawkes, J. & Yates, P. O. (1982). Immunohisto-chemical staining of senile plaques. *Neuropath. Appl. Neurobiol.*, **8**, 55–61.
Markesbery, W. R., Ehmann, W. D., Hossain, T., Alanddin, M. & Goodin, T. (1981). Instrumental neutron activation analysis of brain aluminum in Alzheimer disease and aging. *Ann. Neurol.*, **10**, 511–16.
Masters, C. L., Simms, G., Weinman, N. A., Multhaup, G., McDonald, B. L. & Beyreuther, K. (1985a). Amyloid plaque core proteins in Alzheimer's disease and Down's syndrome. *Proc. Nat. Acad. Sci. USA.*, **82**, 4245–9.
Masters, C. L., Multhaup, G., Simms, G., Pottgiesser, J., Martins, R. W. & Beyreuther, K. (1985b). Neuronal origin of a cerebral amyloid: neurofibrillary tangles of Alzheimer's disease contain the same protein as the amyloid of plaque cores and blood results. *EMBO J.*, **4**, 2757–63.
Matsuyama, H. & Nakamura, S. (1978). Senile changes in the brain in the Japanese: Incidence of Alzheimer's neurofibrillary changes and senile plaques. In *Aging*, vol. 7, ed. R. Katzman, R. Terry & K. Bick, pp. 287–98. New York: Raven Press.
McDermott, J. R., Smith, A. I., Iqbal, K. & Wisniewski, H. M. (1977). Aluminum in Alzheimer's disease. *Lancet*, II, 710–1.
McLachlan Crapper, D. R. & Farnell, B. J. (1986). Cellular mechanisms of aluminum toxicity. *Ann. Ist. Super. Sanita*, (In press.)
Middleton, P. J., Petric, M., Kozak, M., Rewcastle, N. B. & Crapper McLachlan, D. R. (1980). Herpes-simplex viral genome and senile and pre-senile dementia of Alzheimer and Pick. *Lancet*, II, 1038.
Mortimer, S. A., French, R. L., Hutton, J. T. Schumana, L. M. (1985). Head injury as a risk factor for Alzheimer's disease. *Neurol.*, **35**, 264–7.
Nee, L., Polinsky, R. J., Eldridge, R., Weingartner, H., Smallberg, S. & Ebert, M. (1983). A family with histologically confirmed Alzheimer's disease. *Arch. Neurol.*, **40**, 203–8.
Perl, D. & Brody, A. (1980). Alzheimer's disease: X-ray spectrometric evidence of aluminum accumulation in neurofibrillary tangle-bearing neurons. *Science*, **208**, 297–9.
Perl, D., Gajdusek, D. & Garruto, R. (1982). Intraneuronal aluminum accumulation in amyotrophic lateral sclerosis and Guam parkinsonism-dementia of Guam. *Science*, **217**, 053–5.
Perry, G., Rizzuto, N., Autilio-Gambetti, L. & Gambetti, P. (1985). Paired helical filaments from Alzheimer's disease patients contain cytoskeletal components. *Proc. Nat. Acad. Sci. USA*, **82**, 3916–20.
Petit, T. L., Biederman, G. B. & McMuller, P. A. (1980). Neurofibrillary degeneration, dendritic dying back and learning-memory deficits after aluminum administration, implications for brain aging. *Exp. Neurol.*, **67**, 152–62.
Pogo, B. G. T. & Elizan T. S. (1985). Search for viral DNA sequences n Alzheimer brain tissues. *Lancet*, II, 978–9.
Powers, J. M., Schlaeper, W., Willingham, M. C. & Hall, B. S. (1981). An Immunoperoxidased study of senile cerebral amyloidosis with pathogenetic considerations. *J. Neuropath. & Exp. Neurol.*, **40**, 592–612.

Rabe, A., Lei, M., Shek, J. & Wisniewski, H. (1982). Learning deficit in immature rabbits with aluminum-induced neurofibrillary degeneration. *Exp. Neurol.*, **76,** 441–6.

Rasool, C. G., Abraham, C., Anderton, B. H., Haugh, M., Kahn, J. & Selkoe, D. J. (1984). Alzheimer's disease: immunoreactivity of neurofibrillary tangles with anti-neurofilament and anti-paired helical filament antibodies. *Brain Res.*, **310,** 249–60.

Rasool, C. G. & Selkoe, D. (1985). Sharing of specific antigens by degenerating neurons in Pick's disease and Alzheimer's disease. *New Engl. J. Med.*, **312,** 700–5.

Sanderson, C., Crapper McLachlan, D. R. & De Boni, U. (1982). Inhibition of corticosterone binding in vitro in rabbit hippocampus by chromatin bound aluminum. *Acta Neuropathol.*, **57,** 249–54.

Selkoe, D. J. (1985). Structural proteins in Alzheimer's disease. Thirteenth World Congress of Neurology, Hamburg, Abstract 03.01.03.

Somerville, R. A. (1985). Ultra-structural links between scrapie and Alzheimer's disease. *Lancet*, I, 504–6.

Sternberger, N. H., Sternberger, L. A. & Ulrich, J. (1985). Aberrant neurofilament phosphorylation in Alzheimer's disease. *Proc. Nat. Acad. Sci. USA*, **82,** 4274–6.

Taylor, G. R., Crow, T. J., Markakis, D. A., Lofthouse, R., Neeley, S. & Carter, G. I. (1984). Herpes simplex virus and Alzheimer's disease: a search for virus DNA by spot hybridization. *J. Neurol. Neurosurg. Psychiatry*, **47,** 1061–5.

Torack, R. M. & Lynch, R. G. (1981). Cytochemistry of brain amyloid in adult dementia. *Acta Neuropathol. (Berl.)*, **53,** 189–96.

Trapp, G. A., Miner, G. D., Zimmerman, R. L., Master, A. R. & Heston, L. L. (1978). Aluminum levels in brain in Alzheimer's disease. *Biol. Psychiatry*, **13,** 709–18.

Troncoso, J. C., Sternberger, L. A., Sternberger, N. H., Hoffman, P. N. & Prince D. L. (1985). Immunocytochemical studies of neurofilament antigens in the neurofibrillary pathology induced by aluminum. *J. Neuropath. & Exp. Neurol.*, **44,** 332 abstract 77.

VanBerkum, M. F. A., Wong Y. L., Lewis P. N. & McLachlan Crapper D. R. (1986). Total and poly (A) RNA yields during an aluminum encephalopathy in rabbit brains. *Neurochem. Res.*, **2,** 1347–59.

Weiss, A. (1981). Replication and evolution in inorganic systems. *Angew. Chem. Int. Ed. Engl.*, **20,** 850–60.

Weitgrefe, S., Zupancic, M., Huase, A., Chesebras, B., Races, R., Frey, W., Rustan, T. & Friedman, R. (1985). Cloning of gene whose expression is increased in scrapie and in senile plaques in human brain. *Science*, **230,** 1177–81.

Weitkamp, L. R., Nee, L., Keats, B., Polinsky, R. J. & Guttormaen, S. (1983). Alzheimer's disease: evidence for susceptibility loci in chromosome 6 and 14. *Am. J. Hum. Genet.*, **35,** 443–53.

Yase, Y. (1980). The role of aluminum in CNS degeneration with interaction of calcium. *Neurotoxicology*, **1,** 101–10.

Yen, S., Gaskin, F. & Man, S. (1983). Neurofibrillary tangles in senile dementia of the Alzheimer's type share an antigenic determinant with intermediate filaments of the vimentin class. *Am. J. Pathol.*, **113,** 373–81.

Yokel, R. A. (1983). Repeated systemic aluminum exposure effects on classical conditioning of the rabbit. *Neurobehav. Toxicol. Teratol.*, **5**, 41–6.

Yoshimasu F., Yusui, M., Yoshida, H., Yoshida, S., Lebayashi, Y., Yase, Y., Gajdusek, D. C. & Chen, KI. M. (1985). Aluminum in Alzheimer's disease in Japan and Parkinsonism-dementia in Guam. Twelfth World Congress of Neurology, Abstract 15.07.02.

7

Cortical neurotransmitter receptors: distribution and involvement in Alzheimer's disease

E. K. Perry and J. M. Candy

7.1 Introduction

The tremendous surge of current research into the nature and possible cause of Alzheimer's disease (AD) testifies to increasing awareness of the great burden this disease imposes on the sufferer, relatives and society. Obviously the ultimate objective is to devise an effective treatment or, better still, discover a means of prevention. Since the primary clinical characteristic of the disease is a loss of short-term memory an important by-product of Alzheimer research may be to discover the mechanisms of memory in the human brain. In this respect the status of transmitter receptors is an area of great interest since it has long been supposed that the encoding of information in the brain involves an alteration in the function of the synaptic junction between neurons, which is characterized on both the pre- and post-synaptic components by the presence of specific transmitter receptors.

The physiological function of the synapse is principally controlled at two levels: the synthesis and release of transmitter molecules from the nerve terminal on the one hand and, via the transmitter receptor, recognition and translation of this chemical signal on the other hand. Regarding the transmitter molecules themselves, neurochemical research in AD has now uncovered consistent defects, manifest as changes in the levels of transmitters or activities of their synthesizing enzymes, in several cortical systems which arise from subcortical nuclei – cholinergic (Davies & Maloney, 1976; Perry *et al.*, 1977; White *et al.*, 1977), noradrenergic (Perry *et al.*, 1981a) and serotoninergic (Cross *et al.*, 1983). There are also reports that two intrinsic cortical systems are affected – somatostatin (reviewed by Beal *et al.*, 1986) and glutamate (Cross *et al.*, 1987). Surprisingly, few consistent abnormalities in transmitter receptors have been reported, due probably to the limitations of conducting biochemical binding assays on crude tissue homogenates and to problems of differentiating receptor subtypes.

In the human, investigations of receptor function are necessarily restricted by the range of techniques that can be successfully applied. To date these include biochemical and autoradiographic methods for the determination of the numbers, affinities and distribution of receptor binding sites in post-mortem brain tissue and, more recently, the application of positron emission tomography (PET) to study receptor distribution *in vivo*. In AD reports are so far confined to the status of receptor ligand binding sites in autopsy brain (Section 7.3). Autoradiographic studies, mainly at present in animals, have provided much valuable information on the distribution of individual transmitter receptors in the cerebral cortex and these data, mainly relating to laminar distributions, are reviewed in Section 7.2. Whilst information gained from biochemical and autoradiographic approaches has been and will continue to be of great value in determining the status of neurotransmitter binding sites *per se*, it is becoming increasingly apparent that investigations of the actual functioning of receptors, in terms of the status of receptor translation mechanisms, are also necessary in pathological human studies such as AD. These and other more novel approaches, together with the implications of present research for potential drug therapy in AD, are discussed in the final Section 7.4.

7.2 Distribution of neurotransmitter receptors in the cerebral cortex

7.2.1 *Autoradiographic techniques*

The introduction of tritium film autoradiography has provided a powerful tool for receptor binding studies (Penney *et al.*, 1981a; Palacios *et al.*, 1981a). This technique allows receptor densities to be quantified in the different cortical laminae; however, the resolution of this method is not sufficient to enable receptor binding sites to be identified in such minute structures as senile plaques (<200 μm). An alternative autoradiographic approach that has a much higher (2–4 μm) resolution (Rogers, 1979) and permits accurate morphological examination of the distribution of receptor binding sites involves the apposition of emulsion-coated coverslips to ^{3}H or ^{125}I labelled sections (Young & Kuhar, 1979). An inherent problem with both the tritium film and emulsion-coated coverslip techniques is due to the greater absorption by white as opposed to grey matter of the low energy beta particles emitted by tritium. This problem has only recently been appreciated and a compensatory method suggested (Greary *et al.*, 1985).

In general the cortical laminar distribution of binding sites for a number of putative neurotransmitters (see below) has been documented using either the tritium sensitive film or coverslip techniques. Whilst the majority of these studies relate to non-human cerebral cortex, receptor distributions particularly in primate cortex are likely to be broadly similar to those in human. In most neocortical areas affected by Alzheimer type neuropathological abnormalities (senile plaques and neurofibrillary tangles) it is the lower layers (III to V) which are generally, although not invariably, most heavily involved.

7.2.2 *Neuropeptide binding sites*

The presence of three subclasses (designated mu, kappa and delta) of opiate binding sites has been described in the brain (Snyder, 1982). In the rat cerebral cortex mu receptors are concentrated in laminae I and IV (Atweh & Kuhar, 1977; Goodman *et al.*, 1980). In the monkey, Wise & Herkenham (1982) found that the mu laminar binding pattern varies between cortical areas: thus, for example, in the premotor and precentral motor cortex lamina VI contains the highest density of binding sites, whilst in the postcentral somatic sensory areas and striate visual cortex laminae V and VI contain high levels of binding. In the human neocortex the highest density of mu binding sites occurs in laminae I–V, whereas the density of kappa receptors is highest in lamina VI (Maurer *et al.*, 1983). A high density of kappa binding sites has also been found in laminae V and VI of the guinea pig cerebral cortex (Foote & Maurer, 1982; Goodman & Snyder, 1982). In the rat delta sites have been observed in laminae II, III and V (Goodman *et al.*, 1980); however, marked regional variations in the distribution of this receptor have been reported (Perry & Sadee, 1987).

By comparison with the opiate receptor other neuropeptide receptors are less well characterized and consequently not so intensively investigated. Lamina IV of the rat cerebral cortex has been reported to contain the highest density of neurotensin binding sites in most areas although exceptions exist in such regions as medial frontal, anterior cingulate and rhinal sulcus (Young & Kuhar, 1981). High densities of CCK-8 binding sites have also been observed in both rat and guinea pig cerebral cortex (Mantyh & Mantyh, 1985) and high densities of CCK-5 binding sites and of CCK-33 in the pyriform cortex of the rat and in laminae I and III of area 27 (Gaudreau *et al.*, 1983) an of CCK-33 in layers IV and VI (Zarbin *et al.*, 1983). Somatostatin-14 receptors are most densely distributed in deeper layers of the rat cerebral cortex (Tran *et al.*, 1984; Leroux & Pelletier, 1984; Whitford *et al.*, 1987). In rat and human brain two subclasses of somatostatin binding sides are present (Tran *et al.*, 1985; Weightman *et al.*, 1985; Whitford *et al.*, 1986). Binding sites for corticotropin-releasing factor have been reported in rat neocortex with the highest densities in laminae I and IV (De Souza *et al.*, 1984). A moderate density of substance P binding has also been detected autoradiographically in rat frontal cortex (Shults *et al.*, 1982), and a low density of binding sites for vasoactive intestinal polypeptide in rat frontal and parietal cortex (Besson *et al.*, 1984).

7.2.3 *Amino acid binding sites*

Two GABA binding sites are present in rat brain. $GABA_A$ binding sites have been identified in all cortical laminae of the rat; Wamsley *et al.* (1981) reported a slightly higher density in lamina IV, whereas Crossman *et al.* (1983) observed the highest density of $GABA_A$ receptors in laminae I–III of the rat. $GABA_B$ binding sites appear to be concentrated in laminae I and II (Crossman *et al.*, 1983).

Three subclasses of receptors for the excitatory amino acids (glutamate and aspartate) have currently been identified. The best characterized subclass is the *N*-methyl-D-aspartate (NMDA) receptor. The other sites – quisqualate- and kainate-preferring receptors are less well documented (Fagg, 1985). Glutamate binds to all three receptor subclasses, and an additional, pharmacologically distinct binding site, in the presence of chloride and calcium ions (Mena *et al.*, 1982), has been identified in autoradiographic studies. In the rat brain all cortical laminae have been reported to contain a very high density of glutamate binding sites (Halpain *et al.*, 1983; Greenamyre *et al.*, 1983). In the human brain a greater density of glutamate binding sites has, in contrast been found in laminae I and II (Greenamyre, 1985). Monaghan *et al.* (1985) reported that in the absence of calcium, chloride and sodium ions, the majority of glutamate binding is to the NMDA site and that in the rat cerebral cortex the greatest concentration of these sites is present in the outer cortical layers. Regarding the hemispheric distribution of NMDA-sensitive binding sites in the rat brain, the frontal, peripheral, anterior cingulate and pyriform cortices have higher densities compared with the parietal, posterior cingulate and entorhinal cortices (Monaghan *et al.*, 1985). With respect to the distribution of kainate binding sites, the outer and deeper layers of rat cerebral cortex contain more binding sites than the middle layers and the highest densities of kainate binding sites have been observed in the frontal and insular cortices (Monaghan & Cotman, 1982). Quisqualate-like binding sites have also been reported to be present in rat neocortex (Monaghan *et al.*, 1984; Rainbow *et al.*, 1984c) with little regional variation but a distinct laminar distribution, laminae I–III containing a higher density of binding sites (Monaghan *et al.*, 1984).

7.2.4 *Monoamine binding sites*

Two subclasses of serotonin (5-HT) receptors have been identified (Peroutka & Snyder, 1979; see also section 7.3). The highest densities of the S_1 subtype have been variously reported to be present in laminae II and IV (Biegon *et al.*, 1982) and laminae IV–VI (Deshmukh *et al.*, 1983) of the rat cerebral cortex. The S_1 subclass is heterogenous with S_{1a}, S_{1b} and S_{1c} subtypes present in the cerebral cortex of the rat (Marcinkiewicz *et al.*, 1984; Pazos & Palacios, 1985). In human frontal cortex S_{1a} receptors are most dense in layer II (Hoyer *et al.*, 1986a) where S_{1b} binding has not been detected (Hoyer *et al.*, 1986a) and S_{1c} sites are sparse and evenly distributed (Hoyer *et al.*, 1986b). The highest density of S_2 binding sites in the rat has been reported in lamina IV of rat (Slater & Patel, 1983) and in the deeper layers of the human cerebral cortex (Bergnon *et al.*, 1986).

Both α_1- and α_2-adrenergic binding sites are present at a low to moderate density in the rat cerebral cortex. While α_1 binding sites are fairly uniformly distributed in all laminae, α_2 binding sites are more dense in laminae I–III (Young & Kuhar, 1980). β-adrenergic binding sites are also present in all cortical laminae of the rat with the highest densities in laminae I–III (Wamsley *et al.*, 1981). The cortical distribution of the two subtypes of β-receptors has also been investigated and it appears that β_1 binding sites are most concentrated in laminae I and VI, while β_2-receptors are more concentrated in laminae IV and VI of the rat frontoparietal cortex (Rainbow *et al.*, 1984a).

High levels of histamine H_1 binding sites have been observed in the outer layers of the guinea pig cerebral cortex (Palacios *et al.*, 1979), whereas in rat brain these sites are concentrated in lamina IV (Palacios *et al.*, 1981).

7.2.5 *Cholinergic binding sites*

The highest density of muscarinic receptors detected by antagonist binding has been reported in lamina VI of the rat cerebral cortex (Kuhar & Yamamura, 1976). Rotter *et al.* (1979) further observed a high density of muscarinic binding sites in lamina III with a fairly even distribution of binding sites in the other cortical laminae. In other studies a relatively low density of binding sites has been found in lamina V (Kuhar & Yamamura, 1976; Wamsley *et al.*, 1980; Nonaka & Moroji,

1984) and lamina IV (Nonaka & Moroji, 1984). The distribution of high affinity agonist binding sites has also been ivestigated in the rat cerebral cortex, laminae I–III containing the least and lamina IV the highest proportion of the binding sites (Wamsley *et al.*, 1980).

Recently nicotine has been used to label presumed nicotinic binding sites in the rat cerebral cortex such sites being concentrated in lamina IV with a high density also present in laminae I and III of the retrosplenal cortex (Clarke *et al.*, 1984). In contrast in an investigation using acetylcholine to label nicotinic receptors, binding sites have been detected in all laminae of the rat cerebral cortex (Rainbow *et al.*, 1984b; Schwartz, 1986).

7.2.6 *Overview*

These numerous reports on the laminar and regional distribution of various neurotransmitter binding sites in normal cerebral cortex highlight the great potential of the autoradiographic approach in receptor investigations in disease states. Discrete laminar changes in a neurotransmitter binding site, which are unlikely to be reflected in whole homogenate preparations using conventional biochemical binding assays, can be readily quantified using this technique.

While the physiological significance of the laminar distribution of neurotransmitter binding sites is presently uncertain, comparison of the pharmacological profile and distribution of binding sites for drugs which selectively affect a particular neurotransmitter subtype may help elucidate the function of that receptor. Thus, for example, Goodman & Snyder (1982) have proposed that the selective localization of kappa opiate receptors in laminae V and VI may account for the unique selective and analgesic properties of kappa opiate drugs by affecting neurons in lamina VI which project to the thalamus and regulate thalamic sensory input to the cerebral cortex. It is interesting to note that in the cerebral cortex lamina IV has been found to contain a high density of binding sites for a number of different neurotransmitters, perhaps reflecting the complex synaptic connections of granule cells in this cortical layer. There have, however, been few autoradiographic studies of neurotransmitter binding sites in human cerebral cortex and the need for investigations of the laminar distribution in both homotypical and heterotypical areas of human neocortex is obvious, especially in disease conditions such as AD. Changes in the laminar distribution pattern of neurotransmitter binding sites may help to define those neuronal populations specifically involved.

7.3 Status of cortical neurotransmitter receptors in Alzheimer's disease

Investigations of receptor binding sites in pathological conditions such as AD are critically dependent on the availability of specific ligands, which can be used to localize and quantify the receptor binding sites for a particular neurotransmitter and discriminate between the receptor subtypes that may be present. Parallel behavioural studies of the effects of such drugs may provide clues to the function of a receptor or its subtype and such data should be valuable in interpreting the physiological significance of receptor changes observed in AD.

The status in AD of a number of different transmitter receptors and some of their subtypes, identified using currently available radioligands, is summarized in Table 7.1. The majority of reported investigations on autopsy tissue relate to the classical transmitters with reports on cholinergic receptors being the most numerous whereas, with a few exceptions, neuropeptide receptors remain to be investigated.

7.3.1 *Cholinergic receptors*

There is convincing psychopharmacological evidence of a role for the cholinergic system in memory in both man and other primates (Deutsch, 1973; Drachman & Leavitt, 1974). Neurochemical autopsy studies in AD have shown that amongst a range of neurotransmitters investigated pre-synaptic changes in this system are generally the most extensive and consistent (Perry *et al.*, 1981b; Candy *et al.*, 1986). Research on cholinergic receptors is currently complicated by uncertainties regarding the subdivision of muscarinic receptors into agonist and antagonist subtypes (Birdsall *et al.*, 1984) and the identification of nicotinic receptors. In electrophysiological studies although a muscarinic effect of acetylcholine is readily apparent in the cerebral cortex (Krnjevic & Phillis, 1963), a purely nicotinic-like action has not been observed (Krnjevic & Phillis, 1963). Such studies, do however, indicate that a receptor with mixed nicotinic and muscarinic pharmacology is present in the cerebral cortex (Phillis & York, 1968). A major problem in neurochemical investigations of this receptor with intermediate pharmacological characteristics is the availability of suitable ligands (see also Section 7.2.5).

The majority of binding studies of cortical muscarinic sites in both isolated membrane preparations and, *in situ*, by autoradiographic localisation indicate no signficant abnormality in the density of muscarinic binding sites (Table 7.1) using antagonists such as *N*-methylscopolamine (NMS) or quinuclidinyl benzylate (QNB) which do not discriminate between antagonist subtypes. A few investigators have, however, reported moderate reductions, especially in archicortical areas, in total muscarinic binding (Table 7.1). The binding of the muscarinic antagonist pirenzepine, which distinguishes M_1 from M_2 antagonist subtypes in the human brain, has been reported to be unchanged in AD (Caulfield *et al.*, 1982). It has, however, recently been reported that there is a selective reduction of M_2 sites in AD (Mash *et al.*, 1985; Whitehouse *et al.*, 1985), the low affinity state being detected by carbachol displacement of QNB or NMS and the high affinity site by direct binding of oxotremorine. However, it should be noted that M_2 sites probably represent a heterogeneous population (Birdsall *et al.*, 1984). Mash *et al.* (1985) have reported that reductions in M_2 sites correlate with the loss of choline acetyltransferase in AD, although curiously total antagonist binding has been reported to increase as this enzyme decreases (Nordberg *et al.*, 1983). Reductions in both M_2 sites and cholinergic enzyme activities occur in the septally lesioned hippocampus of experimental animals and high as opposed to low affinity carbachol binding sites are said to correlate with the cholinergic innervation of the cortex (McKinney & Coyle, 1982) – suggesting that these receptors may be localized mainly on pre-synaptic cholinergic terminals (Mash *et al.*, 1985). Thus, if the observations in AD are confirmed, then the development of specific M_2 ligands may be useful in the antemortem diagnosis of the disease using PET scanning technique. It should however be noted that Caulfield *et al.* (1982) did not detect changes in the receptor population which was not displaced by pirenzepine (which presumably includes M_2 sites) – a finding due perhaps to the omission of an uncoupling agent such as *N*-ethylmaleimide which in human cortex substantially increases the high affinity agonist sites (C. Smith and E. Perry, unpublished observations).

As noted above (see also Section 7.2.5) the status of the CNS nicotinic receptor is unclear. In AD α-bungarotoxin binding sites are said to be either normal or reduced (Table 7.1) although the inability of this drug to influence the nicotinic response in CNS neurons suggests this site may not be directly related to the nicotinic receptor. Evidence for a high affinity nicotinic-like binding sites for nicotine (Clarke *et al.*, 1984) and two nicotinic-like binding sites for dihydro-β-erythroidine (Williams & Robinson, 1985) suggests these or other ligands may be more useful tools for investigating nicotinic-like binding sites in AD and there is already one report on the normality of nicotine binding in the cortex, despite reductions in subcortical areas in AD (Shimohama *et al.*, 1986), although other groups are now reporting cortical reductions (e.g. Perry *et al.*, 1986).

Table 7.1. *Cortical transmitter receptor binding in Alzheimer's disease*

Receptor	Ligand	Subtype	Binding in Alzheimer's disease	References
Muscarinic	QNB/NMS		Generally normal in neocortex	Perry *et al.*, 1977; Davies & Verth, 1978; Palacios, 1982; Bowen *et al.*, 1983; Lange & Henke, 1983; Jenni-Eiermann *et al.*, 1984; Greenamyre *et al.*, 1985
			Moderate reductions in some limbic areas	Riesine *et al.*, 1978; Nordberg *et al.*, 1983; Mash *et al.*, 1985; Rinne *et al.*, 1985
	Pirenzepine (direct-binding/QNB displacement)	M_1	Normal	Cauldfield *et al.*, 1982; Gulya *et al.*, 1985
	Carbachol inhibition QNB/NMS	M_1 and M_2 low affinity states	Selective loss M_2	Mash *et al.*, 1985; Whitehouse *et al.*, 1985
	Oxotremorine	M_2 high affinity	Decreased	Mash *et al.*, 1985
	Cis-dioxalane	High affinity agonist	Normal	Gulya *et al.*, 1985
Nicotinic?	Bungarotoxin	?	Decreased	Davies & Feissullin, 1981
			Normal	Lang & Henke, 1983
	Nicotine		Normal/Reduced	Shimohama *et al.*, 1985; Perry *et al.*, 1987
Serotonergic	LSD	S_1, S_2	Reduced	Bowen *et al.*, 1979
	Serotonin	S_1	Reduced	Cross *et al.*, 1984b; Perry *et al.*, 1984
	Ketanserin	S_2	Reduced	Cross *et al.*, 1984b; Perry *et al.*, 1984

Adrenergic	WB-4101	α_1	Normal	Cross *et al.*, 1984a
			Increased (some areas)	Jenni-Eiermann *et al.*, 1984
	Rauwolscine	α_2	Normal	Cross *et al.*, 1984a
	Dihydroal-prenalol	β	Normal	Bowen *et al.*, 1983; Cross *et al.*, 1984
			Increased (temporal lobe)	Jenni-Eiermann *et al.*, 1984
Dopaminergic	Spiroperidol		Normal	Reisine *et al.*, 1978
γ-aminobutyric acid	GABA		Reduced	Reisine *et al.*, 1978
			Normal	Cross *et al.*, 1984a
	Muscimol	A	Normal	Reisine *et al.*, 1978; Bowen *et al.*, 1983; Cross *et al.*, 1984; Greenamyre *et al.*, 1985
Benzodiazepine	Diazepam		Normal	Cross *et al.*, 1984a
	Flunitrazepam		Normal	Greenamyre *et al.*, 1985
Glutamate	Glutamate		Normal (amygdala)	Pearce *et al.*, 1984
			Reduced	Greenamyre *et al.*, 1985
Somatostatin	Dicarba analogue CGP, 23 996		Reduced	Gulya *et al.*, 1985
	Leu^8, D Trp^{22}, Tyr^{25} somatostatin 28		Reduced	Beal *et al.*, 1985
	Tyr-11 somatostatin 14		Normal	Crow *et al.*, 1985
Opiate	Naloxone		Normal	Bowen *et al.*, 1979
Cholecystokinin	CCK-33		Normal	Hays & Paul, 1982

Autoradiographic studies in AD have so far mainly used the non-selective muscarinic antagonists NMS or QNB, (Palacios 1982; Lang & Henke, 1983) and, rather surprisingly, indicate no marked variation in tissue heavily populated by senile plaques and neurofibrillary tangles. However, the resolution of the autoradiographic method employed was not sufficient to demonstrate possible alterations at the level of individual senile plaques or neurofibrillary tangle bearing neurones (see Section 7.2.1). One report (Lang & Henke, 1983) suggests that the laminar distribution of muscarinic binding is disrupted – a disruption also apparent in the pre-synaptic cholinergic marker choline acetyltransferase (Perry *et al.*, 1984).

7.3.2 *Serotonergic receptors*

In contrast to cholinergic and other neurotransmitter receptors, serotonergic receptor abnormalities have been consistently detected in AD although the significance of these changes either in terms of clinical symptoms, pathogenesis or possible drug effects is not yet understood. Reductions in both S_1 and S_2 receptor densities are apparent (Table 7.1) although not in all cortical areas affected by senile plaques and neurofibrillary tangles. Both receptor subtypes appear to be post-synaptic to the cortical serotonergic input – lesions of the midbrain raphe nuclei do not significantly alter the density of either in the cerebral cortex (Blackshear *et al.*, 1981). Following lesions of the basal forebrain cholinergic neurones, the density of cortical S_2 binding sites has in contrast been reported to be decreased, suggesting that a portion of S_2 receptors may exist on cholinergic terminals in at least the rat brain (Quirion *et al.*, 1985). The latter observation is, however, inconsistent with the finding in human brain that in cases of Parkinson's disease where there is a marked cholinergic deficit, S_2 binding is unaltered in the cortex (Perry *et al.*, 1984). In AD there is no evidence for a correlation between S_2 reductions and plaques (Cross *et al.*, 1984b) although some evidence of a connection with the density of neurofibrillary tangles exists (Perry *et al.*, 1984). Obviously high resolution autoradiographic investigation of both S_1 and S_2 in AD would help to determine if these abnormalities are closely related to Alzheimer-type pathology.

7.3.3 *Catecholaminergic receptors*

Unlike serotonergic receptors current evidence suggests that catecholaminergic, including noradrenergic α_1- and α_2- and β-adrenergic receptors, are not reduced in AD (Table 7.1). The normality of noradrenergic receptors in the cortex is surprising in view of the assumed degeneration of projecting fibres from the locus coeruleus – both cortical noradrenergic markers and locus coeruleus neuron numbers are reduced in AD (Perry *et al.*, 1981a). Experimental denervation of the cortical noradrenergic input is accompanied by changes in both α_1- and β-adrenergic receptors which appear to be co-regulated (Sutin & Minneman, 1985). The long-term pathological changes of AD are however likely to be distinct from those following short-term experimental lesions. However, one recent report (Jenni-Iermann *et al.*, 1984) has indicated increased α_1- and β-adrenergic receptor binding in specific but not identical areas in AD. Thus, further screening of these receptors in a broader range of cortical areas and at various stages of the disease would clearly be worthwhile.

7.3.4 *Amino acid receptors*

Interest in GABA (inhibitory) and glutamate (excitatory) receptors in AD stems from the relatively high proportion, over 30%, of these transmitter systems in the cortex – mainly associated with intrinsic neurons and far exceeding the combined proportion of the afferent (cholinergic, noradrenergic, dopaminergic and serotonergic) systems. All except one of the reports on the $GABA_A$ receptor and its associated benzodiazepine binding site indicate normality in AD (Table 7.1), although the $GABA_B$ receptor has yet to be investigated. The situation is less clear regarding the glutamate receptor with one report, based on autoradiographic studies, of reductions in glutamate binding in the cortex, said to reflect shrinkage of the cortical dendritic arbor (Greenamyre *et al.*, 1985) not confirmed by others – at least in the amygdaloid nucleus – using isolated membranes (Pearce *et al.*, 1984). The validity of the suggestion (Greenamyre *et al.*, 1985), that PET scanning of glutamate binding sites might provide a diagnostic tool in AD obviously depends on confirmation of disease-related abnormalities.

Glutamate receptors will continue to attract interest in AD on at least two accounts: (i) it has been suggested that during long-term potentiation – a model for memory formation – the binding and release of glutamate is altered (Lynch & Baudry, 1984); (ii) certain glutamate receptor subtypes bind neurotoxic molecules such as kainic acid (see Section 7.2.3) and the possibility arises that endogenous neurotoxins may act similarly in the pathogenesis of degenerative disorders such as AD. Thus the examination of the various glutamate receptor subtypes in key cortical areas subject to degenerative changes needs to be made not only in AD but in other degenerative disorders associated with cortical damage (e.g. Pick's, Gerstmann Straussler, Huntington's and Jakob–Creutzfeldt diseases).

7.3.5 *Neuropeptide receptors*

Neuropeptide receptors, with the exception of opiate receptors, are generally much less well characterized compared with the classical transmitter receptors. Although opiate binding was originally reported to be normal in AD (Table 7.1) the heterogeneity of subtypes (for example, mu, kappa and delta) in human brain (see Section 7.2.2) suggests that further more detailed studies would now be of value. One neuropeptide that has consistently been found to be abnormal in at least some cortical areas in AD is somatostatin and whilst there are now several reports on somatostatin receptors in AD, these are unfortunately contradictory (Table 7.1). This may reflect the different ligands employed and in particular the problem of rapid degradation of certain ligands. In future, sub-populations of this receptor need to be assessed under conditions where degradation of the ligand is minimal. Another neuropeptide now implicated in AD is corticotropin releasing factor (CRF). Reductions in CRF immunoreactivity are reported to be accompanied by increased CRF receptor binding, indicative of receptor supersensitivity (De Souza *et al.*, 1986). Curiously, CRF immunoreactivity in the hippocampus – a key area in the pathology of AD, is apparently normal – an observation which casts some doubt on the prime importance of this peptide abnormality in the disease.

7.4 **Future prospects**

Fascinating as receptor analyses of the human brain are, studies in AD have not so far shed much light on the nature of the disease nor clearly indicated directions for therapy. This partly reflects the limitations of current techniques and several problems or possibilities for future research are outlined below.

7.4.1 *Comparative pathology*

A great deal can be learned concerning the specificity of neurochemical changes in Alzheimer's disease – whether they relate closely to core pathology – by making comparisons with other disorders. Although plaques and tangles may occur separately in a variety of diseases their co-appearance in the cortex in substantial numbers is restricted to AD and Down's syndrome. Little is known of receptor status in Down's syndrome but in a variety of other disorders (Pick's, Gerstmann Straussler and Huntington's diseases) total cortical muscarinic binding has been reported to be normal (Wood *et al.*, 1983; Greenamyre *et al.*, 1985). In Parkinson's disease in which dementia is accompanied by a pre-synaptic cholinergic deficit there is said to be an increase in QNB binding which, when related to the activity of choline acetyltransferase, correlates with the degree of dementia (Ruberg *et al.*, 1982). Possible drug effects complicate this finding since anti-cholinergic agents – sometimes employed in the treatment of Parkinson's disease – are associated with an increase in muscarinic binding. In a more recent Parkinsonian series, increased muscarinic binding (particularly to the low affinity agonist subtype, assessed by carbachol displacement of NMS) was apparently independent of anticholinergic drug treatment (Perry *et al.*, 1986). Such evidence of cholinergic denervation induced muscarinic receptor supersensitivity in Parkinson's but not Alzheimer's disease (Perry *et al.*, 1986) may relate to the lower incidence and lesser severity of dementia in the former compared with the latter.

It is of considerable interest that the serotonergic S_2 receptor reduction of AD may be relatively specific to this disorder. The abnormality has not been observed in Parkinson's disease (Perry *et al.*, 1984) or Huntington's disease (A. Cross, personal communication) and may relate to critical intrinsic cortical changes. This would then seem to be an abnormality worth pursuing in the hope of understanding, perhaps through identification of those neurons bearing S_2 receptors, the nature of intrinsic Alzheimer type abnormalities.

7.4.2 *Drug effects*

Any investigation of receptor binding in human brain tissue is constantly plagued by the possibility that drug regimes – particularly prevalent in hospitalized patients often employed in autopsy investigations – may have influenced binding either by their immediate presence in the preparation or more likely through long-term adaptive processes. In AD although no drug for the treatment of the disorder exists, neuroleptics are commonly administered and have been found in normal human brain samples to increase caudate but not cortical muscarinic binding – an alteration not, curiously enough, seen in AD (Rinne *et al.*, 1985). The question of whether the serotonergic S_2 receptor abnormality may relate to neuroleptic administration has not been specifically addressed although it is known that antidepressant therapy – occasionally employed in AD – can decrease binding. Clearly future receptor analysis in AD need to address this problem, either by seeking drug-free individuals or by conducting parallel animal experiments on drug effects.

7.4.3 *Receptor localization*

Binding studies on isolated membrane preparations and to a lesser extent autoradiographic studies, at least at a low level of resolution, suffer the obvious limitation of failing to localize receptors to specific cell types. Unlike pre-synaptic transmitter activities, generally confined to the neurons of the specific systems involved, receptors are widely distributed not only on different neuronal types but also on glial cells and blood vessels. Thus muscarinic cholinergic binding sites have been identified not only on astrocytes (Repke & Maderspach, 1982) but also in intracerebral blood vessels (Estrada & Krause, 1982). In addition, α_1-, α_2- and β-adrenergic binding sites are associated with glial cells (Maguire *et al.*, 1976) and β-adrenergic receptors with cerebral microvessels (Harik *et al.*, 1980; Peroutka, 1980). Hopefully improvements in high resolution autoradiographic procedures (see Section 7.2.1) will resolve some of these problems of cellular localization, of receptor binding sites.

7.4.4 *Effector mechanisms*

As a complex of molecular entities on the plasma membrane, ligand binding studies so far conducted in AD have examined only the recognition site, leaving the coupling mechanism and transducing system (ultimately mediating the response by the recipient cells to the transmitter signal) as parameters to be explored. Coupled reactions include adenylate cyclase (associated with for example β-adrenergic receptors) and polyphosphoinositide hydrolysis (muscarinic M_1, serotonergic S_2). Preliminary investigations have detected the phosphoinositide response to the muscarinic agonist carbachol in biopsy and optimal autopsy human brain tissue (Candy *et al.*, 1984) but, unfortunately, not in routine autopsy specimens. Presumably adverse pre- or postmortem conditions affect membrane conformation, possibly uncoupling individual components of the receptor complex. Such problems may perhaps only be resolved at present by the use of biopsy tissue although whether the need to determine the integrity of, for example, the muscarinic response in the Alzheimer brain ethically justifies a biopsy operation is another question. It may be just as informative to test patients in the early stages of AD with specific muscarinic agonists which have been shown in cortical cholinergic deafferentated animal brains to restore cholinergic function.

7.4.5 *Drug therapy*

A final question of great importance is what possible therapeutic directions should now be pursued as a result of current receptor and related studies in AD. The most definitive statement that can be made at present relates to the established cholinergic deficit – which probably reflects the degeneration of cortical cholinergic fibres and is related to the memory impairment – appearing to leave the post-synaptic muscarinic receptor relatively intact. If the assumption is correct that pre- and post-synaptic muscarinic receptors possess different binding characteristics (Section 7.3.1) then drugs need to be tailored to interact with the latter but not the former, since stimulation of the former is likely to inhibit the release of acetylcholine from surviving terminals. Even so the involvement of other transmitter systems in AD indicates that cholinergic therapy is only likely to be effective at early stages of the disease and more basic research into the cause of AD is urgently required.

Project grant funding by the Medical Research Council to E. K. Perry and the expert secretarial assistance of Mrs D. Hinds are gratefully acknowledged.

References

Atweh, S. F. & Kuhar, M. J. (1977). Autoradiographic localization of opiate receptors in rat brain. III The telencephalon. *Brain Res.*, **134,** 393–405.

Beal, M. F., Mazurek, M. F., Tran, V. T., Chattha, G., Bird, E. D. & Martin, J. B. (1985). Reduced numbers of somatostatin receptors in the cerebral cortex in Alzheimer's disease. *Science*, **229,** 289–91.

Beal, M. F., Uhl, G., Mazurek, M. F., Kowall, N. & Martin, J. B. (1986). Somatostatin: Alterations in the central nervous system in neurological disorders. In *Neuropeptides in Neurologic and Psychiatric Disease*, ed. J. B. Martin & J. D. Barchas, pp. 215–57. New York: Raven Press.

Beigon, A., Kargman, S., Synder, L. & McEwen, B. S. (1986). Characterisation and localisation of serotonin receptors in human brain postmortem. *Brain Res.*, **363,** 91–8.

Beigon, A., Rainbow, T. C. & McEwen, B. S. (1982). Quantitative autoradiography of serotonin receptors in rat brain. *Brain Res.*, **242,** 197–204.

Besson, J., Dussaillant, M., Marie, J.-C., Rostene, W. & Rosselin, G. (1984). In vitro autoradiographic localization of vasoactive intestinal peptide (VIP) binding sites in the rat central nervous system. *Peptides*, **5,** 339–40.

Birdsall, N. J., Hulme, E. C. & Stockton, J. M. (1984). Muscarinic receptor heterogeneity. *Trends Pharmacol. Sci., Suppl.* 4–8.

Blackshear, M. A., Steranka, L. R. and Sanders-Bush, E. (1981). Multiple serotonin receptors: Regional distribution and effect of raphe lesions. *Eur. J. Pharmacol.*, **76,** 325–34.

Bowen, D. M., Allen, S. J., Benton, J. S., Goodhardt, M. J., Haan, E. A., Palmer, A. M., Sims, N. R., Smith, C. C. T., Spillane, J. A., Esiri, M. M., Neary, D., Snowdon, J. S., Wilcock, G. K. & Davison, A. N. (1983). Biochemical assessment of serotonergic and cholinergic dysfunction and cerebral atrophy in Alzheimer's disease. *J. Neurochem.*, **44,** 266–72.

Bowen, D. M., White, P., Spillane, J. A., Goodhardt, M. J., Curzon, G., Iwangoff, I. P., Deier-Ruge, W. & Davison, A. N. (1979). Accelerated ageing or selective neuronal loss as an important cause of dementia? *Lancet*, I, 11–14.

Candy, J. M., Court, J. A., Perry, R. H. & Smith, C. J. (1984). Carbachol-stimulated phosphatidylinositol hydrolysis in the cerebral cortex after freezing and post mortem delay. *Br. J. Pharmacol.*, **83,** 356P.

Candy, J. M., Perry, E. K., Perry, R. H., Court, J. A., Oakley, A. E. & Edwardson, J. A. (1986). The current status of the cortical cholinergic system in Alzheimer's disease and Parkinson's disease. *Prog. Brain Res.*, in press.

Candy, J. M., Snell, C. R. & Whitford, C. A. (1985). Distribution of high affinity [^{3}H]-somatostatin binding sites in the rat brain. *Br. J. Pharmacol.*, in press.

Caulfield, M. P., Straughan, D. W., Cross, A. J., Cross, T. & Birdsall, N. J. (1982). Cortical muscarinic receptor subtypes and Alzheimer's disease. *Lancet*, II, 1277.

Clarke, P. B. S., Pert, C. B. & Pert, A. (1984). Autoradiographic distribution of nicotine receptors in rat brain. *Brain Res.*, **323,** 390–5.

Cross, A. J., Crow, T. J., Johnson, J. A., Joseph, M. H., Perry, E. K., Perry, R. H., Blessed, G. & Tomlinson, B. E. (1983) Monoamine metabolism in senile dementia of Alzheimer type. *J. Neurol. Sci.*, **60,** 383–92.

Cross, A. J., Crow, T. J., Johnson, J. A., Perry, E. K., Perry, R. H., Blessed, G. & Tomlinson, B. E. (1984a). Studies on neurotransmitter receptor systems in neocortex and hippocampus in senile dementia of the Alzheimer-type. *J. Neurol. Sci.*, **64,** 109–17.

Cross, A. J., Crow, T. J., Ferrier, I. N., Johnson, A., Bloom, S. R. & Corsellis, J. A. N. (1984b). Serotonin receptor changes in dementia of the Alzheimer-type. *J. Neurochem.*, **43,** 1574–81.

Cross, A. J., Slater, P., Candy, J. M., Perry, E. K. & Perry, R. H. (1987). Glutamate uptake sites are reduced in the cortex in Alzheimer type dementia. *J. Neurol. Neurosurg. Psychiatry*, **50,** 357–8.

Crossman, A. R., Latham, A., Patel, S. & Slater, P. (1983). Tritium-film autoradiography $GABA_A$ and $GABA_B$ receptors in rat brain. *Br. J. Pharmacol., 78–80 Supplements*: 532P.

Crow, T. J., Farmery, S. M., Owen, F. & Poulter, M. (1985). Iodinated somatostatin binding to human brain membranes: a comparison of controls and Alzheimer type dementia patients. *Br. J. Pharmacol.*, **84,** 8P.

Davies, P. & Feisullin, S. (1981). Postmortem stability of α-bungarotoxin binding sites in mouse and human brain. *Brain Res.*, **216,** 449–54.

Davies, P. & Maloney, A. J. (1976). Selective loss of cholinergic neurons in Alzheimer's disease. *Lancet*, II, 1403.

Davies, P. & Verth, A. H. (1978). Regional distribution of muscarinic acetylcholine receptors in normal and Alzheimer's type dementia brains. *Brain Res.*, **138,** 385–92.

Deshmukh, P. P., Yamamura, H. I., Woods, L. & Nelson, D. L. (1983). Computer-assisted autoradiographic localization of subtypes of serotonin, receptors in rat brain. *Brain Res.*, **288,** 338–43.

De Souza, E. B., Perrin, M. H., Insel, T. R., Rivier, J., Vale, W. W. & Kuhar, M. J. (1984). Corticotropin-releasing factor receptors in rat forebrain: Autoradiographic identification. *Science*, **224,** 1449–51.

De Souza, E. B., Whitehouse, P. J., Kuhar, M. J., Price, D. L. & Vale, W. W. (1986). Reciprocal changes in corticotropin-releasing factor (CRF)-like immunoreactivity and CRF receptors in cerebral cortex of Alzheimer's disease. *Nature*, **319,** 593–5.

Deutsch, J. A. (1973). The cholinergic synapse and the site of memory. In *The physiological basis of memory*, ed. J. A. Deutsch. pp. 59–74. New York: Academic Press.

Drachman, D. A. & Leavitt, J. (1974). Human memory and the cholinergic system. *Arch. Neurol.*, **30**, 113–21.
Estrada, C. & Krause, D. N. (1982). Muscarinic cholinergic receptor sites in cerebral blood vessels. *J. Pharmacol. Exp. Ther.*, **221**, 85–90.
Fagg, G. E. (1985). L-Glutamate, excitatory amino acid receptors and brain function. *Trends Neurosci.*, **8**, 207–10.
Foote, R. W. & Maurer, R. (1982). Autoradiographic localisation of opiate k-receptors in the guinea-pig brain. *Eur. J. Pharmacol.*, **85**, 99–103.
Gaudreau, P., Quirion, R., St-Pierre, S. & Pert, C. B. (1983). Tritium-sensitive film autoradiography of [^{3}H] cholecytokinin — 5/pentagastrin receptors in rat brain. *Eur. J. Pharmacol.*, **87**, 173–4.
Geary, W. A., Toga, A. W. & Wooten, G. F. (1985). Quantitative film autoradiography for tritium: methodological considerations. *Brain Res.*, **337**, 99–108.
Goodman, R. R. & Snyder, S. H. (1982). Autoradiographic localization of Kappa opiate receptors to deep layers of the cerebral cortex may explain unique sedative and analgesic effects. *Life Sci.*, **31**, 1291–4.
Goodman, R. R., Snyder, S. H., Kuhar, M. J. & Young, W. S. (1980). Differentiation of delta and mu opiate receptor localizations by light microscopic autoradiography. *Proc. Nat. Acad. Sci. USA*, **77**, 6239–43.
Greenamyre, J. T., Penney, J. B., Young, A. B., D'Amato, C. J., Hicks, S. P. & Shoulson, I. (1985). Alterations in L-glutamate binding in Alzheimer's and Huntingdon's diseases. *Science*, **227**, 1496–9.
Greenamyre, J. T., Young, A. B. & Penney, J. B. (1983). Quantitative autoradiography of L-[^{3}H] glutamate binding to rat brain. *Neurosci. Lett.* **37**, 155–60.
Gulya, K., Vickroy, T. W., Watson, M., Roeske, W. R., Perry, E. K., Perry, R. H., Duckles, S. P. & Yamamura, H. I. (1985). Cholinergic and somatostatinergic receptor alterations in senile dementia of the Alzheimer's type (SDAT) and its animal model. *Soc. Neurosci. Abstr.*, **11**, 1119.
Halpain, S., Parson, B. & Rainbow, T. C. (1983). Tritium-film autoradiography of sodium-independent glutamate binding sites in rat brain. *Eur. J. Pharmacol.*, **86**, 313–4.
Harik, S. I., Sharma, V. K., Wetherbee, I. R., Warren, R. H. & Banerjee, S. P. (1980). Adrenergic receptors of cerebral microvessels. *Eur. J. Pharmacol.*, **61**, 207–8.
Hays, S. E. & Paul, S. M. (1982). CCK receptors and human neurological disease. *Life Sci.*, **31**, 319–22.
Hoyer, D., Pazos, A., Probst, A. & Palacios, J. M. (1986a). Serotonin receptors in the human brain. I. Characterisation and autoradiographic localisation of 5-HT_{1A} recognition sites. Apparent absence of 5-HT_{1B} sites. *Brain Res.*, **376**, 85–96.
Hoyer, D., Pazos, A., Probst, A. & Palacios, J. M. (1986b). Serotonin receptors in the human brain. II. Characterisation and autoradiographic localisation of 5-HT_{1C} and 5-HT_2 recognition sites. *Brain Res.*, **376**, 97–107.
Jenni-Eiermann, S., Von Hahn, H. P., Honegger, C. G. & Ulrich, J. (1984). Studies on neurotransmitter binding in senile dementia. *Gerontology*, **30**, 350–8.
Krnjevic, K. & Phillis, J. W. (1963). Pharmacological properties of acetylcholine-sensitive cells in the cerebral cortex. *J. Physiol.*, **166**, 328–50.
Kuhar, M. J. & Yamamura, H. I. (1976). Localization of cholinergic muscarinic

receptors in rat brain by light microscopic radioautography. *Brain Res.*, **110,** 229–43.
Lang, W. & Henke, H. (1983). Cholinergic receptor binding and autoradiography in brains of non-biological and senile dementia of Alzheimer-type patients. *Brain Res.*, **267,** 271–80.
Leroux, P. & Pelletier, G. (1984). Radioautographic localization of somatostatin-14 and somatostatin-28 binding sites in the rat brain. *Peptides*, 5, 503–6.
Lynch, G. & Baudry, M. (1984). The biochemistry of memory: a new and specific hypothesis. *Science*, **224,** 1057–63.
Maguire, M. E., Wiklund, R. A., Anderson, H. J. & Gilman, A. G. (1976). Binding of [^{125}I] iodohydroxybenzylpinodol to putative β-adrenergic receptors of rat glioma cells and other cell clones. *J. Biol. Chem.*, **251,** 1221–31.
Marcinkiewicz, M., Verge, D., Gozlan, H., Pichat, L. & Hamon, M. (1984). Autoradiographic evidence for the heterogeneity of 5-HT_1 sites in the rat brain. *Brain Res.*, **291,** 159–63.
Mantyh, C. R. & Mantyh, P. W. (1985). Differential localization of cholecystokinin-i binding sites in the rat vs the guinea pig brain. *Eur. J. Pharmacol.*, **113,** 137–9.
Mash, D. C., Flynn, D. D. & Potter, L. T. (1985). Loss of M_2 muscarinic receptors in the cerebral cortex in Alzheimer's disease and experimental cholinergic denervation. *Science*, **228,** 1115–17.
Maurer, R., Cortes, R., Probst, A. & Palacios, J. M. (1983). Multiple opiate receptors in human brain: An autoradiographic investigation. *Life Sci.*, **33,** 231–4.
McKinney, M. & Coyle, J. T. (1982). Regulation of neocortical muscarinic receptors: Effects of drug treatment and lesions. *J. Neurosci.*, **2,** 97–105.
Mena, E. E., Fagg, G. E. & Cotman, C. W. (1982). Chloride ions enhance L-glutamate binding to rat brain synaptic membranes. *Brain Res.*, **243,** 378–81.
Monaghan, D. T. & Cotman, C. W. (1982). The distribution of [^{3}H] kainic acid binding sites in rat CNS as determined by autoradiography. *Brain Res.*, **252,** 91–100.
Monaghan, D. T., Yao, D. & Cotman, C. W. (1984). Distribution of [^{3}H] AMPA binding sites in rat brain as determined by quantitative autoradiography. *Brain Res.*, **324,** 160–4.
Monaghan, D. T., Yao, D. & Cotman, C. W. (1985). L-[^{3}H] glutamate binds to kainate-, NMDA- and AMPA-sensitive binding sites: an autoradiographic analysis. *Brain Res.*, **340,** 378–83.
Nonaka, R. & Moroji, T. (1984). Quantitative autoradiography of muscarinic receptors in the rat brain. *Brain Res.*, **296,** 295–303.
Nordberg, A., Larsson, C., Adolfsson, R., Alafuzoff, I. & Winblad, B. (1983). Muscarinic receptor compensation in hippocampus of Alzheimer patients. *J. Neural Transm.*, **56,** 13–19.
Palacios, J. M. (1982). Autoradiographic localization of muscarinic cholinergic receptors in the hippocampus of patients with senile dementia. *Brain Res.*, **243,** 173–5.
Palacios, J. M., Niehoff, D. L. & Kuhar, M. J. (1981a). Receptor autoradiography with tritium-sesnstive film: potential for computerized densitometry. *Neurosci. Lett.*, **25,** 101–5.
Palacios, J. M., Young, W. S. & Kuhar, M. J. (1979). Autoradiographic

localization of H_1-histamine receptors in brain using ^{3}H-mephyramine: Preliminary studies. *Eur. J. Pharmacol.*, **58,** 295–304.
Palacios, J. M., Wamsley, J. K., & Kuhar, M. J. (1981b). The distribution of histamine-H_1 receptors in the rat brain: an autoradiographic study. *Neuroscience*, **6,** 15–37.
Pazos, A. & Palacios, J. M. (1985). Quantitative autoradiographic mapping of serotonin receptors in the rat brain. 1. Serotonin-1 receptors. *Brain Res.*,**346,** 205–30.
Pearce, B. R., Palmer, A. M., Bowen, D. M., Wilcock, G. K., Esiri, M. M. & Davison, A. N. (1984). Neurotransmitter dysfunction and atrophy of the caudate nucleus in Alzheimer's disease. *Neurochem. Pathol.*, **2,** 221–32.
Penney, J. B., Frey, K. & Young, A. B. (1981a). Quantitative autoradiography of neurotransmitter receptors using tritium-sensitive film. *Eur. J. Pharmacol.*, **72,** 421–2.
Peroutka, S. J., Moskowitz, M. A., Reinhard, F. and Snyder, S. H. (1980). Neurotransmitter receptor binding in bovine cerebral microvessels. *Science*, **208,** 610–2.
Peroutka, S. J. and Snyder, S. H. (1979). Multiple serotonin receptors: differential binding of ^{3}H-5-hydroxytryptamine, ^{3}H-lysergic acid diethylamide and ^{3}H-spiroperidol. *Mol. Pharmacol.*, **16,** 687–99.
Perry, D. C. & Sadee, W. (1986). Autoradiography of λ binding sites in rat brain. *Eur. J. Pharmacol.*, **129,** 147–58.
Perry, E. K., Atack J. R., Perry, R. H., Hardy, J. A., Dodd, P. R., Edwardson, J. A., Blessed, G., Tomlinson, B. E. & Fairbairn, A. F. (1984). Intralaminar neurochemical distributions in human mid temporal cortex: comparisons between Alzheimer's disease and the normal. *J. Neurochem.*, **42,** 1402–10.
Perry, E. K., Blessed, G., Tomlinson, B. E., Perry, R. H., Crow, T. J., Cross, A. J., Dockray, G. J., Dimaline, R. & Arregui, A. (1981b). Neurochemical activities in human temporal lobe related to aging and Alzheimer-type changes. *Neurobiol. Aging*, **2,** 251–6.
Perry, E. K., Curtis, M., Dick, D. J., Candy, J. M., Atack, J. R., Bloxham, C. A., Blessed, G., Fairbairn, A. & Tomlinson, B. E. (1985). Cholinergic correlates of cognitive impairment in Parkinson's disease: comparisons with Alzheimer's disease. *J. Neurol. Neurosurg. Psychiatry*, **48,** 413–21.
Perry, E. K., Perry, R. H., Blessed, G. & Tomlinson, B. E. (1977). Necropsy evidence of central cholinergic deficits in senile dementia. *Lancet*, I, 189.
Perry, E. K., Perry, R. H., Candy, J. M., Fairbairn, A. F., Blessed, G., Dick, D. J. & Tomlinson, B. E. (1984). Cortical serotonin-S_2 receptor binding abnormalities in patients with Alzheimer's disease: comparisons with Parkinson's disease. *Neurosci. Lett.*, **51,** 353–7.
Perry, E. K., Perry, R. H., Smith, C. J., Purohit, D., Bonham, T., Dick, D. J., Candy, J. M., Edwardson, J. A. & Fairbairn, A. (1986). Cholinergic receptors in cognitive disorders. *Can. J. Neurol. Sci.*, **13,** 521–7.
Perry, E. K., Tomlinson, B. E., Blessed, G., Perry, R. H., Cross, A. J. & Crow, T. J. (1981a). Neuropathological and biochemical observations on the noradrenergic system in Alzheimer's disease. *J. Neurol. Sci.*, **51,** 279–87.
Phillis, J. W. & York, D. H. (1968). Pharmacological studies on a cholinergic inhibition in the cerebral cortex. *Brain Res.*, **10,** 297–306.
Quirion, R., Richard, J. & Dam, T. V. (1985). Evidence for the existence of serotonin type-2 receptor on cholinergic terminals in rat cortex. *Brain Res.*, **333,** 345–9.
Rainbow, T. C., Parsons, B. & Wolfe, B. B. (1984a). Quantitative

autoradiography of β_1 and β_2-adrenergic receptors in rat brain. *Proc. Nat. Acad. Sci. USA*, **81,** 1585—9.
Rainbow, T. C., Schwartz, R. D., Parsons, B. & Kellar, K. J. (1984b). Quantitative autoradiography of nicotinic [^{3}H] acetylcholine binding sites in rat brain. *Neurosci. Lett.*, **50,** 193–6.
Rainbow, T. C., Wieczorek, C. M. & Halpain, S. (1984c). Quantitative autoradiography of binding sites for [^{3}H] AMPA, a structural analogue of glutamic acid. *Brain Res.*, **309,** 173–7.
Reisine, T. D., Yamamura, H. I., Bird, E. D., Spokes, E. & Emna, S. J. (1978). Pre- and post-synaptic neurochemical alterations in Alzheimer's disease. *Brain Res.*, **159,** 477–81.
Repke, H. & Maderspach, K. (1982). Muscarinic acetylcholine receptors on cultured glia cells. *Brain Res.*, **232,** 206–11.
Rinne, J. O., Laakso, K., Lonnberg, P., Molsa, P., Paljarvi, L., Rinne, J. K., Sako, E. & Rinne, UK (1985) Brain muscarinic receptors in senile dementia. *Brain Res.*, **336,** 19–35.
Rogers, A. W. (1979). *Techniques of autoradiography*, 3rd edn, pp. 1–429. Amsterdam: Elsevier/North Holland Biomedical Press.
Rotter, A., Birdsall, N. J. M., Burgen, A. S. V., Field, P. M., Hulme, E. C. & Raisman, G. (1979). Muscarinic receptors in the central nervous system of the rat. I. Techniques for autoradiographic localization of the binding of [^{3}H] propylbenzilylcholine mustard and its distribution in the forebrain. *Brain Res. Rev.*, **1,** 141–65.
Ruberg, M., Ploska, A., Javoy-Agid, F. & Agid, Y. (1982). Muscarinic binding and choline acetyltransferase activity in Parkinsonian subjects with reference to dementia. *Brain Res.*, **232,** 129–39.
Schwartz, R. D. (1986). Autoradiographic distribution of high affinity muscarinic and nicotinic cholinergic receptors labeled with [^{3}H]acetylcholine in rat brain. *Life Sci.*, **38,** 2111–19.
Shimohama, S., Taniguchi, T., Fujiwara, M. & Kameyama, M. (1986). Changes of nicotinic and muscarinic cholinergic receptors in senile dementia of the Alzheimer-type. *J. Neurochem.*, **46,** 288–93.
Shults, C. W., Quirion, R., Jensen, R. T., Moody, T. W., O'Donohue, T. L. and Chase, T. N. (1982). Autoradiographic localization of substance P receptors using ^{125}I substance P. *Peptides,* **3,** 1073–5.
Slater, P. & Patel, S. (1983). Autoradiographic distribution of serotonin$_2$ receptors in rat brain. *Eur. J. Pharmacol.*, **92,** 297–8.
Snyder, S. H. (1982). Drug and neurotransmitter receptors in the brain. *Science*, **224,** 22–31.
Sutin, J. & Minneman, K. P. (1985). α_1- and β-adrenergic receptors are coregulated during both noradrenergic denervation and hyperinnervation. *Neuroscience,* **14,** 973–80.
Tran, V. T., Beal, M. F. & Martin, J. B. (1985). Two types of somatostatin receptors differentiated by cyclic somatostatin analogues. *Science*, **228,** 492–5.
Tran, V. T., Uhl, G. R., Perry, D. C., Manning, D. C., Vale, W. W., Perrin, W. H., Rivier, J. E., Martin, J. B. & Snyder, S. H. (1984). Autoradiographic localization of somatostatin receptors in rat brain. *Eur. J. Pharmacol.*, **101,** 307–9.
Wamsley, J. K., Palacios, J. M., Young, W. S. & Kuhar, M. J. (1981). Autoradiographic determination of neurotransmitter receptor distributions in the cerebral and cerebellar cortices. *J. Histochem. Cytochem.*, **29,** 125–35.
Wamsley, J. K., Zarbin, M. A., Birdsall, N. J. M. & Kuhar, M. J. (1980).

Muscarinic cholinergic receptors: Autoradiographic localization of high and low affinity agonist binding sites. *Brain Res.*, **200,** 1–12.

Weightman, D. R., Whitford, C. A., Snell, C. R., Hirst, B. H., Brundish, D. E. & Kendall-Taylor, P. A. (1985). Rat brain possesses two high-affinity binding sites for [^{3}H]somatostatin. *Neurosci. Lett.*, **55,** 161–6.

White, P., Hiley, C. R., Goodhardt, M. J., Carrasco, L. H., Keet, J. P., Williams, I. E. & Bowen, D. M. (1977) Neocortical cholinergic neurons in elderly people. *Lancet*, I, 668–70.

Whitehouse, P. J., Kopajtic, T. J., Jones, B. C., Kuhar, M. J. & Price, D. L. (1985). An in vitro receptor autoradiographic study of muscarinic cholinergic receptor subtypes in the amygdala and neocortex of patients with Alzheimer's disease. *Neurology,* **35,** *(Suppl. 1)*, 217.

Whitford, C. A., Bloxham, C. A., Snell, C. R., Candy, J. M. & Hirst, B. H. (1986). Regional distribution of high affinity ^{3}H-somatostatin binding sites in the human brain. *Brain Res.*, **398,** 141–7.

Whitford, C. A., Candy, J. M., Snell, C. R., Hirst, B. H., Oakley, A. E., Johnson, M. & Thompson, J. E. (1987). Autoradiographic visualisation of binding sites for [^{3}H] somatostatin in the rat brain. *Eur. J. Pharmacol.*, **138,** 327–33.

Williams, M. & Robinson, J. L. (1985). Binding of the nicotinic cholinergic antagonist, dihydro-β-erythroidine (DBE) to rat brain tissue. *J. Neurosci.*, in press.

Wise, S. P. & Herkenham, M. (1982). Opiate receptor distribution in the cerebral cortex of the rhesus monkey. *Science*, **218,** 387–9.

Wood, P. L., Etienne, P., Lal, S., Nair, N. P., Finlayson, M. H., Gauthier, S., Palo, J., Haltia, M., Paetau, A. & Bird, E. D. (1983). A post mortem comparison of the cortical cholinergic system in Alzheimer's disease and Pick's disease. *J. Neurol. Sci.*, **62,** 211–7.

Young, W. S. and Kuhar, M. J. (1979). A new method for receptor autoradiography: [^{3}H] opioid receptors in rat brain. *Brain Res.*, **179,** 255–70.

Young, W. S. & Kuhar, M. J. (1980). Noradrenergic α_1 and α_2 receptors: Light microscopic autoradiographic localization. *Proc. Nat. Acad. Sci. USA*, **77,** 1696–700.

Young, W. S. & Kuhar, M. J. (1981). Neurotensin receptor localization by light microscopic autoradiography in rat brain. *Brain Res.*, **206,** 273–85.

Zarbin, M. A., Innis, R. B., Wamsley, J. K., Snyder, S. H. & Kuhar, M. J. (1983). Autoradiographic localization of cholecystokinin receptors in rodent brain. *J. Neurosci.*, **3,** 877–906.

8

Neurotransmitter receptors in normal human aging and Alzheimer's disease

David G. Morgan, Patrick C. May and Caleb E. Finch

8.1 Introduction

Interest in the biochemistry of dementia disorders has blossomed over the last decade because of new neurochemical techniques, and a greater availability of postmortem brain samples from diseased and control subjects. A number of neurotransmitter and neuropeptide systems are compromised in Alzheimer-type dementias in both cortical and subcortical brain regions (for review see Davies, 1983; Perry & Perry, 1985). In most cases of Alzheimer's disease (AD), the cholinergic innervation of cerebral cortex has degenerated, and, in some cases, the noradrenergic and serotonergic innervation is also reduced. This review will focus exclusively on changes in brain neurotransmitter receptors associated with both normal (non-pathological) human aging, and in AD.

8.2 Considerations in experimental design

In general, the literature on receptors in AD and human aging presents many interpretive problems and gaps of information. A substantial portion of the reports failed to present important methodological details, such as the compound used to define non-specific binding of the radioligand, or the concentrations of radiolabeled compound used. These basic methodological variables need to be in the report itself, rather than a secondary reference, to allow critical appraisal of the methodology in the light of more recent developments.

We also were disappointed that few researchers performed full range saturation analyses on their samples. Many reports are based on single concentration measurements. In this regard, the human literature is less rigorous than the experimental animal literature, where full saturation analysis of receptor binding sites is the norm. Obviously, the guidelines presented below will be difficult for all researchers to follow due to various constraints (time, tissue availability, expense). Indeed, our own studies occasionally fail to meet these criteria. However, attempts to achieve these ideal assay conditions may help to alleviate some of the ambiguity in the literature, and, in any case, will produce more reliable data.

8.2.1 *Saturation analyses*

In general, the studies reviewed here measured radioligand binding sites at a single radioligand concentration. The major problem with such analyses is that any differences between groups may result from differences in the actual number of receptors (receptor density, B_{max}) or a change in the affinity of the receptor for the radioligand (equilibrium dissociation constant, K_d). It is impossible to discriminate these two possibilities from single concentration data, yet the implications are widely different. A change in receptor density implies that the maximal *capacity* of the system to respond to a neurotransmitter (or drug) is different, i.e. a change in responsivity. In contrast, a change in affinity implies that the *sensitivity* of the system to a neurotransmitter or drug is altered. From a pharmacologist's viewpoint, selective changes in these parameters would have considerably different therapeutic consequences.

In most instances, changes in single concentration analyses are interpreted as differences in B_{max}, which is probably correct. Real differences in receptor affinity would imply an altered molecular entity and few, if any, instances of this type have been reported. However, drugs used to treat patients, particularly patients with neurological disorders, can interfere with the radioligand binding if residual drug is present in the *in vitro* assay. A full saturation analysis (five or more radioligand concentrations, with specific binding at the highest concentration reaching 90% of B_{max}) can discriminate the influence of residual drug from an authentic change in receptor density, since the drug would change K_d but not B_{max} (assuming competitive interactions). However, the single concentration analysis would simply detect a decrease in binding, and could falsely interpret this as a receptor loss.

A second difficulty in single concentration analyses occurs when a radioligand binds to membranes with more than one affinity. A prime example in this regard is the binding of GABAergic radioligands, which have at least two binding affinities (Olsen *et al.*, 1980). Changes in a single concentration analysis may represent interconversion of low affinity and high affinity sites, with no change in receptor number. Again, a saturation analysis would discriminate an interconversion from a true change in receptor density.

Finally, the single concentration analysis is not as precise as a saturation analysis. Saturation analyses will use 24 or more measurements to obtain B_{max} and K_d values, while single concentration analyses will use 6–10 determinations. Thus, errors in a single tube due to pipeting or contamination are less likely to influence the final result in a saturation analysis.

Admittedly, a saturation analysis is more costly in terms of time, tissue, and radioisotopes. However, the benefits far outweigh these savings. It is surprising that rodent studies, where brain tissue is considerably less abundant, typically employ saturation analyses, even when subjects must be pooled to obtain sufficient material; whereas human brain studies, where tissue samples are measured in grams instead of milligrams, often perform analyses at only a single radioligand concentration. Thus, tissue quantity is not a major limitation for studies of most human brain regions. In addition, assay time is now less of a problem with the introduction of multiport cell harvesters for receptor filtration assays. It is feasible to run 800 tube assays (up to 32 saturation analyses) in a single afternoon with these filtration devices.

Finally, we plead that all reports include the basic parameters of their assays in the Methods section or figure captions. The information provided should minimally include, in addition to the radioligand concentration, the compound used to estimate non-specific binding and its concentration, the affinity of the radioligand for the receptor being measured, the percentage of total binding which is specific (at apparent K_d, if a saturation analysis), and the amount of tissue or protein present in each assay tube. It is rare for two laboratories to have the same K_d estimates (some K_d estimates in the literature range over an order of magnitude). It is not acceptable to assume that the affinity of a radioligand for a receptor is the same as in another laboratory. Each laboratory must characterize its system. In addition, advances in receptor binding techniques and pharmacology continually redefine the optimal method of measuring a given receptor site. Often what appears to be a single site by saturation analysis is subsequently demonstrated to be an aggregate of two or more sites with similar affinities for the radioligand. Knowledge of the compound and concentration used to estimate non-specific binding will allow future readers to appraise critically data obtained using less precise methodology. In most cases, using the same compound as both radioligand and to estimate non-specific binding is a mistake, since non-specific, but saturable, binding may be displaced. Whenever possible, the radioligand and displacing compound should be of different chemical classes to reduce this problem. We recommend using an antagonist radioligand and agonist displacer whenever possible, although in many instances suitable radioligand antagonists are not available (as in the GABA or glutamate systems). In any case, the compound used as a displacer should be specified.

8.2.2 *Normalization*

In the data reviewed here, three methods of data normalization were used. In most cases, estimates of the protein concentration of the membrane preparation are used. In others, data are expressed on a gram wet weight basis. We favor normalization by protein content, which accounts for possible differences in subcellular fractionation that might occur as a function of neuronal atrophy or changes in membrane properties during aging or in disease conditions. However, even the protein content may be influenced by shifts in the ratio of neurons to glia or changes in vascularization accompanying infarcts. A similar, more pronounced, difficulty is encountered in studies of brain development. Here, data are often expressed on *both* a protein and wet weight basis. Perhaps a similar resolution would be appropriate for studies of aging brain or neurodegenerative disease. Normalizing data on a per structure basis will probably result in increased variance due to dissection variability, and is also sensitive to subcellular fractionation differences.

8.2.3 *Multiple tissue sources*

While not imperative, the testing of tissue from several sources would increase the generalizability of the results obtained. If the same effects are obtained in tissues from subjects in the United States, Britain, and Germany, the results are unlikely to be a population specific phenomenon. Such analysis is more convincing than simply increasing the number of subjects from single region. Obviously, it is not easy to find multiple sources of human material and the hazards associated with transporting precious, heat-sensitive samples must be considered. However, exchanging samples is one potential method of resolving conflicting data from different laboratories. The regional Alzheimer's Disease Centers in the United States, recently established to collect and distribute human brain material, may facilitate this exchange in the future.

8.2.4 *Donor criteria*

The quality of human brain material is potentially a major source of variability in studies of human neurochemistry. The genetic and

Table 8.1. *Cholinergic receptors in normal aging and AD*

(a) Cholinergic receptor changes in normal aging brain

Receptor	Ligand	NSB	[S.P.]	Sat'n	*n*	Age range	Region	Change	Reference
Muscarinic	QNB	Atropine	0.4 nM	0	11	55–85	Hippocampus		Nordberg & Winblad (1981)
							Anterior	↓ 30–40%	
							Posterior	0	
Muscarinic	QNB	Atropine	10 nM	Some	13	46–79	Caudate	0	Davies & Verth (1978)
							Frontal CX	0	
							Hippocampus	0	
Muscarinic	QNB	Atropine	—	All	8	43–82[a]	Hippocampus	↓ 60%	Tollefson & Gade (1983)
Muscarinic	QNB	Oxotremorine	2 nM	Some	15	50–90	Temporal lobe[b]	0	Allen *et al.* (1983)
					9	50–90	Caudate	0	
Muscarinic	QNB	?	1 nM	0	11	22–76	Frontal CX	0	Bennett *et al.* (1979)
					10	17–78	Frontal CX	0	
Muscarinic	Atropine	?	?	0	23	65–90	Frontal CX	↓ 30%	White *et al.* (1977)
Muscarinic	?	?	?	?	16	63–92	Temporal CX	↓ 20%	Perry (1980)

(b) Cholinergic receptor changes in AD

Receptor	Ligand	NSB	[S.P.]	Sat'n	CTL(*n*)	AD(*n*)	Region	Change	Reference
Muscarinic	QNB	Atropine	10 nM	Some	11	5	Caudate	0	Davies & Verth (1978)
					7	5	Thalamus	0	
					11	5	Frontal CX		
							Orbital	0	
							Convexity		
					11	5	Parietal CX	0	
					10	4	Hippocampus	0	
					11	5	Temporal gyrus	0	
Muscarinic	QNB	?	0.14 nM	Some	4	6	Caudate	0	Reisine *et al.* (1978)
					3	5	Putamen	0↓	
					3	4	Frontal CX	0	
					5	4	Hippocampus	↓ 55%	
Muscarinic	QNB	?	1 nM	0	12	9	Temporal CX	0	Jenni-Eiermann *et al.* (1984)
					9	10	Thalamus	0↑	

					11	6	Putamen	0↓	
					10	4	Caudate	0	
					8	5	Hippocampus	0	
Muscarinic	QNB	?	—	All	5	13	Frontal CX	0↓	Wood *et al*. (1983)
Muscarinic	QNB	?	?[c]	0	13	8	Frontal CX	↓20%	Mash *et al*. (1985)
					8	7	Infratemporal CX	↓25%	
Muscarinic	QNB	?	?	0	14	6	Temporal lobe[b]	0	Bowen *et al*. (1983)
Muscarinic	QNB	?	0.2 nM	0	10	8	Hippocampus	0	Nordberg *et al*. (1983)
Muscarinic	QNB	?	?[c]	0	5	5	Cortex	0	Greenamyre *et al*. (1985b)
M_1	QNB	Carbachol	?[c]	0	3	3	Frontal CX	0	Mash *et al*. (1985)
M_2	QNB	Carbachol	?[c]	0	3	3	Frontal CX	↓80%	Mash *et al*. (1985)
Muscarinic	NMS	Atropine	?[c]	0	4	4	Hippocampus	0	Palacios (1982)
Muscarinic	NMS	?	?	0	9	6	Parietal CX	0	Perry *et al*. (1977)
					6	5	Caudate	0	
Muscarinic high/low	NMS	Pirenzepine	10 nM	0	3	3	Temporal CX	0	Caulfield *et al*. (1982)
Muscarinic	Atropine	?	?	0	14	8	Frontal CX	0	White *et al*. (1977)
Muscarinic	Oxotremorine	?	—	All	5	6	Frontal CX	0↓	Wood *et al*. (1983)
Muscarinic	?	?	?	0	16	16	Temporal CX	0	Perry (1980)
Nicotinic	^{125}I-BTX	BTX	0.2 nM	0	10	8	Frontal CX	0↓	Davies & Feisullin (1981)
					10	9	Mid-temporal	↓40%	

[a]The 4 young subjects were normal and the 4 aged subjects were demented.
[b]Data were normalized per structure.
[c]Autoradiographic analysis.
Abbreviations used in column headings: Receptor = common designation of the binding site being labeled given our present understanding of receptor pharmacology; Ligand = the radiolabeled compound (^{3}H, unless specified) used in the binding assay; NSB = compound used to estimate non-specific binding of the radioligand; '?' indicates not given in the primary reference; [S.P.] = concentration of radioligand used for single point estimates of receptor binding; '—' indicates no single point data are presented; Sat'n = indicates whether full saturation analyses were performed; n = number of subjects; if a range was presented in the reference, the lowest n is presented; change = 0 means no detectable change; 0↓ indicates non-significant difference of >20%; ↓50% indicates a significant decrease of 50%.
Other abbreviations: QNB = quinuclidinyl benzilate; NMS = *N*-methyl-scopolamine; CX = cortex.

environmental control available in animal studies is not possible in human studies. While we recognize that in most instances, the neurochemist is not able to dictate the premorbid conditions and postmortem handling of samples, the following variables should be considered in data analysis as independent variables along with age or disease condition.

Premorbid state

In human studies, there is no control over the time or reason for death of the donor. Prolonged hospitalization may influence a number of biochemical parameters, even those as general as tissue pH (Hardy *et al.*, 1985). Obviously, if all the control subjects died rapidly from myocardial infarcts or accidents, and the diseased patients died from prolonged bouts of pneumonia or cachexia, the study would be hopelessly confounded. Wherever possible, subjects should have similar premorbid states, or be equally distributed in control and diseased populations with respect to these variables. It is particularly difficult to satisfy this criterion in studies of normal aging, since most young donors die from accidents, suicides or drug overdose, and older donors die from various disease states. A similar problem exists in studies of AD patients, who frequently suffer from pneumonia and cachexia; these problems are not prevalent in the neurologically normal elderly population. There is no immediate solution to this problem, but analysis of premorbid state as an independent variable should be included in all studies using human material. In most of the studies reviewed here, these variables were considered and tested for their influence.

Drug history

Most hospitalized patients are treated with drugs at some time in their therapy. Animal studies have revealed that most psychoactive drugs do influence receptor density. In most cases, controls for AD studies do not have neurological or psychiatric problems and do not receive psychoactive medication, although opiates may be prescribed in some cases and some hypertension medications may have CNS effects. Most AD patients do receive some psychoactive compounds in the terminal stages of their disease. In addition to interfering with the receptor binding assay *in vitro* (see above), these drugs may cause up- or down-regulation of receptor sites in the CNS. Thus, drug history must also be analyzed as an independent variable wherever possible, psychoactive drug therapy should be discontinued when death is imminent. Again, most studies reviewed here have considered the possible effects of premorbid drug history.

Postmortem interval and tissue storage

Some neurochemical parameters are not stable postmortem (for review, see Hardy & Butterworth, 1983). Ideally, postmortem intervals should be as short as possible (4–12 h practically) and, more importantly, similar between control and diseased groups. Most studies reviewed here analyzed their dependent measures for an influence of postmortem interval. However, if the range of postmortem intervals is narrow, or the number of donors is small, an influence of postmortem interval may not be detected. One method of testing for the effects of postmortem interval on neurochemical variables is to cool rodent brains at the same rate as measured postmortem in humans by Spokes & Koch (1978). This is readily accomplished by submersing brains in a container with 30 l of 37 °C water and moving the container from ambient temperature into a 4 °C cold room after four hours.

Tissue storage should be as cold as possible for as short as possible. Storage below the crystallization temperature of water (−120 °C) may be important for some variables. Again, storage interval should be balanced among experimental groups. Very few instances of significant storage effects have been reported.

Neuropathological diagnosis

The diagnosis of AD must be based on histopathological criteria obtained postmortem. All papers reviewed here used histopathological and clinical criteria to evaluate AD and control brains. Unfortunately, the histopathology protocols and rating scale criteria are often not stated in the reports. Typically, several brain regions are examined for senile plaques and neurofibrillary tangles and a rating between 0–3 or 0–4 is assigned. However, the actual number of plaques or tangles required for each score are infrequently given in the methods sections. This information is needed to make inter-laboratory comparisons of results. New histology methods are continually developed to stain plaques and tangles, and to discriminate multi-infarct dementia from AD. These may yield quantitatively different results than the older methods, yet indicate the same disparity between AD and control material. More details of the histopathological criteria would help the reader in interpreting the results.

We conclude that the editorial criteria for journal publication should be upgraded for human studies to the level now current for studies in animal tissues.

Table 8.2. *Serotonin receptors in normal aging and AD*

(a) Serotonin receptor changes in normal aging brain

Receptor	Ligand	NSB	[S.P.]	Sat'n	*n*	Age range	Region	Change	Reference
S_1	5-HT	?	?	0	11	22–76	Frontal CX	0	Bennett *et al*. (1979)
					9	20–66	Frontal CX	0	
S_1	5-HT	5-HT	8 nM	Some	11	70–85	Frontal CX	↓ 50%	Allen *et al*. (1983)
					11	55–90	Temporal CX	↓ 70%	
S_1	5-HT	5-HT	—	All	20	19–100	Frontal CX	↓ 30%	Marcusson *et al*. (1984a)
					13	19–100	Hippocampus	↓ 35%	
					20	19–100	Putamen	↑ 25%	
S_1 & S_2	LSD	?	2 nM	0	11	22–76	Frontal CX	↓ 45%	Bennett *et al*. (1979)
					9	20–66	Frontal CX	0	
					10	17–78	Frontal CX	↓ 75%	
S_1 & S_2	LSD	LSD	8 nM	Some	14	50–90	Temporal lobe[a]	↓ 30%	Allen *et al*. (1983)
					9	50–90	Caudate[a]	0	
S_2	^{11}C-methyl-SPIP	Frontal CX–cerebellum	—	—	43	19–73	Frontal CX	↓ 25–35%	Wong *et al*. (1985)
S_2	SPIP	KET	—	All	19	19–100	Frontal CX	↓ 50%	Marcusson *et al*. (1984b)
					21	19–100	Hippocampus	↓ 35%	
S_2	KET	?	1.6 nM	0	29	?	Frontal CX	↓ 25%	Reynolds *et al*. (1984)
Uptake	Imipramine	?	?	0	12	50–90	Temporal CX	0	Allen *et al*. (1983)
Uptake	Imipramine	Desipramine	—	All	23	19–100	Frontal CX	↑ 130%	Severson *et al*. (1985)
					23	19–100	Hypothalamus	↑ 85%	

(b) Serotonin receptor changes in AD

Receptor	Ligand	NSB	[S.P.]	Sat'n	CTL(*n*)	AD(*n*)	Region	Change	Reference
S_1	5-HT	5-HT	2 nM	Some	6	6	Parietal CX	↓ 25%	Perry *et al*. (1984)
S_1	5-HT	?	2 nM	0	11	10	Frontal pole	0	Jenni-Eiermann *et al*. (1984)
					12	5	Gyrus rectus	0	
					11	5	Parietal lobe	↓ 45%	
					11	9	Temporal lobe	↑ 50%	
S_1	5-HT	?	1 & 8 nM	0	7	13	Temporal CX	0 ↓	Bowen *et al*. (1983)
			8 nM	0	6	5	Temporal CX	↓ 40%	
			8 nM	0	5	6	Temporal CX (Biopsy)	0	
			8 nM	0	12	8	Frontal CX	↓ 45%	
			1 & 8 nM	0	5	4	Temporal CX[b]		
S_1	LSD	5-HT	5 nM	Some	17	13	Hippocampus	↓ 45%	Cross *et al*. (1984a)
					13	14	Temporal CX	↓ 30%	
					14	15	Frontal CX	↓ 25%	
S_1	5-HT	LSD	4 nM	Some	10	12	Hippocampus	↓ 40%	Cross *et al*. (1984b)
					11	10	Temporal CX	↓ 45%	
					12	11	Frontal CX	0	
					12	10	Cingulate CX	0 ↓	
					12	12	Amygdala	↓ 50%	
					11	12	Caudate	0	
S_1 & S_2	LSD	?	8 nM	0	6	7	Temporal lobe[a]	0	Bowen *et al*. (1983)
S_1 & S_2	LSD	?	2 nM	0	10	7	Frontal pole	↓ 35%	Jenni-Eiermann *et al*. (1984)
					8	5	Gyrus rectus	0	
S_1 & S_2	LSD	SPIP & 5-HT	5 nM	0	17	13	Hippocampus	↓ 50%	Cross *et al*. (1984a)
					12	14	Temporal CX	↓ 30%	
					14	15	Frontal CX	↓ 25%	

(b) Serotonin receptor changes in AD

Receptor	Ligand	NSB	[S.P.]	Sat'n	CTL(*n*)	AD(*n*)	Region	Change	Reference
S_2	SPIP	?	0.5 nM	0	10	10	Frontal pole	0	Jenni-Eiermann *et al.* (1984)
					11	6	Gyrus rectus	0	
S_2	LSD	SPIP	5 nM	Some	17	13	Hippocampus	↓ 60%	Cross *et al.* (1984a)
					13	14	Temporal CX	↓ 35%	
					14	15	Frontal CX	↓ 30%	
S_2	KET	KET	1 nM	Some	7	8	Entorhinal CX	↓ 60%	Perry *et al.* (1984)
					6	6	Parietal CX	↓ 35%	
S_2	KET	LSD	1 nM	Some	12	12	Hippocampus	0 ↓	Cross *et al.* (1984b)
					11	10	Temporal CX	↓ 65%	
					12	12	Frontal CX	↓ 45%	
					12	9	Cingulate CX	0 ↓	
					12	12	Amygdala	↓ 40%	
S_2	KET	?	0.3 nM & 1.1 nM	0	30	34	Frontal pole	↓ 35%	Reynolds *et al.* (1984)
Uptake	Imipramine	?	2 nM	0	7	13	Temporal CX	↓ 18%	Bowen *et al.* (1983)
			1 nM & 2 nM	0	6	5	Temporal CX	↓ 25%	
			2 nM	0	6	7	Temporal CX[b]	0	
	5-HT	?	40 nM	—	5	6	Temporal CX (biopsy)	↓ 70%	

See Table 8.1 for explanation of column headings.
[a]Data are normalized per structure.
[b]AD subjects are late-onset form of the disorder.
Abbreviations: 5-HT = 5-hydroxytryptamine (serotonin); LSD = lysergic acid diethylamide; SPIP = spiperone; KET = ketanserin; CX = Cortex.

8.3 Specific changes in receptor binding properties with normal aging and AD

Most research in this area has focused on the cholinergic and monoaminergic receptor systems. These systems are probably the best characterized of the CNS neurotransmitter receptor systems, and represent pathways reported to degenerate in AD (Perry & Perry, 1985). By comparison, the major neurotransmitters in brain (GABA and glutamate) have been largely neglected and further research in these systems is called for.

We have attempted to review all receptor studies on both normal human aging and AD, but may have missed some in our computer database search. Our tables include what we consider to be the minimal information required to evaluate critically the assay techniques used. Too often we were not able to obtain this methodological information in the original paper, and time did not permit us to obtain the manuscripts referenced by the authors in the Methods. The field of receptor binding has advanced rapidly; often a single site is resolved into two distinct sites, or two apparent sites are found to be high and low affinity states of the same molecular entity. Whenever possible, we will interpret the results in light of the advanced understanding of the assay system being studied. The effects of normal aging and AD on specific neurotransmitter systems follow below.

8.3.1 *Acetylcholine receptors*

The vast majority of CNS cholinergic receptors are of the muscarinic type (as opposed to nicotinic). Thus, most studies of CNS cholinergic receptors have examined muscarinic receptor selective radioligands.

Normal human aging was examined in seven reports on muscarinic receptors. Most studies found no significant change with age (Table 8.1(*a*)). The single report indicating a large loss of muscarinic sites with age in hippocampus (Tollefson & Gade, 1983) is confounded by the fact that all older donors were demented, while all younger donors were neurologically normal. However, Nordberg & Winblad (1981) found a significant loss in anterior regions of the hippocampus, but not posterior regions. Thus, some loss of muscarinic receptors with age in restricted regions cannot be excluded. However, a general loss of muscarinic sites with age appears unlikely.

In AD, muscarinic sites also appear to be stable (Table 8.1(*b*)). Two studies (Reisine *et al.*, 1978; Mash *et al.*, 1985) report significant but small losses in cortical areas, and several others indicate non-significant declines, but never approaching the extensive loss of the pre-synaptic cholinergic marker, choline acetyltransferase (CAT). Of interest is the report of Nordberg *et al.* (1983), who found an inverse correlation between CAT levels and muscarinic receptor binding in hippocampus of AD subjects (although no difference was found between AD and control samples). This suggests that the loss of pre-synaptic cholinergic input in AD leads to muscarinic receptor up-regulation. Others have speculated that this response occurs in AD, since one would expect a loss of muscarinic sites due to cortical atrophy. Thus, the reasoning follows that the lack of a difference in AD versus control samples represents up-regulation of muscarinic sites on the remaining cortical neurons in AD. Conceivably, high resolution autoradiographic studies of muscarinic receptors would indicate whether more receptors per cell are present in AD brain.

Mash *et al.* (1985) reported that there is a significant loss of the cortical muscarinic sites which function as autoreceptors on cholinergic terminals (designated M_2 muscarinic receptors). The number of these sites were positively correlated with CAT levels in their study, suggesting M_2 sites can serve as pre-synaptic markers for the cholinergic system. However, the characterization of the methodology used has yet to be published in detail or confirmed by others.

Only one report of nicotinic receptors in AD has appeared (Davies & Feisullin, 1981). A significant reduction of these sites was found in the temporal gyrus, and a non-significant decline was found in frontal cortex, raising the possibility that CNS nicotinic receptors do not up-regulate in response to denervation.

8.3.2 *Serotonin receptors*

Serotonin receptor sites have been divided into two classes, referred to here as S_1 and S_2, and by others as 5-HT_1 and 5-HT_2 (Peroutka & Snyder, 1979). Radiolabeled LSD binds to both sites, while [^{3}H]serotonin is S_1 selective (in nM concentrations) and [^{3}H]ketanserin and [^{3}H]spiperone are S_2 selective (under appropriate assay conditions; Morgan *et al.*, 1984). To our knowledge, the discrimination of S_1 sites into S_{1A} and S_{1B} sites, as found in rodent brain (Pedigo *et al.*, 1981) has not been attempted in human brain.

Two reports found age-related reductions of S_1 binding sites in cortical areas (Allen *et al.*, 1983; Marcusson *et al.*, 1984a). In one report these losses exceeded 50% over a narrow age range (Table 8.2(*a*)). A third

Table 8.6. *Excitatory amino acid receptor changes in AD*

Receptor	Ligand	NSB	[S.P.]	Sat'n	CTL(*n*)	AD(*n*)	Region	Change	Reference
Glutamate	GLU	GLU	0.3 & 1 μM	Some	12	13	Caudate	↑ 60–30%	Pearce *et al*. (1984)
							Putamen	0	
							Amygdala	0	
							Thalamus	0	
Glutamate	GLU	Quisqualate	200 nM[a]	Some	5	5	Superior temporal gyrus (low affinity quisqualate)	↓ 55%	Greenamyre *et al*. (1985b)
					5	5	Cortex	↓ 45%	
					5	5	Caudate	0	
					5	5	Putamen	0	
					5	5	Nucleus basalis	0	
Kainate	KA	KA	—	All	8	8	Caudate	0	Pearce & Bowen (1984)

See Table 8.1 for explanation of column headings.
[a]Autoradiographic analysis.
Abbreviations: GLU = glutamic acid; KA = kainic acid.

already been used to sample a normal aging human population. The major advantages of this technique are that the populations studied are living individuals whose general health and neuropsychiatric conditions can be carefully monitored, even after testing, and the technique can be applied more than once on the same individual. The possibility of following longitudinal changes in receptor sites with normal aging and/or disease holds tremendous promise. The use of living subjects, instead of relying on postmortem material, removes many of the confounding variables potentially influencing most human receptor studies (postmortem interval, cause of death, drug effects). These advantages far outweigh the current criticisms of dependence on uniform blood flow and poor definition of non-specific binding.

8.5 Conclusions

Our impressions of the consensus concerning the influence of normal aging and AD on receptor sites are presented in Table 8.7. In no instance is there a large (75%) loss of receptors with either aging or AD. During the usual course of aging without overt neurologic disease, there is a 30–50% loss of D_2 dopamine receptors (in caudate nucleus), S_2 serotonergic receptors, and S_1 serotonergic receptors. Indications that GABA receptors, imipramine binding sites, and D_1

Table 8.7. *Summary of receptor changes during normal aging and AD*

Receptor	Aging	AD
Muscarinic	0	0[a]
Serotonin$_1$	↓ ↓	↓ ↓ ↓
Serotonin$_2$	↓ ↓	↓ ↓ ↓
Imipramine	↑ ↑	↓ ↓
β-adrenergic	0	0
α-adrenergic	?	0
D_1	↑ ↑	0
D_2	↓ ↓	↓
GABA	↑ ↑ ↑	0
Glutamate	?	0[a]

Aging refers to normal aging change (number of arrows indicates amount) AD refers to changes in Alzheimer's disease relative to age matched control subjects.
[a]Selected subtypes of this general receptor class may decrease substantially.

dopamine receptors increase with normal human aging require corroboration. The muscarinic cholinergic receptors, and the β-adrenergic receptors are stable throughout normal aging.

In AD, the post-synaptic muscarinic cholinergic receptors and β-adrenergic receptors are unchanged compared to age-matched controls, or reduced only slightly. On the other hand, both S_1 and S_2 receptors are reduced in AD beyond the reductions that usually accompany aging. Similarly, a small reduction in D_2 dopamine receptors in AD in addition to the loss of these sites with normal aging seems likely.

The effects of AD on GABA and glutamate sites cannot be confidently summarized at this time. More detailed analyses will be required before any consensus is reached. Most probably, there will be small- to medium-sized reductions of selected subtypes of binding sites for these neurotransmitters.

These data have significant implications for pharmacologic intervention in AD symptomology. Presumably, any drug or combination of drugs substituting for a degenerated neurotransmitter system will require an intact post-synaptic network to mediate its effects. The first step in drug action is, presumably, binding to an appropriate receptor. Of the three neurotransmitter systems reported to degenerate in AD, the cholinergic and adrenergic systems are the most likely targets of pharmacotherapies. Approaches using serotonergic drugs may suffer from the absence of serotonin receptors occurring as a result of normal aging and the additional reduction present in AD.

Thus, the best available evidence would suggest that pharmacologic intervention in AD should concentrate on drugs with noradrenergic agonist, or cholinomimetic properties, since the post-synaptic receptors for these transmitters appear unaffected by either aging or disease.

We thank Charlene Williams for her superb clerical assistance. DGM was supported by a French Foundation Fellowship. PCM was supported by NRSA fellowship AG 05329.

Note added in proof. This review was composed in August 1985. An update will appear in Banbury Report #27, *The Molecular Neuropathology of Aging*, P. Davies & C. E. Finch (eds), Cold Spring Harbor Laboratories Press, 1987, in press.

References

Allen, S. J., Benton, J. S., Goodhardt, M. J., Haan, E. A., Sims, N. R., Smith, C. C. T., Spillane, J. A., Bowen, D. M. & Davison, A. N. (1983). Biochemical evidence of selective nerve cell changes in the normal ageing human and rat brain. *J. Neurochem.*, **41**, 256–65.

Bennett, J. P., Jr, Enna, S. J., Bylund, D. B., Gillin, J. C., Wyatt, R. J. & Snyder, S. H. (1979). Neurotransmitter receptors in frontal cortex in schizophrenics. *Arch. Gen. Psychiatry*, **36,** 927–34.

Bondareff, W., Mountjoy, C. Q. & Roth, M. (1982). Loss of neurones of adrenergic projection to cerebral cortex (locus coeruleus) in senile dementia. *Neurology*, **32,** 164–9.

Bowen, D. M., Allen, S. J., Goodhardt, M. J., Haan, E. A., Palmer, A. M., Sims, N. R., Smith, C. C. T., Spillane, J. A., Esiri, M. M., Neary, D., Snowden, J. S., Wilcock, G. K. & Davison, A. N. (1983). Biochemical assessment of serotonergic and cholinergic dysfunction and cerebral atrophy in Alzheimer's disease. *J. Neurochem.*, **411,** 266–72.

Bylund, D. B. & U'Prichard, D. C. (1983). Characterization of alpha-1 and alpha-2 adrenergic receptors. *Int. Rev. Neurobiol.*, **24,** 343–431.

Caulfield, M. P., Straughan, D. W., Cross, A. J., Crow, T. & Birdsall, N. J. M. (1982). Cortical muscarinic receptor subtypes and Alzheimer's disease. *Lancet*, II, 1277.

Cross, A. J., Crow, T. J., Ferrier, I. N., Johnson, J. A., Bloom, S. R. & Corsellis, J. A. N. (1984). Serotonin receptor changes in dementia of the Alzheimer type. *J. Neurochem.*, **43,** 1574–81.

Cross, A. J., Crow, T. J., Johnson, J. A., Perry, E. K., Perry, R. H., Blessed, G. & Tomlinson, B. E. (1984). Studies on neurotransmitter receptor systems in neocortex and hippocampus in senile dementia of the Alzheimer-type. *J. Neurol. Sci.*, **64,** 109–17.

Cross, A. J., Crow, T. J., Ferrier, I. N., Johnson, J. A. & Markakis, D. (1984). Striatal dopamine receptors in Alzheimer-type dementia. *Neurosci. Lett.*, **52,** 1–6.

Crow, T. J., Cross, A. J., Cooper, S. J., Deakin, J. F. W., Ferrier, I. N., Johnson, J. A., Joseph, M. H., Owen, F., Poulter, M., Lofthouse, R., Corsellis, J. A. N., Chambers, D. R., Blessed, G., Perry, E. K., Perry, R. H. & Tomlinson, B. E. (1984). Neurotransmitter receptors and monoamine metabolites in the brains of patients with Alzheimer-type dementia and depression, and suicides. *Neuropharmacology*, **23,** 1561–9.

Davies, P. (1983). The neurochemistry of Alzheimer's disease and senile dementia. *Medicinal Res. Rev.*, **3,** 221–36.

Davies, P., & Feisullin, S. (1981). Postmortem stability of alpha-bungarotoxin binding sites in mouse and human brain. *Brain Res.*, **216,** 449–54.

Davies, P. & Verth, A. H. (1978). Regional distribution of muscarinic acetylcholine receptor in normal and Alzheimer's-type dementia brains. *Brain Res.*, **138,** 385–92.

Fagg, G. E. & Matus, A. (1984). Selective association of N-methyl aspartate and quisqualate types of L-glutamate receptor with brain postsynaptic densities. *Proc. Nat. Acad. Sci. USA*, **81,** 6876–80.

Finch, C. E., Marshall, J. F. & Randall, P. K. (1981). Aging and basal gangliar functions. *Ann. Rev. Geront. Geriat.*, **2,** 49–87.

Greenamyre, J. T., Olson, J. M. M., Penney, J. B., Jr & Young, A. B. (1985a). Autoradiographic characterization of *N*-methyl-D-aspartate-, quisqualate-, and kainate-sensitive glutamate binding sites. *J. Pharmacol. Exp. Ther.*, **233,** 254–63.

Greenamyre, J. T., Penney, J. B., Young, A. B., D'Amato, C. J., Hicks, S. P. & Shoulson, I. (1985b). Alterations in L-glutamate binding in Alzheimer's and Huntington's diseases. *Science*, **227,** 1496–9.

Hardy, J. A. & Dodd, P. R. (1983). Metabolic and functional studies on post-mortem human brain. *Neurochem. Int.*, **5,** 253–66.

Hardy, J. A., Wester, P., Winblad, B., Gezelius, C., Bring, G. & Eriksson, A. (1985). The patients dying after long terminal phase have acidotic brains – Implications for biochemical measurements on autopsy tissue. *J. Neural Transm.*, **61,** 253–64.

Jenni-Eiermann, S., von Hahn, H. P., Honeggar, C. G. & Ulric, J. (1984). Studies on neurotransmitter binding in senile dementia. Comparison of Alzheimer's and mixed vascular dementias. *Gerontology*, **30,** 350–8.

Maggi, A., Schmidt, M. J., Ghetti, B. & Enna, S. J. (1979). Effect of aging on neurotransmitter receptor binding in rat and human brain. *Life Sci.*, **24,** 367–74.

Marcusson, J., Oreland, L. & Winblad, B. (1984). Effect of age on human brain serotonin (S-1) binding sites. *J. Neurochem.*, **43,** 1699–705.

Marcusson, J. O., Morgan, D. G., Winblad, B. & Finch, C. E. (1984). Serotonin receptors in aging human brain. Selective reduction of S-2A receptors in frontal cortex and hippocampus. *Brain Res.*, **311,** 51–7.

Marcusson, J., Fowler, C. J., Hall, H., Ross, S. B. & Winblad, B. (1985). 'Specific' binding of [^{3}H]imipramine to protease-sensitive and protease-resistant sites. *J. Neurochem.*, **44,** 705–11.

Mash, D. C., Flynn, D. D. & Potter, L. T. (1985). Loss of M2 muscarine receptors in the cerebral cortex in Alzheimer's disease and experimental cholinergic denervation. *Science*, **228,** 1115–7.

Minneman, K. P., Dibner, M. D., Wolfe, B. B. & Molinoff, P. B. (1979). Beta-1 and beta-2-adrenergic receptors in rat cerebral cortex are independently regulated. *Science*, **204,** 866–8.

Monaghan, D. T., Holts, V. R., Toy, D. W. & Cotman, C. W. (1983). Anatomical distributions of 4 pharmacologically distinct (^{3}H)L-glutamate binding sites. *Nature*, **306,** 176–9.

Morgan, D. G., Marcusson, J. O. & Finch, C. E. (1984a). Contamination of serotonin-2 binding sites by an alpha-1 adrenergic component in assays with (^{3}H)spiperone. *Life Sci.*, **34,** 2507–14.

Morgan, D. G., Marcusson, J. O., Winblad, B. & Finch, C. E. (1984b). Reciprocal changes in D-1 and D-2 binding sites in human caudate nucleus during normal aging. *Soc. Neurosci Abstr.*, **10,** 445.

Morgan, D. G., May, P. C. & Finch, C. E. (1987a). Dopamine and serotonin systems in human and rodent brain. Effects of age and neurodegenerati disease. *J. Amer. Geriat. Soc.*, **35,** 334–45.

Morgan, D. G., Marcusson, J. O., Nyberg, P., Wester, P., Winblad, B., Gordon, M. N. & Finch, C. E. (1987b). Divergent changes in D-1 and D-2 dopamine binding sites in human brain during aging. *Neurobiol. Aging*, **8,** 195–201.

Nordberg, A., Larsson, C., Adolfsson, R., Alafuzoff, I. & Winblad, B. (1983). Muscarinic receptor compensation in hippocampus of Alzheimer patients. *J. Neural Transm.*, **56,** 13–19.

Nordberg, A. & Winblad, B. (1981). Cholinergic receptors in human hippocampus. Regional distribution and variance with age. *Life Sci.*, **29,** 1937–44.

O'Boyle, K. M. & Waddington, J. L. (1984). Loss of rat striatal dopamine receptors with ageing is selective for D-2 but not D-1 sites: Association with increased nonspecific binding of the D-1 ligand (^{3}H)piflutixol. *Eur. J. Pharmcol.*, **105,** 171–4.

Olsen, R. W., Van Ness, P., Napias, C., Bergman, M. & Tourtellotte, W. W. (1980). GABA receptor binding and endogenous inhibitors in normal human brain and Huntington's disease. In *Receptors for Neurotransmitters and Peptide Hormones*, ed. G. Pepeu *et al.*, pp. 451–60. New York: Raven Press.

Owen, F., Poulter, M., Waddington, J. L., Mashal, R. D. & Crow, T. J. (1983). (^{3}H)RO5-4864 and (^{3}H)flunitrazepam binding in kainate lesioned rat striatum and in temporal cortex of brains from patients with senile dementia of the Alzheimer type. *Brain Res.*, **278**, 373–5.

Palacios, J. M. (1982). Autoradiographic localization of muscarinic cholinergic receptors in the hippocampus of patients with senile dementia. *Brain Res.*, **243**, 173–5.

Pearce, B. R. & Bowen, D. M. (1984). (^{3}H)Kainic acid binding and choline acetyltransferase activity in Alzheimer's dementia. *Brain Res.*, **310**, 376–8.

Pearce, B. R., Palmer, A. M., Bowen, D. M., Wilcock, G. K., Esiri, M. M. & Davison, A. N. (1984). Neurotransmitter dysfunction and atrophy of the caudate nucleus in Alzheimer's disease. *Neurochem. Pathol.*, **2**, 221–32.

Pedigo, N. W., Yamamura, H. I. & Nelson, D. L. (1981). Discrimination of multiple ^{3}H-5-hydroxytryptamine binding sites in rat brain by neuroleptics. *J. Neurochem.*, **36**, 220–66.

Peroutka, S. J. & Snyder, S. H. (1979). Multiple serotonin receptors. Differential binding of 5-hydroxytryptamine, lysergic acid diethylamide, and spiroperidol. *Mol. Pharmacol.*, **16**, 687–99.

Perry, E. K. (1980). The cholinergic system in old age and Alzheimer's disease. *Age Aging*, **9**, 1–8.

Perry, E. K. & Perry, R. H. (1985). A review of neuropathological and neurochemical correlates of Alzheimer's disease. *Dan. Med. Bull.*, **32** (Suppl. 1), 27–34.

Perry, E. K., Perry, R. H., Blessed, G. & Tomlinson, B. E. (1977). Necropsy evidence of central cholinergic deficits in senile dementia. *Lancet*, I, 189.

Perry, E. K., Perry, R. H., Candy, J. M., Fairbairn, A. F., Blessed, G., Dick, D. J. & Tomlinson, B. E. (1984). Cortical serotonin S-2 receptor binding abnormalities in patients with Alzheimer's disease: Comparisons with Parkinson's disease. *Neurosci. Lett.*, **51**, 353–7.

Reisine, T. D., Yamamura, H. I., Bird, E. D., Spokes, E. & Enna, S. J. (1978). Pre- and postsynaptic neurochemical alterations in Alzheimer's disease. *Brain Res.*, **159**, 477–81.

Reynolds, G. P., Arnold, L., Rossor, M. N., Iverson, L. L., Mountjoy, C. Q. & Roth, M. (1984). Reduced binding of (^{3}H)ketanserin to cortical 5-HT_2 receptors in senile dementia of the Alzheimer type. *Neurosci. Lett.*, **44**, 47–51.

Riederer, P. & Jellinger, K. (1982). Morphological and biochemical changes in the aging brain: Pathophysiological and possible therapeutic consequences. *Exp. Brain Res., Suppl*, **5**, 158–66.

Severson, J. A., Marcusson, J., Winblad, B. & Finch, C. E. (1982). Age-correlated loss of dopaminergic binding sites in human basal ganglia. *J. Neurochem.*, **39**, 1623–31.

Severson, J. A., Marcusson, J. O., Osterburg, H. H., Finch, C. E. & Winblad, B. (1985). Elevated density of (^{3}H)imipramine binding in aged human brain. *J. Neurochem.*, **45**, 1382–9.

Spokes, E. G. S. & Koch, D. J. (1978). Post-mortem stability of dopamine glutamate decarboxylase, and choline acetyltransferase in the mouse brain

under conditions simulating the handling of human autopsy material. *J. Neurochem.*, **31**, 381–3.
Stone, E. A. & U'Prichard, D. C. (1981). (^{3}H)Dihydroalprenolol binding in the rat brainstem. *Eur. J. Pharmacol.*, **75**, 159–61.
Tollefson, F. D. & Gade, J. (1983). A comparison of human muscarinic cholinergic receptor properties subsequent to alcohol abuse and senescene. *Biol. Psychiatry*, **18**, 481–91.
White, P., Hiley, C. R., Goodhardt, M. J., Carrasco, L. H., Keet, J. P., Williams, I. E. I. & Bowen, D. M. (1977). Neocortical cholinergic neurons in elderly people. *Lancet*, I, 668–71.
Wong, D. F., Wagner, H. N., Jr, Daniels, R. F., Links, J. M., Frost, J. J., Ravert, H. T., Wilson, A. A., Rosenbaum, A. E., Gjedde, A., Douglass, K. H., Petronis, J. D., Folstein, M. F., Toung, J. K. T., Burns, H. D. & Kuhar, M. J. (1984). Effects of age on dopamine and serotonin receptors measured by positron tomography in the living human brain. *Science*, **226,** 1393–6.
Wood, P. L., Etienne, P., Lal, S., Nair, N. P. V., Finlayson, M. H., Gautheir, S., Palo, J., Haltia, M., Paetau, A. & Bird, E. D. (1983). Post-mortem comparison of the cortical cholinergic system in Alzheimer's disease and Pick's disease. *J. Neurol. Sci.*, **62**, 211–17.

9

Acetylcholine receptor in myasthenia gravis

R. J. Boegman and K. K. Wan

9.1 Introduction

Myasthenia gravis (MG), a disease associated with weakness of skeletal muscle after repetitive use, followed by recovery after rest, was first described by Willis in 1672 (quoted by Viets, 1953). Jolly, in case reports presented in 1895, gave the name 'myasthenia gravis' to the disease (Jolly, 1895).

The prevalence of MG in the population is 1:10 000 to 1:50 000, affecting all races with a medial onset age of 20 years (Simpson, 1974). Females are affected twice as often as males. Onset of the disease can be sudden, being precipitated by such factors as fever or stress. Remissions can occur, being more frequent in younger patients. The most active stage of the disease occurs between four to seven years after onset, with most deaths being reported during the first year.

An abnormality in the function of the neuromuscular junction (NMJ) in MG was suggested because of the similarity between MG and curare poisoning and the response of certain patients to anticholinesterase drugs. This was supported by the observation that patients with MG show reduced miniature end-plate potentials (Elmquist *et al.*, 1964) thought to be due to a reduction in the number of acetylcholine (ACh) molecules released at the NMJ. With the introduction and application of neurotoxins to the isolation of the nicotinic acetylcholine receptor (AChR) (Eldefrawi *et al.*, 1975; Drachman *et al.*, 1979; Sobel *et al.*, 1979; Changeux *et al.*, 1984), the site of the abnormality at the NMJ could be identified as the AChR on the post-synaptic membrane. Support for this conclusion was obtained by the observation that patients with MG show a 70–90% reduction in the number of AChR per muscle end-plate (Fambrough *et al.*, 1973). The relative importance of the AChR in MG was demonstrated by Patrick and Lindstrom who showed that rabbits developed symptoms similar to those seen in MG following immunization with AChR purified from electric eel (Patrick & Lindstrom, 1973). This observation directed research into studies of the autoimmune nature of the disease. Antibodies to AChR have been detected in 87% of patients with MG. However, the antibody titer does not necessarily reflect the clinical state of the patient. Very little is known about events surrounding initiation of the immune response in MG. The thymus, however, may play a role since cells capable of differentiating into muscle cells are present in the thymus, and MG patients show a high incidence of thymic abnormalities. According to Compston *et al.* (1981), MG patients can be divided into the following clinical groups:

Group 1 (10–20%): Thymoma, high titer of autoantibodies to AChR, anti-bodies to muscle striations, no other autoantibodies.

Group 2 (20–30%): Females less than 40 years old, moderate level of autoantibodies to AChR, few antibodies to muscle striations, presence of other autoantibodies, presence of certain chromosomal markers (HLA-A1, B8 and/or DRW3).

Group 3 (30–40%): Males, low level of autoantibodies to receptor, high frequency of other autoantibodies, presence of HLA-A3, B7 and/or DRW2.

Group 4: Neonatal MG.

Group 5: ξ-penicillamine-induced MG (in rheumatoid arthritis patients).

9.2 Acetylcholine receptor

9.2.1 *Synaptic organization*

Receptors are densely packed at the tips of junctional folds in the post-synaptic membrane of skeletal muscle fibers (Fig. 9.1). The receptor packing density on the junctional folds is estimated to be about $10^4/\mu m^2$ and there are approximately 10^7 receptors per junction (Fambrough *et al.*, 1973; Ito *et al.*, 1978). On the extracellular surface a plaque of basal lamina consisting of heparin sulfate proteoglycan, which might play a role in synaptic molecular organization, interacts with the receptor (Sanes *et al.*, 1978; Anderson & Fambrough, 1983; Fallon *et al.*, 1985). It is thought that the main immunogenic (MIR) of the receptor complex might be the recognition site for interaction of the receptor with components of the basal lamina (Tzartos *et al.*, 1981). On the cytoplasmic surface, the receptor is closely associated with a group of M_r 43 000 dalton proteins (43 K proteins) which could be important in the structural organization of the receptor and enzymatic functions mediated by the receptor (Sobel *et al.*, 1977; Neubig *et al.*, 1979; Moore *et al.*, 1979; Klymkowsky *et al.*, 1980; Froehner, 1981; Gysin *et al.*, 1983; Barrantes *et al.*, 1983; Giraudat *et al.*, 1984). In addition to the 43 K proteins, the sub-synaptic surface of the receptor is supported by a network of

Fig. 9.1. The neuromuscular junction and the acetylcholine receptor. Acetylcholine released from vesicles in the nerve ending interacts with receptors (AChR) concentrated on junctional folds. The AChR consists of protein subunits (α, β, γ, δ), contains carbohydrate (CHO) and is attached to the cytoskeleton. Cytoplasmic domains of the receptor are associated with a group of M_r 43 000 proteins (43K), in addition to other proteins of the cytoskeleton.

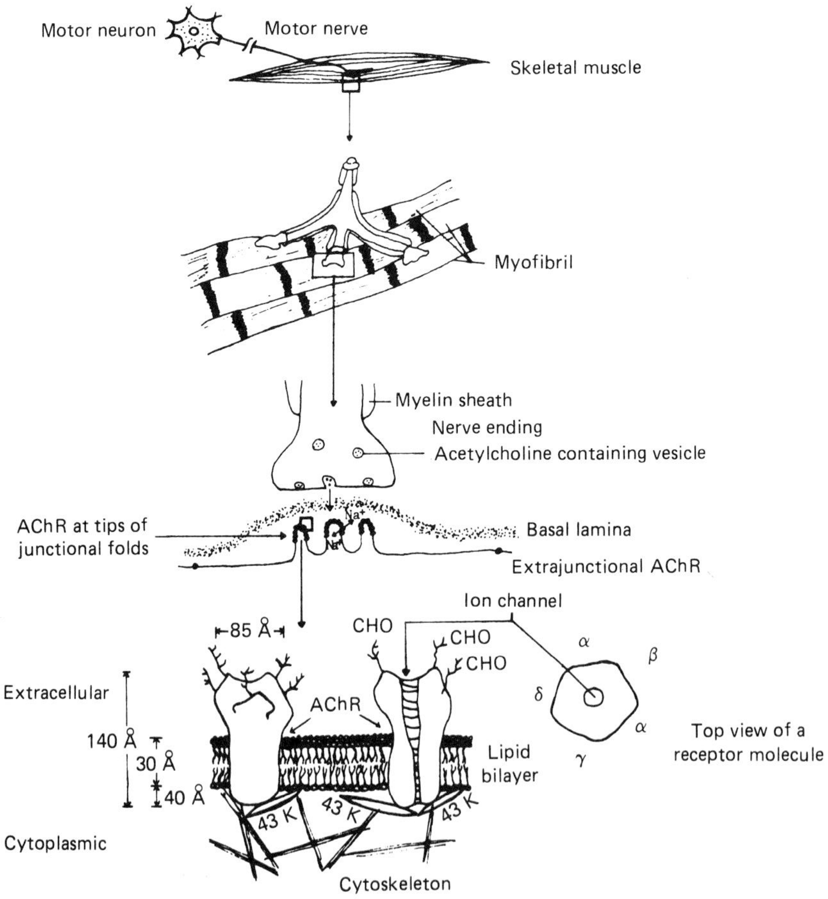

cytoskeletal filaments (Hirokawa & Heuser, 1982), an arrangement common in other receptor post-synaptic complexes (Gulley & Reese, 1981). It is clear from these studies that the post-synaptic membrane is highly organized and alterations in its integrity at any point by neurogenic, myogenic or humoral factors could have profound influences on the normal functions of the receptor at the neuromuscular junction leading to disease states.

9.2.2 *Function*

The function of the receptor is to bind ACh released from the nerve ending in response to an action potential. ACh is exocytosed from active zones in the pre-synaptic nerve membrane (Heuser *et al.*, 1979) adjacent to the tips of the junctional folds where the receptors are concentrated (Heuser & Salpeter, 1979). Recent studies have shown that the active zones represent voltage-sensitive calcium channels (Lang *et al.*, 1984; Fukunaga *et al.*, 1982). The ACh is released in discrete amounts (quanta) although non-quantal release has also been described (del Castillo & Katz, 1954; Tauc, 1982). Binding of ACh to the receptor triggers a conformational change and transiently opens a cation-specific channel leading to local depolarization of the postsynaptic membrane that can trigger an action potential which is propagated along the sarcolemma leading to contraction. Two ACh molecules are thought to be required to activate a receptor whose channel remains open for about 1 msec allowing passive diffusion of about 5×10^4 monovalent cations (Katz & Miledi, 1965; Sakmann, 1978; Sine & Steinbach, 1984).

Receptor activation is terminated by hydrolysis and diffusion of ACh. Hydrolysis of ACh is mediated by esterase located in the basal lamina between the nerve ending and the post-synaptic membrane (Rosenberry, 1982). Continuous exposure of the receptor to ACh or other agonists results in desensitization (Katz & Thesleff, 1957). The desensitized state of the receptor is characterized by a closed channel and increased binding affinity for agonists. A large safety factor is built in, in terms of the amount of ACh being released and in terms of efficient activation of the receptor, to ensure effective transmission. However, when the number of receptors are reduced as in MG, or when the amount of ACh released from the nerve is decreased as in Lambert–Eaton syndrome, transmission in many muscle fibers is likely to fail.

9.2.3 *Structure*

Structural information on the ACh receptor has come mainly from studies of receptors isolated from fish electric organs, e.g. *Torpedo californica* or *Electrophorus electricus* (for reviews see Karlin, 1980; Conti-Tronconi and Raftery, 1982; Barrantes, 1983; Changeux *et al.*, 1984; Wan and Lindstrom, 1984). Biochemical studies on the AChR have been greatly facilitated by the use of toxins from snake venom. The toxins are small (M_r 6000–8000 daltons) basic proteins which bind nearly irreversibly and with great specificity to the AChR binding sites and thereby block their function (Lee, 1970). Examples are α-bungarotoxin from *Bungarus multicinctus* (Chang & Lee, 1963) and cobratoxin from *Naja naja siamensis* (Karlsson *et al.*, 1971). Radioactive-labeled toxin receptor complexes are often used to assay for anti-receptor antibodies in serum from MG patients (Lindstrom, 1977). As shown in Fig. 9.1, the fish receptor when viewed from the top is a 80–90 Å doughnut-shaped particle containing a 30 Å wide central hole (Brisson & Unwin, 1985). Longitudinally, the receptor is approximately 140 Å high, protrudes 70 Å above the extra-cellular membrane surface, and projects about 35–45 Å into the cytoplasmic space (Brisson & Unwin, 1985). The ion channel within the receptor is funnel-shaped with the stem toward the cytoplasm and traverses the membrane through the center of the receptor. At its narrowest, the stem is only 7 Å wide (Kistler *et al.*, 1982).

Each *Torpedo* electric organ receptor complex consists of five subunits, two copies of α, and one each of β, γ, and δ subunit ($\alpha_2\beta\gamma\delta$). Bovine muscle AChR has two types of subunit structure, $\alpha_2\beta\gamma\delta$ ($AChR_\gamma$) and $\alpha_2\beta\varepsilon\delta$ ($AChR_\varepsilon$). Electrophysiological and developmental studies suggest $AChR_\varepsilon$ and $AChR_\gamma$ correspond to the adult and fetal form of mammalian muscle AChR respectively (Reynolds & Karlin, 1978; Lindstrom *et al.*, 1979; Raftery *et al.*, 1980; Claudio *et al.*, 1983; Noda *et al.*, 1983, 1983a; Takai *et al.*, 1985; Mishina *et al.*, 1986). Amino acid sequences of these subunits have been obtained by N-terminal analysis (Raftery *et al.*, 1980; Conti-Tranconi *et al.*, 1982) and by cDNA studies (Claudio *et al.*, 1983; Devillers-Thiery *et al.*, 1983; Noda *et al.*, 1983a,b; LaPolla *et al.*, 1984; Takai *et al.*, 1985; Boulter *et al.*, 1985). Alignment of these sequences shows extensive homology among the subunits which are thought to be the result of gene duplication. Primary sequences of fish and mammalian receptor subunits also show high degrees of homology, which is consistent with biochemical and immunochemical studies (Noda *et al.*, 1983a,b; Takai *et al.*, 1985; LaPolla *et al.*, 1984; Boulter *et al.*, 1985; reviewed by Wan Lindstrom, 1984). Despite these similarities most, but not all, anti-subunit antibodies are specific for a single subunit and some are species-specific (Tzartos & Lindstrom, 1980; Dwyer *et al.*, 1981; Mochly-Rosen & Fuchs, 1981; Tzartos *et al.*, 1981a; Gullick &

Lindstrom, 1983; Souroujon *et al.*, 1983; Froehner *et al.*, 1983). Each subunit is glycosylated, presumably on its extracellular surface (Lindstrom *et al.*, 1979; Vandlen *et al.*, 1979; Anderson & Blobel, 1983); at least some have covalently bound lipid (Olson *et al.*, 1984), and some or all are phosphorylated at the cytoplasmic surface (Saitoh & Changeux, 1980; Davies *et al.*, 1982; Huganir & Greengard, 1983). The subunits have their N-termini exposed on the extracellular surface of the membrane and their C-termini on the cytoplasmic surface (Lindstrom *et al.*, 1984). Up to seven α-helical transmembranous domains are thought to exist in each unit (Guy, 1983; Claudio *et al.*, 1983; Finer-Moore & Stroud, 1984; Criado *et al.*, 1985). It is suggested that the subunits group around the cation channel like the staves of a barrel (Finer-Moore & Stroud, 1984) and are probably arranged as $\alpha\beta\alpha\gamma\delta$ (Kistler *et al.*, 1982; Zingsheim *et al.*, 1982; Hamilton *et al.*, 1985) leading to pentagonal symmetry (Brisson & Unwin, 1985).

The functional role of receptor subunits is not well understood; however, reconstitution of purified receptors into model membranes indicates that the $\alpha_2\beta\gamma\delta$ complex constitutes the basic functional unit (Huganir *et al.*, 1979; Lindstrom *et al.*, 1980; Wu & Raftery, 1981; Popot *et al.*, 1981). When mRNAs for each subunit are translated in various combinations in *Xenopus* oocytes, functional receptors are produced only when all four mRNAs are present (Mishina *et al.*, 1984; Sakmann *et al.*, 1985). Each of the two α-subunits contains the physiologically significant ACh binding site, and thus there are two ACh binding sites in each receptor molecule. Recently the ACh binding sites have been shown to be near cysteine-192 which participates in a disulfide bond with one of the other three cysteines in the N-terminal end of the α-subunit (Kao *et al.*, 1984). Interestingly, a major determinant of the bungarotoxin binding site on the α-subunit has been located to residues 173–204, which should then encompass the ACh binding site (Wilson *et al.*, 1985).

Studies with antipeptide antibodies are consistent with this finding (Neumann *et al.*, 1985; Ratnam *et al.*, 1985). However, the two α-subunits are nonequivalent in terms of molecular weights, chemical reactivity and affinity for d-tubocurarine (Damle & Karlin, 1978; Moore *et al.*, 1979; Neubig *et al.*, 1979; Sine and Taylor, 1980; Gullick *et al.*, 1981; Conti-Tronconi *et al.*, 1984). This is attributed to differences in post-translational modification of the α-units such as glycosylation (Ratnam *et al.*, 1985). Site-directed mutagenesis in cDNA studies have shown that some regions in the α-subunit other than the ACh binding site are also important in ACh and α-bungarotoxin binding and ion gating of the channel (Mishina *et al.*, 1985).

The physiological roles of the other subunits (β, γ, δ) in receptor functions are not yet clear. However, it has been shown that monoclonal antibodies directed at cytoplasmic determinants of the β- and γ-subunits can interfere with receptor functions (ligand binding and cation flux) (Wan & Lindstrom, 1985), although these cytoplasmic-directed antibodies should not be pathologically significant. Recently, Huganir *et al.*, (1986) similarly showed that phosphorylation of the subunits by cyclic AMP dependent protein kinases caused desensitization of the receptor. Since physiological phosphorylation occurs on cytoplasmic determinants of the receptor, these studies taken together suggest cytoplasmic mechanisms also play important roles in receptor regulations.

9.2.4 *Metabolism*

Studies with cultured BC3H-1 non-fusing mouse muscle cells showed that, like other membrane proteins, receptor subunits are synthesized by membrane-bound ribosomes and are co-translationally glycosylated in the endoplasmic reticulum (Anderson *et al.*, 1982; Merlie *et al.*, 1983). After conformational maturation, the individual subunits assemble to form the receptor molecule which is then transported to the surface membrane via the Golgi system (Merlie *et al.*, 1983). Localization of the receptor at the tips of junctional folds is probably maintained by association with other peripheral proteins (e.g. 43 K protein), the cytoskeleton and basal lamina (Fig. 9.1).

Degradation of the receptor involves endocytosis and lysosomal proteolysis (reviewed in Pumplin & Fambrough, 1982). Fig. 9.2 shows a proposed mechanism of receptor destruction. The rate-limiting step appears to be endocytosis (Lindstrom & Einarson, 1979). Cross-linking of receptors by antibodies, which occurs in MG (Drachman *et al.*, 1978) and its animal model (Lindstrom & Einarson, 1979), produces receptor aggregates which facilitate receptor endocytosis. Endocytosis is not closely linked to lysosomal degradation (Libby *et al.*, 1980); thus, even if lysosomal proteolysis is inhibited, receptors continued to be internalized at the same rate.

Chromosomal localization of the genes encoding the four subunits of mouse muscle nicotinic receptor has been determined (Heidmann *et al.*, 1986). The α-subunit genes cosegregates with the α-cardiac actin gene on chromosome 17, the β-subunit gene is located on chromosome 11 linked to the different isoforms of the myosin heavy chain genes, and the γ- and δ-subunit genes co-segregate and are located on chromosome 1 linked to the genes of the fast skeletal muscle isoform of myosin alkaline light chain. Nef *et al.* (1984) showed that, in the chick, the

γ- and δ-subunit genes are separated by only 740 bp on the chromosome. The chromosomal separation of the four subunit genes suggests that their expression is regulated by *trans*-acting elements rather than by cis-acting elements. It is also interesting to note that the genes of the AChR subunits co-segregate with genes for contractile proteins that are expressed coordinately with them at the onset of myotube formation. However, the subunit genes and the contractile protein genes may not form chromatin domains to allow co-regulation because of the genetic distances separating them (5–20 centiMorgan) (Heidmann *et al.*, 1986).

9.3 Acetylcholine receptor antibodies and experimental autoimmune myasthesia gravis

Binding of antibodies to the ACh receptor causes MG (reviewed by Engel, 1979; Vincent, 1980; Drachman, 1983; Lindstrom, 1985). This is based on: (i) the demonstration of IgG and complement deposits at

Fig. 9.2. Catabolism of AchR in the presence of specific antibody. Endocytosis is initiated by cross-linking receptors with antibodies. Internalized receptors are then destroyed by lysosomal proteolysis and the degradation products are released to the extracellular space. These processes can be followed by labeling the receptors in culture with [^{125}I]α-bungarotoxin (Devreotes & Fambrough, 1975).

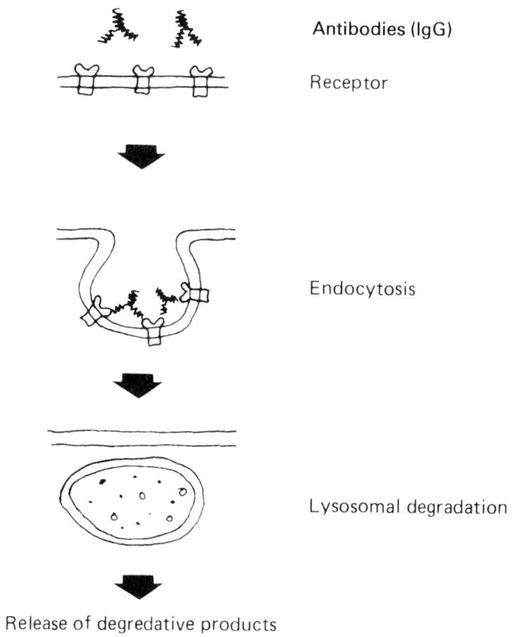

the neuromuscular junction without a lymphocytic cellular response (Engel *et al.*, 1977a, 1978); (ii) inhibition of α-bungarotoxin binding by MG serum; (iii) passive transfer of the myasthenic syndrome with IgG in experimental autoimmune myasthenia gravis (EAMG) and neonatal MG (Toyka *et al.*, 1978; Keesey *et al.*, 1977); (iv) reproduction of MG syndromes in experimental animals by injection of purified ACh receptor (Patrick & Lindstrom, 1973); and (v) the beneficial effect of plasmaphoresis (Dau, 1980).

Impairment of neuromuscular transmission by anti-receptor antibodies is due to receptor loss and blockade of receptor function. Loss of functional receptors causes loss of sensitivity to ACh released from the nerve and is the major contributing factor responsible for the weakness and fatiguability which characterizes MG (Fambrough *et al.*, 1973; Engel *et al.*, 1979). ACh receptor loss is due to cross-linking of receptors by antibody (antigenic modulation) which accelerates AChR internalization and degradation (Merlie *et al.*, 1979; Fumagalli *et al.*, 1983; Stanley & Drachman, 1983). Complement-mediated focal lysis (complement fixation) is probably the primary mechanism leading to alterations in the morphology of the post-synaptic membrane (Engel *et al.*, 1977b). Neither complement fixation nor antigenic modulation can deplete AChR if the loss is compensated for by new receptor synthesis and insertion. Increased receptor turnover at the denervated NMJ (Levitt & Salpeter, 1981) and in passively transferred MG in mice (Wilson *et al.*, 1983a,b) has been observed. It is possible that the result of inserting new AChR is nullified by the reduction of membrane surface available due to complement attack. In MG patients, budding of the nerve terminal probably occurs in response to post-synaptic damage, resulting in the increased release of ACh (Molenaar *et al.*, 1981). The anti-receptor antibodies in MG are usually not just curare-like competitive antagonists. Antibodies blocking receptor function (ligand binding and cation flux) have been detected in 10–88% of MG sera although in most cases these specific antibodies account for less than 1% of all anti-receptor antibodies (Mittag *et al.*, 1981; Drachman *et al.*, 1982; Lennon *et al.*, 1983; Vincent *et al.*, 1983; Tzartos *et al.*, 1983). This explains why MG patients or mice receiving serum from these patients do not succumb within hours, as do animals injected with monoclonal antibodies to the ACh binding sites (Gomez & Richman, 1983). However, receptor blocking antibodies could contribute to further reducing the number of functional receptors. Thus, anti-acetylcholine-site antibodies and some anti-α-bungarotoxin-site antibodies have been shown to reduce miniature end-plate potentials (Albuquerque *et al.*, 1976).

The antibody response in MG and EAMG is polyclonal. The specificity of anti-receptor antibodies in EAMG has been studied using monoclonal antibodies. More than 50% of the monoclonal antibodies made to solubilized intact receptors are directed to a region on the extracellular surface of α-subunits, the 'main immunogenic region' (MIR). Other antibodies bind to a variety of sites on the receptor, while a small proportion bind to the agonist site (James *et al.*, 1980; Tzartos & Lindstrom, 1980; Mochly-Rosen & Fuchs, 1981; Tzartos *et al.*, 1981a, 1983; Gomez & Richman, 1983; Watters & Maelicke, 1983). Monoclonal antibodies made to SDS-denatured purified receptor subunits are directed to the cytoplasmic surface and obviously do not play a significant role in the pathology of MG (Froehner *et al.*, 1983; Sargent *et al.*, 1984). These antibodies might be important in the regulatory mechanism of receptor function (Wan & Lindstrom, 1985). In contrast, antibodies to the MIR are highly significant because they can passively transfer the myasthenic syndrome by causing complement fixation and antigenic modulation of receptors (Tzartos & Lindstrom, 1980; Seybold & Lindstrom, 1981). The reason for the high immunogenicity of the MIR is not known. A recent study by Lennon and co-workers (1985) has localized a myasthenogenic region to peptide 125–147 on the α-subunit. The synthetic peptide 125–147 belongs to the extracellular domain of the receptor, binds anti-receptor autoantibodies, induces EAMG, T-cell responses and modulating autoantibodies. It does not inhibit toxin binding, which is expected because the toxin binding domain has been located to peptide 173–204 of the α-subunit (Wilson *et al.*, 1985).

The specificity of anti-receptor antibodies in MG patients has been studied using monoclonal antibodies as competitive inhibitors (Tzartos *et al.*, 1981b). These studies indicate that the average spectrum of anti-receptor antibody specificity in all patient groups was the same and very similar to those observed in animals immunized with ACh receptors. Most of the antibodies were made against the MIR, whereas determinants on the subunits were sometimes recognized. These results show that MG patients do not, in general, have anti-receptor antibodies of unusual specificity. Furthermore, the spectrum of anti-receptor specificities in most patients remains constant over years despite changes in the clinical state and antibody titer (Tzartos *et al.*, 1981b). Interestingly, in one case a MG patient was found to have a monospecific response to galactosamine, with antibodies appearing to recognize one of the two α subunits, binding close to the ACh binding site and recognize only a particular developmental stage of the receptor (Hall *et al.*, 1983). Apparently, the triggering mechanism for the monospecific response is different from that of the polyclonal response seen in most patients. Some MG patients make antibodies specific for determinants present only on extrajunctional receptors (Weinberg & Hall, 1979) which may reflect the origin of the immunogen in these patients. The avidity, subclass and interspecies cross-reaction of anti-receptor antibodies from various patient groups have been examined (Lindstrom *et al.*, 1978; Mittag *et al.*, 1981, 1984; Conti-Tronconi *et al.*, 1981; Garlepp *et al.*, 1981; Vincent & Newsome-Davis, 1982a,b; Bray & Drachman, 1982; Drachman *et al.*, 1982). These data suggest that these antibodies are polyclonal, heterogeneous, and generally of high affinity.

The titer of anti-receptor antibodies in MG patients varies over a wide range (e.g. 0.6–1000 nM of toxin binding sites in the serum) with an average of 50 nM (Lindstrom *et al.*, 1976). The titer in ocular muscle weakness is lower than that with generalized muscle weakness. A patient's titer does not correlate closely with the severity of muscle weakness, although relative changes in an individual's titer can be correlated with changes in severity in muscle weakness (Lindstrom *et al.*, 1976; Dau *et al.*, 1977; Compston *et al.*,1981; Konishi *et al.*, 1981; Limberg *et al.*, 1983). The lack of a general correlation between antibody titer and muscle weakness probably reflects the polyclonal nature of the response, the multiple mechanism by which antibodies to receptors can impair neuromuscular transmission, the safety factor for transmission, and the multiple compensatory mechanisms for maintaining this safety factor.

Anti-receptor antibodies are predominantly of the IgG_1 and IgG_2 subclasses and are relatively enriched in the κ-light-chain moiety (Vincent & Newsome-Davies, 1981; Lefvert, 1981). Patients with ocular MG have a significantly greater proportion of κ-light-chain and IgG_3 subclass antibodies. However, no differences in the distribution of IgG-light-chains and subclasses were observed in generalized MG. Some antibody characteristics may change with the duration of the disease. For example, the percentage of κ-light-chain antibodies and anti-receptor avidity are lower in patients with recent onset MG; whether spontaneous or penicillamine-associated, than in generalized MG of more than one year's duration (Vincent & Newsome-Davies, 1982a).

Antibodies can be assayed by indirect immune precipitation of [^{125}I] α-bungarotoxin-labeled receptors prepared from muscle (Lindstrom, 1977). The antigen giving the best results in these assays is human muscle AChR (Lindstrom *et al.*, 1976, 1978; Savage-Marengo *et al.*, 1979; Garlepp *et al.*, 1981). An ELISA (Enzyme Linked ImmunoSorbent Assay)

assay for anti-receptor antibodies in MG patient sera has also been developed (Dwyer *et al.*, 1983).

Naturally-occurring anti-idiotype antibodies have been detected in MG patients (Dwyer *et al.*, 1983). Using MIR monoclonal antibodies as the antigen, anti-idiotype antibodies were produced in rats (Lennon *et al.*, 1983; Killen *et al.*, 1985). However, there is little cross-reaction between anti-idiotype antibodies to one MIR antibody and another (Killen *et al.*, 1985). In addition, these anti-idiotype antibodies do not protect animals from developing EAMG when immunized with purified receptor (Lennon & Lambert, 1980; Barkas & Simpson, 1981; Killen *et al.*, 1985). Antibodies directed against Bis Q (a structurally-constrained receptor agonist) can induce EAMG when injected into rabbits (Wasserman *et al.*, 1982), suggesting that the binding sites of antibodies to Bis Q resemble ACh binding sites on receptors. These studies indicate that an autoimmune anti-receptor disease could originate from an anti-idiotypic response to a receptor ligand; however, its significance in the pathogenesis of MG is unclear.

9.4 Immunopathogenesis

The immunopathogenesis of MG is unknown. Viral transformation and genetic predisposition to MG, such as association of some forms of MG with specific HLA genotypes, remain of interest (Christadoss *et al.*, 1981; Korn & Abramsky, 1981; Pirskanen *et al.*, 1981). Alterations in T-cell sub-populations have been reported (Sagar *et al.*, 1980; Skolnik *et al.*, 1982; Miller *et al.*, 1982; Hohlfeld *et al.*, 1982, 1984; Lisak *et al.*, 1983, Berrih *et al.*, 1984); however, the significance of these studies is not yet clear. In lymphocyte cultures from MG patients, addition of *Torpedo* ACh receptor causes thymidine incorporation and addition of pokeweed mitogen stimulates anti-receptor antibody synthesis (Abramsky *et al.*, 1975; Conti-Tranconi *et al.*, 1979; Richman *et al.*, 1979; McLachlan *et al.*, 1981). The involvement of the thymus continues to attract attention. Myoid cells are formed in the thymus and muscle cells can be grown out of thymus culture (Wekerle *et al.*, 1981). A small amount of acetylcholine receptor can be extracted from thymus (Kao & Drachman, 1976). It has also been observed that anti-receptor antibodies are released from the thymus (Scadding *et al.*, 1981) and thymic lymphocytes exhibit anti-receptor antibody synthesis even without mitogen stimulation (McLachlan *et al.*, 1981; Newsome-Davis *et al.*, 1981). In addition, the presence of thymoma in some MG patients and the beneficial effects of thymectomy suggest that the thymus might play a significant role in the pathogenesis of MG.

9.5 Therapy

The treatment of patients with MG has been reviewed by Drachman (1978). Jolly, who commented on the similarity between curare poisoning and MG, proposed the use of physostigmine in the treatment of MG. The beneficial effect of anticholinesterase drugs was reported in 1934 (Walker, 1934). By increasing the concentration of ACh at the NMJ, more AChRs are activated leading to muscle contraction. Inhibitors of acetylcholinesterase have become the standard form of therapy in MG. Overdosage with anticholinesterase drugs may lead to muscle weakness due to progressive accumulation of inactive desensitized AChR. In addition, muscle necrosis has been observed following prolonged AChR activation (Wecker *et al.*, 1978).

Treatment of MG with corticosteroids leads to improvement in 70–100% of patients. In order to maintain a beneficial effect, steroid therapy must be continued indefinitely, raising the potential of adverse side effects. Steroids exert a direct effect on neuromuscular transmission and suppress the immune response. Medication with anticholinesterases should be continued, especially during initiation of steroid therapy. Steroids may be indicated for any patient whose muscle weakness is difficult to control with anticholinesterases or thymectomy.

In addition, corticosteroids have been used with thymectomy since both result in immunosuppression.

Since the thymus plays an important role in mediating the immune response, it is not surprising that removal of the thymus gland leads to improvement in 50–80% of patients with MG. The main advantage of thymectomy lies in the possibility that permanent remission or improvement may occur.

The immunosuppressive drugs, azathioprine and 6-mercaptopurine, have been helpful in the treatment of MG. Serious side effects such as bone marrow depression limit the prolonged use of immunosuppressive therapy.

Plasma exchange and thoracic duct drainage used to deplete serum antibodies have been used in some patients.

We would like to thank Mrs J. LeSarge for help in preparing this review.

References

Abramsky, O., Aharonov, A., Webb, C. & Fuchs, S. (1975). Cellular immune response to acetylcholine receptor-rich fraction in patients with myasthenia gravis. *Clin. Exp. Immunol.*, **19**, 11.

Albuquerque, E. X., Rash, J. E., Mayer, R. F. & Satterfield, J. R. (1976). An electrophysiological study of the neuromuscular junction in patients with myasthenia gravis. *Exp. Neurol.*, **51,** 536.
Anderson, D. & Blobel, G. (1983). Molecular events in the synthesis and assembly of nicotinic acetylcholine receptor. *Cold Spring Harbor Symp. Quant. Biol.,* XLVIII, 125.
Anderson, D. J., Walter, P. & Blobel, G. (1982). Signal recognition protein is required for the integration of acetylcholine receptor δ subunit, a transmembrane glycoprotein, into the endoplasmic reticulum membrane. *J. Cell Biol.*, **93,** 501.
Anderson, M. J. & Fambrough, D. M. (1983). Aggregates of acetylcholine receptors are associated with plaques of a basal lamina heparan sulfate proteoglycan on the surface of skeletal muscle fibers. *J. Cell Biol.*, **97,** 1396.
Barkas, T. & Simpson, J. (1981). Lack of inter-animal crossreaction of anti-acetylcholine receptor antibodies at the receptor binding site as demonstrated by heterologous anti-idiotype antisera: Implications for immunotherapy of myasthenia gravis. *Clin. Exp. Immunol.*, **47,** 119.
Barrantes, F.J. (1983) Recent developments in the structure and function of the acetylcholine receptor. *Int. Rev. Neurobiol.*, **24,** 259.
Barrantes, F. J., Mieskes, G., Wallimann, T. (1983). Creatine kinase activity in the Torpedo electrocyte and in the nonreceptor, peripheral proteins from acetylcholine receptor-rich membranes. *Proc. Nat. Acad. Sci. USA* **80,** 5440.
Berrih, S., Morel, E., Gaud, C., Baimond, F., LeBrigand, H. & Bach, J. (1984). Anti-AChR antibodies, thymic histology and T-cell subsets in myasthenia gravis. *Neurology*, **34,** 66.
Boulter, J., Luyten, W., Evans, K., Mason, P., Ballivet, M., Goldman, D., Stengelin, S., Martin, G., Heinemann, S. & Patrick, J. (1985). Isolation of a clone coding for the α-subunit of a mouse acetylcholine receptor. *J. Neurosci.*, **5,** 2545.
Bray, J. & Drachman, D. (1982). Binding affinities of anti-acetylcholine receptor autoantibodies in myasthenia gravis. *J. Immunol.*, **128,** 105.
Brisson, A. & Unwin, P. N. T. (1985). Quaternary structure of the acetylcholine receptor. *Nature*, **315,** 474.
Chang, C. C. & Lee, C. Y. (1963). Isolation of neurotoxins from the venom of *Bungarus multicinctus* and their modes of neuromuscular blocking action. *Arch. Int. Pharmacodyn. Ther.,* **144,** 241.
Changeux, J.-P., Devillers-Thiery, A. & Chemovilli, P. (1984). Acetylcholine receptor: An allosteric protein. *Science*, **225,** 1335.
Christadoss, P., Lennon, V., Krco, C., Lambert, E. & David, C. (1981). Genetic control of autoimmunity to acetylcholine receptors: Role of Ia molecules. *Ann. NY Acad. Sci.*, **377,** 258.
Claudio, T., Ballivet, M., Patrick, J. & Heinemann S. (1983). Nucleotide and deduced amino acid sequences of *Torpedo californica* acetylcholine receptor γ subunit. *Proc. Nat. Acad. Sci. USA*, **80,** 1111.
Compston, D., Vincent, A., Newsome-Davis, J. & Batchelor, J. (1981). Clinical pathological, HLA antigen and immunological evidence for disease heterogeneity in myasthenia gravis. *Brain*, **103,** 579.
Conti-Tronconi, B., Brigonzi, A., Fumagalli, G., Sher, M., Cosi, Y., Piccolo, G. & Clementi, F. (1981). Antibody-induced degradation of acetylcholine receptor in myasthenia gravis: Clinical correlates and pathogenetic significance. *Neurology*, **31,** 1440.
Conti-Tronconi, B. M., Hunkapieller, M. W. & Raftery, M. A. (1984). Molecular weight and structural non-equivalence of the mature α-subunits

of *Torpedo californica* acetylcholine receptor. *Proc. Nat. Acad. Sci. USA*, **81,** 2631.
Conti-Tronconi, B., Morgutti, M., Sghirlanzoni, A. & Clementi, F. (1979). Cellular immune response against acetylcholine receptor in myasthenia gravis: Relevance to clinical course and pathogenesis. *Neurology*, **29,** 496.
Conti-Tronconi, B. M. & Raftery, M. A. (1982). The nicotinic cholinergic receptor: Correlation of molecular structure with functional properties. *Annu. Rev. Biochem.*, **51,** 491.
Criado, M., Hochschwender, S., Sarin, V., Fox, J. L. & Lindstrom, J. (1985). Evidence for unpredicted transmembrane domains in acetylcholine receptor subunits. *Proc. Nat. Acad. Sci. USA*, **82,** 2004.
Damle, V. & Karlin, A. (1978). Affinity labelling of 1 of 2 α-neurotoxin binding sites in acetylcholine receptor from Torpedo californica *Biochemistry*, **17,** 2039.
Dau, P., Lindstrom, J. M., Cassell, C. K., Denys, E. H. Spitter, L. E. (1977). Plasmapheresis and immunosuppressive drug therapy in myasthenia gravis. *New Engl. J. Med.*, **297,** 1134.
Dau, P. C. (1980). Plasmapheresis therapy in myasthenia gravis. *Muscle & Nerve*, **3,** 468.
Davis, C., Gordon, A. & Diamond, I. (1982). Specificity and localization of the acetylcholine receptor kinase. *Proc. Nat. Acad. Sci. USA*, **79,** 3666.
del Castillo, J. & Katz, B. (1954). Quantal components of the endplate potential. *J. Physiol.*, **124,** 560.
Devillers-Thiery, A., Giraudat, J., Dentaboulet, M. & Changeux, J.-P. (1983). Complete messenger RNA coding sequence of the acetylcholine binding α-subunit of *Torpedo mamorata* acetylcholine receptor: A model for the transmembrane organization of the polypeptide chain. *Proc. Nat. Acad. Sci. USA*, **80,** 2067.
Devreotes, P. N. & Fambrough, D. M. (1975). Acetylcholine receptor turnover in membranes of developing muscle fibers. *J. Cell Biol.*, **65,** 335.
Drachman, D. B. (1978). Myasthenia gravis. *New Engl. J. Med.*, **298,** 136 & 186.
Drachman D. B. (1983). Myasthenia gravis: Immunology of receptor disorder. *Trends Neurosci.,* Nov, 446.
Drachman, D., Adams, R., Josifek, L. & Self, S. (1982). Functional activities of autoantibodies to acetylcholine receptors and the clinical severity of myasthenia gravis. *New Engl. J. Med.*, **307,** 769
Drachman, D. B., Angus, C. W., Adams, R. N., Michel, J. D. & Hoffman, G. J. (1978). Myasthenic antibodies crosslink acetylcholine receptors to accelerate degradation. *New Engl. J. Med.*, **298,** 1116.
Drachman, D. B., Pestronk, A. & Stanley, E. F. (1979). Pathogenesis of myasthenia gravis as a disorder of acetylcholine receptors. In *Advances in Cytopharmacology*, vol. 3, ed. B. Ceccarelli & F. Clementi, p. 237. New York: Raven Press.
Dwyer, D., Bradley, R., Urquhart, C. & Kearney, J. (1983). An enzyme-linked immunoabsorbent assay for measuring antibodies against muscle acetylcholine receptor. *J. Immunol. Methods*, **57,** 111.
Dwyer, D., Kearney, J., Bradley, R., Kemp, G. & Oh, S. (1981). Interaction of human antibody with muscle acetylcholine receptor. *Ann. NY Acad. Sci.*, **37,** 143.
Eldefrawi, M. E., Eldefrawi, A. T. & Shamoo, A. E. (1975). Molecular and functional properties of the acetylcholine receptor. *Ann. NY Acad. Sci.*, **264,** 183.

Elmquist, D., Hoffman, W. W., Kugelberg, J. & Quastel, D. M. J. (1964). An electrophysiological investigation of neuromuscular transmission in myasthenia gravis. *J. Physiol.*, **174,** 417.

Engel, A. (1979). Myasthenia gravis. In *Handbook of Clinical Neurology*, vol. 41, pt. II ed. P. Vinken & G. Bruyn, p. 95.

Engel, A., Lambert, E. & Howard, G. (1977a). Localization of acetylcholine receptors, antibodies, and complement at endplates of patients with myasthenia gravis. *Mayo Clin. Proc.*, **52,** 267.

Engel, A. G., Lindstrom, J. M., Lambert, E. H. & Lennon, V. A. (1977b). Ultrastructural localization of the acetylcholine receptor in myasthenia gravis and its experimental autoimmune model. *Neurology*, **27,** 307.

Engel, A., Sahashi, K., Lambert, E. & Howard, F. (1979). The ultrastructural localization of the acetylcholine receptor, immunoglobulin G, and the third and ninth complement components at the motor endplate and the implications for the pathogenesis of myasthenia gravis. *Excerpta Medica International Congress*, **455,** 111.

Engel, A., Sakakibara, H., Sahashi, K., Lindstrom, J., Lambert, E. & Lennon, V. (1978). Passively transferred experimental autoimmune myasthenia gravis. *Neurology*, 29, 179.

Fallon, J. R., Nitkin, R. M., Reist, N. E., Wallace, B. G. & McMahan, U. J. (1985). Acetylcholine receptor aggregating factor is similar to molecules concentrated at neuromuscular junctions. *Nature*, **315,** 571.

Fambrough, D. M., Drachman, D. B. & Satyamutti, S. (1973) Neuromuscular junction in myasthenia gravis: Decreased acetylcholine receptors. *Science*, **182,** 293.

Finer-Moore, J. & Stroud, R. (1984). Amphipathic analysis and possible formation of the ion channel in an acetylcholine receptor. *Proc. Nat. Acad. Sci. USA*, **81,** 155.

Froehner, S. C. (1981). Identification of exposed and buried determinants of the membrane-bound acetylcholine receptor from *Torpedo californica. Biochemistry*, **20,** 4905.

Froehner, S. C., Douville, E., Klink, S. & Culps, W. J. (1983). Monoclonal antibodies to cytoplasmic domains of the acetylcholine receptor. *J. Biol. Chem.*, **258,** 7112.

Fukunaga, H., Engel, A., Osame, M. & Lambert, E. (1982). Paucity and disorganization of presynaptic membrane active zones in the Lambert–Eaton Myasthenic Syndrome. *Muscle & Nerve*, **5,** 686.

Fumagalli, G., Engel, A. G. & Lindstrom, J. (1983). Ultrastructural aspects of acetylcholine receptor turnover at the normal end-plate and in autoimmune myasthenia gravis. *J. Neuropathol. & Exp. Neurol.*, **44,** 567.

Garlepp, M., Kay, P., Dawkins, R., Bucknold, R. & Kemp, A. (1981). Cross-reactivity of anti-acetylcholine receptor antibodies. *Muscle & Nerve*, **4,** 282.

Giraudat, J., Devillers-Thiery, A., Perriard, J.-C. & Changeux, J.-P. (1984). Complete nucleotide sequence of Torpedo marmorata m-RNA coding for the 43,000 daltion V_2 protein: Muscle specific creatine kinase. *Proc. Natl. Acad. Sci. USA*, **81,** 7313.

Gomez, C. & Richman, D. (1983). Anti-acetylcholine receptor antibodies directed against the α-bungarotoxin binding site induce a unique form of experimental myasthenia. *Proc. Nat. Acad. Sci. USA*, **80,** 4089.

Gulley, R. L. & Reese, T. S. (1981). Cytoskeletal organization at the postsynaptic complex. *J. Cell Biol.*, **91,** 298.

Gullick, W. J. & Lindstrom, J. M. (1983). Structural similarities between acetylcholine receptors from fish electric organs and mammalian muscle. *Biochemistry,* **22,** 3801.
Gullick, W. J., Tzartos, S. & Lindstrom, J. (1981). Monoclonal antibodies as probes of acetylcholine receptor structure. I. Peptide mapping. *Biochemistry,* **20,** 2173.
Guy, R. (1983). A structural model of the acetylcholine receptor channel based on partition energy and helix packing calculations. *Biophys. J.*, **45,** 249.
Gysin, R., Wirth, M. & Flanagan, S. D. (1983). Structural heterogeneity and subcellular distribution of nicotinic synapse-associated proteins. *J. Biol. Chem.,* **256,** 11373.
Hall, Z., Roisin, M., Gu, Y. & Gorin, P. (1983). A developmental change in the immunological properties of acetylcholine receptors at the rat neuromuscular junction. *Cold Spring Harbor Symp. Quant. Biol.*, XLVIII, 101.
Hamilton, S. L., Pratt, D. R. & Eaton, D. C. (1983). Arrangement of the subunits of the nicotinic acetylcholine receptor of *Torpedo californica* as determined by α-neurotoxin cross-linking. *Biochemistry*, **24,** 2210.
Heidmann, O., Buonanno, A., Geoffroy, B., Robert, B., Guenet, J.-L., Merlie, J. P. & Changeux, J.-P. (1986). Chromosomal localization of muscle nicotinic acetylcholine receptor genes in the mouse. *Science*, **234,** 866.
Heuser, J. E., Reese, T. S., Dennis, M. J., Jan, Y., Jan, L. & Evans, L. (1979). Synaptic vesicle exocytosis captured by quick freezing and correlated with quantal transmitter release. *J. Cell Biol.*, **81,** 275.
Heuser, J. E. & Salpeter, S. R. (1979). Organization of acetylcholine receptors in quick-frozen, deep-etched and rotary-replicated *Torpedo* postsynaptic membrane. *J. Cell Biol.*, **82,** 150.
Hirokawa, N. & Heuser, J. E. (1982). Internal and external differentiation of the postsynaptic membrane at the neuromuscular junction. *J. Neurocytol.*, **11,** 487.
Hohlfeld, R., Kalies, I. & Ernst, M. (1982). T-lymphocytes in experimental autoimmune myasthenia gravis. *J. Neurol. Sci.*, **57,** 265.
Hohlfeld, R., Toyka, K. V., Heiminger, K., Crosse-Wilde, H. & Kalies, I. (1984). Autoimmune human T lymphocytes specific for acetylcholine receptor. *Nature*, **310,** 244.
Huganir, R. L., Dekour, A. H., Greengard, P. & Hess, G. (1986). Phosphorylation of the nicotinic acetylcholine receptor regulates its rate of desensitization. *Nature*, **321,** 774.
Huganir, R. L. & Greengard, P. (1983). cAMP-dependent protein kinase phosphorylates the nicotinic acetylcholine receptor. *Proc. Nat. Acad. Sci. USA*, **80,** 1130.
Huganir, R. L., Schell, M. A. & Racker, E. (1979). Reconstitution of the purified acetylcholine receptor from *Torpedo californica. FEBS Lett.*, **108,** 155.
Ito, Y., Miledi, R. & Molenaar, P. C. (1978). Acetylcholine receptors and end-plate physiology in myasthenia gravis. *Brain*, **101,** 345.
James, R., Kato, A., Rey, M. & Fulpius, B. (1980). Monoclonal antibodies directed against the neurotransmitter binding site of nicotinic acetylcholine receptor. *FEBS Lett.*, **120,** 145.
Jolly, F. (1895). Pseudoparalysis myasthenica. *Neurol. Zentralbl.*, **14,** 34.
Kao, I. & Drachman, D. (1976). Thymic muscle cells bear acetylcholine receptors: Possible relation to myasthenia gravis. *Science*, **195,** 74.

Kao, P. N., Dwork, A. J., Kaldany, R. R. J., Stein, S. & Karlin, A. (1984). Identification of the α-subunit half-cysteine specifically labelled by an affinity reagent for the acetylcholine receptor binding site. *J. Biol. Chem.*, **259,** 11662.

Karlin, A. (1980). Molecular properties of nicotinic acetylcholine receptors. In *The Cell Surface and Neuronal Function*, ed. G. Poste, G. Nicolson & C. Cotman, p. 191. New York: Elsevier/North Holland Biomedical Press.

Karlsson, E., Arnberg, H. & Eaker, D. (1971). Isolation of the principal neurotoxins of two *Naja naja* subspecies. *Eur. J. Biochem.,* **21,** 1.

Katz, B. & Miledi, R. (1965). The measurement of synaptic delay, and the time course of acetylcholine release at the neuromuscular junction. *Proc. R. Soc. Lond. B*, **161,** 483.

Katz, B. Thesleff, S. (1957). A study of the 'desentitization' produced by acetylcholine at the motor end-plate. *J. Physiol.*, **138,** 63.

Keesey, J., Lindstrom, J., Cokely, H. & Herrmann, C. (1977). Anti-acetylcholine receptor antibody in neonatal myasthenia gravis. *New Engl. J. Med.*, **296,** 55.

Killen, J., Hochschwender, S. & Lindstrom, J. (1985). The main immunogenic region of acetylcholine receptor does not provoke the formation of antibodies of a predominant idiotype. *J. Neuroimmunol.*, **9,** 229.

Kistler, J., Stroud, R. M., Klymkowsky, M. W., Lalancette, R. A. & Fairclough, R. H. (1982). Structure and function of an acetylcholine receptor. *Biophys. J.*, **37,** 371.

Klymkowsky, M. W., Heuser, J. E. & Stroud, R. M. (1980). Protease effects on the structure of acetylcholine receptor membranes from *Torpedo californica. J. Cell Biol.*, **85,** 823.

Konishi, T., Nishitani, H., Matsubara, F. & Ohta, M. (1981). Myasthenia gravis: Relation between jitter in single fiber EMG and antibody to acetylcholine receptor. *Neurology*, **31,** 386.

Korn, I. L. & Abramsky, O. (1981). Myasthenia gravis following viral infection. *Eur. Neurol.*, **20,** 435.

Lang, B., Molenaar, P., Newsome-Davis, J. & Vincent, A. (1984). Passive transfer of Lambert-Eaton Myasthenic Syndrome in mice: Decreased rates of resting and evoked release of acetylcholine from skeletal muscle. *J. Neurochem.*, **42,** 658.

LaPolla, R. J., Mayne, K. M. & Davidson, N. (1984). Isolation and characterization of a cDNA clone for the complete coding region of the δ subunit of the mouse acetylcholine receptor. *Proc. Nat. Acad. Sci. USA*, **81,** 7970.

Lee, C. Y. (1970). Elapid neurotoxins and their mode of action. *Clin. Toxicol.*, **3,** 456.

Lefvert, A. (1981). Anti-idiotypic antibodies against the receptor antibodies in myasthenia gravis. *Scand. J. Immunol.*, **13,** 493.

Lennon, V. A., Jones, G. & Howard, F. M. (1983). Autoantibodies to acetylcholine receptors in myasthenia gravis. *New Engl. J. Med.*, **308,** 402.

Lennon, V. & Lambert, E. (1980) Myasthenia gravis induced by monoclonal antibodies to acetylcholine receptor. *Nature*, **285,** 238.

Lennon, V. A., McCormick, D. J., Lambert, E. H., Griesmann, G. E. & Atassi, M. Z. (1985). Region of peptide 125–147 of acetylcholine receptor α-subunit is exposed at neuromuscular junction and induces experimental autoimmune myasthenia gravis, T-cell immunity, and modulating autoantibodies. *Proc. Nat. Acad. Sci. USA,* **82,** 8805.

Levitt, T. A. & Salpeter, M. M. (1981). Denervated end-plates have a dual population of junctional acetylcholine receptors. *Nature*, **291,** 239.

Libby, P., Buraztajn, S. & Goldberg, A. L. (1980). Degradation of the acetylcholine receptor in cultured muscle cells: Selective inhibitors and the fate of undegraded receptors. *Cell*, **19,** 481.

Limburg, P. C., The, T. H. & Hummel-Tappel, E. (1983). Anti-acetylcholine receptor antibodies in myasthenia gravis. Part 1. Relation to clinical parameters in 250 patients. *J. Neurol. Sci.*, **58,** 357.

Lindstrom, J. (1977). An assay for antibodies to human acetylcholine receptor in serum from patients with myasthenia gravis. *Clin. Immunol. Immunopathol.*, **7,** 36.

Lindstrom, J. (1985). Immunobiology of myasthenia gravis, experimental autoimmune myasthenia gravis and Lambert–Eaton syndrome. *Annu. Rev. Immunol.*, **3,** 109.

Lindstrom, J., Anhold, R., Einarson, B., Engel, A., Osame, M. & Montal, M. (1980). Purification of acetylcholine receptors, reconstitution into lipid vesicles, and study of agonist-induced cation channel regulation. *J. Biol. Chem.*, **255,** 8340.

Lindstrom, J., Criado, M., Hochschwender, S., Fox, J. L. & Sarin, V. (1984). Immunochemical tests of acetylcholine receptor subunit models. *Nature*, **311,** 573.

Lindstrom, J. M. & Einarson, B. (1979). Antigenic modulation and receptor loss in EAMG. *Muscle & Nerve*, **2,** 173.

Lindstrom, J., Einarson, B. & Merlie, J. (1978). Immunization of rats with polypeptide chains from *Torpedo* acetylcholine receptor causes an autoimmune response to receptors in rat muscle. *Proc. Nat. Acad. Sci. USA*, **75,** 769.

Lindstrom, J., Merlie, J. & Yogeeswaran, G. (1979). Biochemical properties of acetylcholine receptor subunits from *Torpedo californica. Biochemistry*, **18,** 4465.

Lindstrom, J., Seybold, M. E., Lennon, V. A., Whittingham, S. & Duane, D. (1976). Antibody to acetylcholine receptor in myasthenia gravis: Prevalence, clinical correlates and diagnostic view. *Neurology*, **26,** 1054.

Lisak, R., Zweimann, B., Skolnik, P., Levinson, B., Moskovitz, A. & Guerrero, F. (1983). Thymic lymphocyte subpopulations in myasthenia gravis. *Neurology*, **33,** 868.

McLachlan, S., Nicholson, L., Venables, G., Mastalgia, F., Bates, D., Ross Smith, B., & Hall, R. (1981). Acetylcholine receptor antibody synthesis in lympocyte cultures. *J. Clin. Lab. Immunol.*, **5,** 137.

Merlie, J., Sebbane, R., Gardner, S., Olson, E. & Lindstrom, J. (1983). The regulation of acetylcholine receptor expression in mammalian muscle. *Cold Spring Harbor Symp. Quant. Biol.,* XLVIII, 135.

Merlie, J. P., Heinemann, S. J. & Lindstrom, J. M. (1979) Acetylcholine receptor degradation in adult rat diaphragms in organ culture and the effect of anti-acetylcholine receptor antibodies. *J. Biol. Chem.*, **254,** 6320.

Miller, A., Hudson, J. & Tindall, R. (1982). Immune regulation in myasthenia gravis: Evidence for an increased suppressor T-cell population. *Ann. Neurol.*, **12,** 341.

Mishina, M., Kurosaki, T., Tobimatsu, T., Morimoto, Y., Noda, M., Yamamoto, T., Terao, M., Lindstrom, J., Takahashi, T., Kuno, M. & Numa, S. (1984). Expression of functional acetylcholine receptor from cloned cDNAs. *Nature*, **307,** 604.

Mishina, M., Tobimatsu, T., Imoto, K., Tanaka, K-I., Fugita, Y., Fukuda, K., Kureasaki, M., Takahashi, H., Morimoto, Y., Hirose, T., Inayama, S., Takahashi, T., Kuno, M. & Numa, S. (1985). Location of functional regions of acetylcholine receptor α-subunit by site-directed mutagenesis. *Nature*, **313**, 364.

Mittag, T., Massa, T., Kornfeld, P., Papatistas, A., Bender, A. & Genkins, G. (1981). Multiple forms of anti-acetylcholine receptor antibody in myasthenia gravis. *Muscle & Nerve,* **4**, 16.

Mittag, T., Xu, X., Moshoyiannis, H., Kornfeld, P. & Genkins, G. (1984). Analysis of false negative results in the immunoassay for anti-acetylcholine receptor antibodies in myasthenia gravis. *Clin. Immunol. Immunopathol.,* **31,** 191.

Mochly-Rosen, D. & Fuchs, S. (1981). Monoclonal anti-acetylcholine receptor antibodies directed against the cholinergic binding site. *Biochemistry*, **20,** 5920.

Mishina, M., Takai, T., Imoto, K., Noda, M., Takahashi, T., Numa, S., Methfessel, C. & Sakmann, B. (1986). Molecular distinction between fetal and adult forms of muscle acetylcholine receptor. *Nature*, **321,** 406.

Molenaar, P., Newsome-Davis, J., Polak, R. & Vincent, A. (1981). Choline acetyltransferse in skeletal muscle from patients with myasthenia gravis. *J. Neurochem.*, **37,** 1081.

Moore, H.-P., Hartig, P. R. & Raftery, MA. (1979). Correlation of polypeptide composition with functional events in acetylcholine receptor-enriched membranes from *Torpedo californica. Proc. Nat. Acad. Sci. USA*, **76,** 6265.

Nef, P., Mauron, A., Stalder, R., Alliod, C. & Ballivet, M. (1984). Structure linkage and sequences of the two genes encoding the δ and γ subunits of the nicotinic acetylcholine receptor. *Proc. Nat. Acad. Sci. USA*, **81,** 7975.

Neubig, R. R., Krodel, E. K., Boyd, N. D. & Cohen, J. B. (1979). Acetylcholine and local anesthetic binding to *Torpedo* nicotinic postsynaptic membranes after removal of nonreceptor peptides. *Proc. Nat. Acad. Sci. USA*, **76,** 690.

Neumann, D., Gershani, J. M., Fridkin, M. & Fuchs, S. (1985). Antibodies to synthetic peptides as probes for the binding site on the α-subunit of the acetylcholine receptor. *Proc. Nat. Acad. Sci USA*, **82,** 3490.

Newsome-Davis, J., Willcox, N. & Calder, L. (1981). Thymus cells in myasthenia gravis selectively enhance production of anti-acetylcholine receptor antibody by autologous blood lymphocytes. *New Engl. J. Med.*, **305,** 1313.

Noda, M., Futurani, Y., Takahashi, H., Toyosato, M., Tanabe, T., Shimizu, S., Kikyotani, S., Kayano, T., Hirose, T., Inayama, S. & Numa, S. (1983b). Cloning and sequence analysis of calf cDNA and human genomic DNA encoding α-subunit precursor of muscle acetylcholine receptor. *Nature*, **305,** 818.

Noda, M., Takahashi, H., Tanabe, T., Toyosato, M., Kikyotami, S., Furutani, Y., Hirose, T., Takashima, H., Inayama, S., Miyata, T. & Numa, S. (1983a). Structural homology of *Torpedo californica* acetylcholine receptor subunits. *Nature*, **302,** 528.

Olson, E., Glaser, L. & Merlie, J. (1984). α and β subunits of the nicotinic acetylcholine receptor contain covalently bound lipid. *J. Biol. Chem.*, **259,** 5364.

Patrick, J. C. & Lindstrom, J. (1973). Autoimmune response to acetylcholine receptor. *Science*, **180,** 871.

Pirskanen, R., Bergstrom, K. & Hammarstrom, L. (1981). Neuromuscular safety margin: Genetical, immunological, and electrophysiological determinants in relatives of myasthenic patients: A preliminary report. *Ann. NY Acad. Sci.*, **377**, 606.

Popot, J-L., Cartaud, J. & Changeux, J.-P. (1981). Reconstitution of a functional acetylcholine receptor: Incorporation into artificial lipid vesicles and pharmacology of the agonist-controlled permeability changes. *Eur. J. Biochem.*, **118**, 203.

Pumplin, D. W. & Fambrough, D. M. (1982). Turnover of acetylcholine receptors in skeletal muscle. *Annu. Rev. Physiol.*, **44**, 319.

Raftery, M. A., Hunkapiller, M. W., Strader, C. D. & Hood, L. E. (1980). Acetylcholine receptor: Complex of homologous subunits. *Science*, **208**, 1454.

Ratnam, M., Gullick, W., Speiss, J., Wan, K. K., Criado, M. & Lindstrom J. (1986). Non-equivalence of the two α subunits of *Torpedo* acetylcholine receptor. *Biochemistry*, **15**, 4268.

Reynolds, J. A. & Karlin, A. (1978) Molecular weight in detergent solution of acetylcholine receptor from *Torpedo californica. Biochemistry*, **17**, 2035.

Richman, D., Antel, J., Patrick, J. Arnason, B. (1979). Cellular immunity to acetylcholine receptor in myasthenia gravis: Relationship to histocompatability type and antigenic site. *Neurology,* **29**, 291.

Rosenberry, T. (1982). Acetylcholinesterase: The relationship of protein structure to cellular localization. In *Critical Reviews in Membrane Transport,* ed. A. Martonosi, p. 339. New York: Plenum Press.

Sagar, J. H., Davies-Jones, G. A. B. & Allonby, I. D. (1980). Clinical and immunological associations in myasthenia gravis. 2. Cell-mediated immunity. *J. Neurol. Neurosurg. Psychiatry*, **43**, 971.

Saitoh, T. & Changeux, J.-P. (1980). Phosphorylation *in vitro* of membrane fragments from *Torpedo marmorata* electric organ: Effect on membrane solubilization by detergents. *Eur. J. Biochem.*, **105**, 51.

Sakmann, B. (1978). Acetylcholine-induced ionic channels in rat skeletal muscle. *Fed. Proc.*, **37**, 2654.

Sakmann, B., Methfessel, C., Mishina, M., Takahashi, T., Takai, T., Kurasaki, M., Fukuda, K. & Numa, S. (1985). Role of acetylcholine receptor subunits in gating of the channel. *Nature*, **318**, 538.

Sanes, J. R., Marshall, L. M. & McMahan, U. J. (1978). Reinnervation of muscle fiber basal lamina after removal of myofibers: Differentiation of regenerating axons at original synaptic sites. *J. Cell Biol.*, **78**, 38.

Sargent, P., Hedges, B. E., Tsavaler, L., Clemmons, L., Tzartos, S. & Lindstrom, J. M. (1984). Structure and transmembrane nature of the acetylcholine receptor in amphibian skeletal muscle as revealed by crossreacting monoclonal antibodies. *J. Cell Biol.*, **98**, 609.

Savage-Marengo, T., Harrison, R., Lunt, G. G. & Behan, P. (1979). Rat or human acetylcholine receptor antigen for investigation of myasthenia gravis. *Lancet*, 442.

Scadding, G. K., Vincent, A. & Newsom-Davis, J. (1981). Acetylcholine receptor antibody synthesis by thymic lymphocytes: Correlation with thymic histology. *Neurology*, **31**, 935.

Seybold, M. & Lindstrom, J. (1981). Patterns of acetylcholine receptor antibody fluctuation in myasthenia gravis. *Ann. NY Acad. Sci.*, **377**, 292.

Simpson, J. A. (1960). Myasthenia gravis: A new hypothesis. *Scott. Med. J.*, **5**, 419.

Sine, S. & Steinbach, J. (1984). Activation of a nicotinic acetylcholine receptor. *Biophys. J.*, **45**, 175.

Sine, S. M. & Taylor, P. (1980). The relationship between agonist occupation and the permeability response of the cholinergic receptor reviewed by bound cobra α-toxin. *J. Biol. Chem.*, **255,** 10144.

Skolnik, P., Lisak, R. & Zweiman, B. (1982). Monoclonal antibody analysis of blood T-cell subsets in myasthenia gravis. *Ann. Neurol.*, **11,** 170.

Sobel, A., Hofler, T., Heidmann, T. & Changeux, J.-P. (1979). Structural and functional properties of the acetylcholine regulator. In *Advances in Cytopharmacology*, vol. 3, ed. B. Ceccarelli & F. Clementi, p. 191. New York: Raven Press.

Sobel, A., Weber, M. & Changeux, J.-P. (1977). Large-scale purification of the acetylcholine receptor protein in its membrane-bound and detergent-extracted forms from *Torpedo marmorata* electric organ. *Eur. J. Biochem.*, **80,** 215.

Souroujon, M., Mochly-Rosen, D., Gordon, A. & Fuchs, S. (1983). Interaction of monoclonal antibodies to Torpedo acetylcholine receptor with the receptor of skeletal muscle. *Muscle & Nerve*, **6,** 303.

Stanley, E. F. & Drachman, D. B. (1983). Rapid degradation of 'new' acetylcholine receptors at neuromuscular junctions. *Science*, **222,** 67.

Takai, T., Noda, M., Futurani, Y., Takahashi, H., Notake, M., Shimizu, S., Kayano, T., Tanabe, T., Tanaka, K.-I., Hirose, T., Inayama, S. & Numa, S. (1984). Primary structure of γ subunit precursor of calf-muscle acetylcholine receptor deduced from the cDNA sequence. *Eur. J. Biochem.*, **143,** 109.

Tauc, L. (1982). Nonvesicular release of neurotransmitter. *Physiol. Rev.*, **62,** 857.

Toyka, K. V., Birmberger, K. L., Anzil, A. P., Schlegel, C., Besinger, V. & Struppler, A. (1978). Myasthenia gravis: Further electrophysiological and ultrastructural analysis of transmission failure in the mouse passive transfer model. *J. Neurol. Neurosurg. Psychiatry*, **41,** 746.

Tzartos, S., Langeberg, L., Hochschwender, S. & Lindstrom, J. (1983). Demonstration of a main immunogenic region on acetylcholine receptors from human muscle using monoclonal antibodies to human receptor. *FEBS Lett.*, **158,** 116.

Tzartos, S. J. & Lindstrom, J. M. (1980). Monoclonal antibodies used to probe acetylcholine receptor structure: Localization of the main immunogenic region and detection of similarities between subunits. *Proc. Nat. Acad. Sci. USA*, **77,** 755.

Tzartos, S. J., Rand, D. E., Einarson, B. L. & Lindstrom, J. M. (1981a). Mapping of surface structures of *Electrophorus* acetylcholine receptor using monoclonal antibodies. *J. Biol. Chem.*, **256,** 8635.

Tzartos, S. J., Seybold, M., Lindstrom, J. (1981b). Specificity of antibodies to acetylcholine receptors in sera from myasthenia gravis patients measured by monoclonal antibodies. *Proc. Nat. Acad. Sci. USA*, **79,** 188.

Vandlen, R. L., Wu, W. C.-S., Eisenach, J. C. & Raftery, M. A. (1979). Studies of the composition of purified *Torpedo californica* acetylcholine receptor and of its subunits. *Biochemistry*, **18,** 1845.

Viets, J. R. (1953). A historical review of myasthenia gravis from 1672 to 1900. *J. Am. Med. Assoc.*, **153,** 1273.

Vincent, A. (1980). Immunology of acetylcholine receptors in relation to myasthenia gravis. *Physiol. Rev.*, **60,** 757.

Vincent, A. & Newsome-Davis, J. (1982a). Acetylcholine receptor antibody characteristics in myasthenia gravis. I. Patients with generalized myasthenia or disease restricted to ocular muscles. *Clin. Exp. Immunol.*, **49,** 256.

Vincent, A. & Newsome-Davis, J. (1982b). Acetylcholine receptor antibody characteristics in myasthenia gravis. II. Patients with penicillamine-induced myasthenia or idiopathic myasthenia of recent onset. *Clin. Exp. Immunol.*, **49,** 266.

Vincent, A., Newsome-Davis, J. & Newton, P. (1983). Acetylcholine receptor antibody and clinical response to thymectomy in myasthenia gravis. *Neurology*, **33,** 1276.

Walker, M. B. (1934). Treatment of myasthenia gravis with physostigmine. *Lancet*, I, 1200.

Wan, K. K. & Lindstrom, J. (1984). Nicotinic acetylcholine receptor. In *The Receptors*, vol. 1, ed. M. Coon, pp. 377–430. New York: Academic Press.

Wan, K. K. & Lindstrom, J. M. (1985). Effect of monoclonal antibodies on the function of acetylcholine receptors purified from *Torpedo californica* and reconstituted into vesicles. *Biochemistry*, **24,** 1212.

Wasserman, N., Penn, A., Freimuth, P., Treptow, S., Wentzel, S., Cleveland, W. & Erlanger, B. (1982). Anti-idiotypic route to anti-acetylcholine receptor antibodies and experimental myasthenia gravis. *Proc. Nat. Acad. Sci. USA*, **79,** 4810.

Watters, D. & Maelicke, A. (1983). Organization of ligand binding sites at the acetylcholine receptor: A study with monoclonal antibodies. *Biochemistry*, **22,** 1811.

Wecker, L., Laskowski, M. B. & Dettbarn, W.-D. (1978). Neuromuscular dysfunction induced by acetylcholinesterase inhibition. *Fed. Proc.*, **37,** 2818.

Weinberg, C. G. & Hall, Z. W. (1979). Antibodies from patients with myasthenia gravis recognize determinants unique to extrajunctional acetylcholine receptors. *Proc. Nat. Acad. Sci. USA*, **76,** 504.

Wekerle, H., Hohfeld, R., Ketelson, V., Kolden, J. & Kalies, I. (1981). Thymic myogenesis T-lymphocytes and the pathogenesis of myasthenia gravis. *Ann. NY Acad. Sci.*, **377,** 455.

Wilson, P. T., Lentz, T. L. & Hawrot, E. (1985). Determination of the primary amino acid sequence specifying the α-bungarotoxin binding site on the α subunit of the acetylcholine receptor from Torpedo californica. *Proc. Nat. Acad. Sci. USA*, **82,** 8790.

Wilson, S., Vincent, A. & Newsome-Davis, J. (1983a). Acetylcholine receptor turnover in mice with passively transfered myasthenia gravis. I. Receptor degradation. *J. Neurol. Neurosurg. Psychiatry,* **46,** 377.

Wilson, S., Vincent, A. & Newsome-Davis, J. (1983b). Acetylcholine receptor turnover in mice with passively transfered myasthenia gravis. II. Receptor synthesis. *J. Neurol. Neurosurg. Psychiatry*, **46,** 383.

Wu, W. C. S. & Raftery, M. A. (1981). Reconstitution of acetylcholine receptor function using purified receptor protein. *Biochemistry*, **20,** 694.

Zingsheim, H. P., Barrantes, F. J., Frank, J., Jaenicke, W. & Neugebauer, D.-C. (1982). Direct structural localization of two toxin-recognition sites on an ACh receptor protein. *Nature (Lond.)*, **299,** 81.

Addendum

Recently, isolation of putative neuronal nicotinic AChR subunits has been reported by Boulter *et al.* (1986) (*Nature*, **319,** 368) and by Whiting & Lindstrom 1986). (*Biochemistry*, **25,** 2082, and (1986) J. Neurosci. 6:3061).

10

Receptor binding in the kindling model of epilepsy

W. M. Burnham

10.1 The kindling model of epilepsy

10.1.1 *Epilepsy – the disorder and its causes*

Epilepsy is a disorder of the central nervous system (CNS) characterized by a chronic low seizure threshold and spontaneous, recurring seizures. It is one of the commonest of the CNS disorders, occurring in approximately one out of every 200 people. In most patients, epilepsy is a permanent condition (see Marsden, 1976, for discussion).

The causes of epilepsy are, as yet, unknown. In some patients, seizures are associated with pathological brain abnormalities – infections, tumors, scars, etc. In many other patients, however, the brain appears to be entirely free of gross pathology (Mathieson, 1975). The occurrence of epilepsy in such pathology-free patients suggests that the basic causes of the disorder may be biochemical in nature, perhaps involving a mismatch in excitatory and inhibitory transmitter systems. A number of biochemical hypotheses of epilepsy have therefore been proposed, the GABA hypothesis being the most popular in the recent literature (Meldrum, 1975; Tower, 1976; Lloyd *et al.*, 1981; Olsen, 1981b).

10.1.2 *Biochemical analysis of epileptic human brains*

The most direct way to search for the biochemical causes of epilepsy would be to assay tissue from epileptic and normal human brains. For a variety of reasons, both ethical and practical, this sort of work progresses very slowly. Although samples of epileptic tissue can be obtained from the brains of patients undergoing seizure surgery, the quantity of tissue is small, the areas from which tissue can be excised are limited, and satisfactory control tissue (normal human brain) is unavailable. Work involving postmortem brains would avoid many of these problems – and be valid within limits – but epileptic patients seldom die in hospital, and epileptic brains rarely find their way into brain banks. In either case, human epileptic brains have usually been subjected to years of drug therapy, with unknown results. For these reasons, studies of the biochemistry of epilepsy usually involve brain tissue taken from 'epileptic' animal subjects. One animal preparation used extensively for such studies has been the 'kindling' model of epilepsy.

10.1.3 *The kindling model of epilepsy*

The basic preparation

The kindling model is an animal preparation in which low-intensity epileptogenic stimulation is repeatedly administered to circumscribed regions of the forebrain. Most commonly, low-intensity electrical stimulation is used, and it is applied to rat brains via chronically implanted bipolar electrodes. At the beginning of the kindling procedure, the low-intensity kindling stimulus triggers only brief localized discharges, which have little or no effect on the subject's behaviour. When the stimulus is repeated at spaced (e.g. daily) intervals, however, secondary generalization begins to develop, and eventually each focal seizure is accompanied by a full-scale generalized convulsive attack. These convulsions are classified according to Racine's (1972b) schema, in which Stages 4 and 5 are generalized attacks marked by rearing (stage 4) or rearing and falling (stage 5). After Stage 4–5 convulsions have developed, the animal is usually considered to be 'kindled'. At this relatively early stage, spontaneous seizures do not occur – all early convulsions being 'stimulus locked'. Spontaneous interictal spikes are seen quite early, however, and eventually, after a very large number of stimulations, spontaneous generalized convulsions – and even status epilepticus – are observed. (For reviews of kindling, see Goddard *et al.*, 1969; Racine, 1978; McNamara *et al.*, 1980; Goddard, 1983; Racine & Burnham, 1984.)

The development of generalized seizures in the kindling model appears to reflect the development of widespread and permanent changes in the subjects' brains (Racine, 1978). The basic nature of these changes is still unknown. Anatomical studies, however, have failed to reveal significant structural abnormalities in kindled tissue (Racine & Burnham, 1984). This suggests that the basic changes in kindling may be biochemical in nature (Burnham, 1986). In electrophysiological studies, the presence of these abnormalities is indicated by the occurrence of a lowered afterdischarge threshold in the focus (Racine, 1972a), modified evoked potentials in extrafocal sites (Racine *et al.*, 1972), and interictal spiking in both (Racine, 1972b; Kairiss *et al.*, 1984; Racine & Burnham, 1984).

Relevance to human epilepsy

How do the changes induced by kindling relate to the abnormalities in the brains of human epileptic patients? This is a crucial question if the kindled brain is to serve as a model for the human epileptic brain. At the present time, we can offer no definite answer to this question, since we do not understand the nature of either abnormality. We can, however, note that the two different sorts of abnormalities have very similar effects on brain function. In human epileptic patients, a low chronic seizure threshold is associated with interictal spiking, increased responsiveness to chemical convulsants, and occasional spontaneous seizures. In kindled subjects, we also find a chronic low threshold (Racine, 1972a), interictal spiking (Racine, 1972b, etc.), increased sensitivity to chemical convulsants (Kalichman & Burnham, 1980; Kalichman, 1982a), and – after many stimulations – spontaneous attacks. While this formal resemblence does not prove identity, it provides a strong rationale for the study of the permanent changes in kindled brains, and the hope that such an investigation may offer clues to the nature of epileptogenesis in human epileptic patients.

Technical advantages

Beyond its clinical parallels, the kindling preparation offers certain technical features which make it very useful for biochemical investigations. It is possible, for instance, to specify the exact focus of seizure activity and the exact amount of seizure development which has taken place. In addition, it is possible to perform assays in the absence of confounding factors such as scarring or recent seizure activity.

This last point deserves special consideration, since it is of particular importance. When epileptic brain tissue is analyzed, it is crucial to distinguish between those abnormalities which are causally related to seizure activity and those which result from it or are irrelevant. In many animal models, the focus is produced by some sort of toxic agent (e.g. metallic ions, freezing). These agents scar the brain, producing structural changes such as necrosis, gliosis and morphological abnormalities in the cells. They also tend to produce spontaneous seizures which occur aperiodically for long periods. Since structural abnormalities and seizure activity are both associated with biochemical abnormalities unrelated to epileptogenesis, the presence of these features complicates the search for biochemical changes specific to epilepsy. In the kindling model, however, long-lasting epileptogenic changes occur in the absence of structural changes (Goddard *et al.*, 1969; Racine, 1978) or – early in kindling –

of spontaneous seizure activity. This greatly simplifies the search for abnormalities directly related to seizure production.

10.1.4 *Biochemical analysis of kindled brains – the role of binding studies*

A large number of biochemical studies of kindled brain tissue have now been done. These have involved investigations of most of the well-known putative transmitters, including acetylcholine, the catecholamines, serotonin, and the amino acids (GABA, glutamate). Recently, the peptides (endorphins, somatostatin, vasopressin and thyrotrophin-releasing hormone) have also been studied, as well as the cyclic nucleotides, calcium-binding protein and certain of the ion species. No complete review of this complex field exists, but partial reviews may be found in Kalichman (1982b), Peterson & Albertson (1982), and McNamara (1984).

A variety of different assay techniques have been used in these experiments, including procedures designed to measure neurotransmitter levels, release, turnover, metabolites, and synthetic and degradative enzymes. The most popular technique, however, has been the receptor binding assay. The popularity of binding assays has stemmed in part from their speed and simplicity, and in part from the glamour attached to a procedure which has revolutionized modern pharmacology. Fortunately, the assays also provide a meaningful and useful approach to the initial investigation of biochemical abnormalities in epileptic tissue.

The *initial* goal in biochemical studies of brain dysfunction is to identify *a system* (or systems) which is abnormal. Once an abnormal *system* has been identified, subsequent studies can determine the exact nature of the abnormality, and attempt to establish casual relationships, if any. Initial screening studies, therefore, should involve a parameter which is a sensitive indicator of changes throughout the system. Receptor binding is one such parameter. Receptors are homeostatically up- and down-regulated in response to a variety of changes in synaptic transmission (Lefkowitz *et al.*, 1984). In addition, they may be altered independently of the rest of the system, presumably as an attempt to up- or down-regulate neural activity (Dasheiff *et al.*, 1981). Thus, receptor binding reflects a number of changes within neural systems, and provides a useful index for initial studies of transmitter abnormalities. Ultimately, other indices may be found which are even more useful. A downstream parameter closely related to neural response would be ideal – e.g. receptor-specific ion flux or electrical response within post-synaptic membranes. At present, however, receptor binding is the most meaningful parameter for which there is a simple standardized assay. The technique, therefore, represents an excellent approach to the initial identification of abnormal systems in dysfunctional brains.

Before leaving the topic of binding assays, however, it is necessary to add a word of caution. Receptor binding is a useful index for initial screening *because* it reflects changes in a wide variety of parameters. This same characteristic necessitates great care in the interpretation of binding data. If abnormal binding is found in a dysfunctional brain, it does not immediately follow that the disorder is a 'receptor disease'. The abnormal binding may reflect another abnormality somewhere else within the system. Binding data, in fact, do not even provide a secure index of the functional nature of the abnormality. Elevated binding may be found either in a hyperfunctional system, or, in its compensatory role, in a system which is hypofunctional. The binding technique, therefore, is useful in locating abnormal systems, but it is wisest to defer interpretation until a full range of physiological, anatomical and biochemical studies have characterized the exact nature of the abnormality.

10.1.5 *Experimental parameters in kindling studies*

Kindling/binding studies have varied on a number of technical parameters. Some of these have probably been of little importance. The development of kindled convulsions, for instance, seems to be relatively unaffected by variations in intensity, frequency or duration of the electrical current used for stimulation (Goddard *et al.*, 1969; Racine, 1972b). Other parameters must be kept in mind, however – particularly in cases of conflicting results – since they have a known effect on kindling/binding data. Among these are: (i) species and strain of subject, (ii) site of stimulation, (iii) interval between stimulations, (iv) kindling criterion reached before sacrifice, (v) area assayed, and (vi) assay technique. These are specified later in Tables 10.1–10.3 for the studies considered below.

In addition, there is one parameter which must *always* be kept in mind when considering kindling/assay data – the interval between the last kindled seizure and the time of sacrifice. The kindling procedure causes a variety of changes in brain function – some temporary and others permanent. Assays performed at different post-kindling intervals reflect different proportions of these temporary and permanent changes. Those performed shortly after the last seizure primarily reflect short-term changes, whereas those performed at long post-kindling intervals primarily reflect permanent alterations. A failure to appreciate this difference caused considerable confusion in the interpretation of the early kindling/binding studies.

10.2 Receptor binding in kindled brains

Sections 10.2.1–10.2.4 consider the kindling/binding data which are currently available. Experimental details are summarized in Tables 10.1–10.3 below. Because of the importance of the kindling/sacrifice interval, studies have been classified as 'short-term', 'intermediate-term', or 'long-term'. Obviously, a biochemical change related to the persistence of the kindling effect must be a long-term change, observable at even the longest post-kindling intervals. Studies conducted at shorter post-kindling intervals provide data on transient changes, and target the systems which are candidates for long-term study. A description of the electrophysiological abnormalities known to exist at each post-kindling interval precedes each discussion section. Due to space limitations, only full publications – with complete methods sections – have been considered.

Most of the studies described below have followed a standard format, which is assumed in the following discussion. Rats have been implanted with chronic indwelling electrodes in either the amygdala or the entorhinal cortex/angular bundle, and, after a period of post-surgical recovery, electrically kindled to a criterion of 1–6 Stage 4–5 convulsions. (Amygdala kindling and entorhinal kindling seem to have roughly equivalent effects – at least on the hippocampus, a favorite site for assays.) Implanted and handled, but non-stimulated, rats have served as controls. After the kindled animals have reached criterion, all subjects have been set aside for a longer or shorter post-kindling period, and then paired kindled and control subjects have been sacrificed by decapitation and the brains removed and frozen. Subsequently, specific brain areas have been subjected to assay, using the filter, centrifugation or autoradiographic techniques. Generally, single-point assays have been done at first, with subsequent Scatchard analyses being performed on those areas which showed significant differences. (Scatchard analysis discriminates between changes in receptor number (B_{max}) and receptor affinity (K_d).) Data have been expressed as percent change in kindled brains from the paired control baseline. So far, all of the systems modified by kindling have shown changes in B_{max}. In a few systems, K_d changes have been seen as well.

10.2.1 *Ultra short-term studies (30 minutes)*

The studies done in the 'short-term' period fall into two distinct groups: those in which subjects were sacrificed at roughly 30 min after the last seizure and those in which subjects were sacrificed at roughly 24 h. These have been termed 'ultra short-term' and 'short-term' studies in the present review. They have been discussed separately, since they have produced different results.

Electrophysiological abnormalities

At 'ultra short' intervals after the last kindled seizure, a wide variety of kindling-induced electrophysiological abnormalities are found in subjects' brains. Presumably these include the 'long-term' changes observed at later time periods (e.g. focal threshold drop, enhanced seizure spread). In addition, there seem to be a series of other changes – the short-term sequelae of seizure activity – which peak and decay in the immediate post-ictal period. Just after seizures, these short-term phenomena may mask the long-term electrophysiological changes associated with kindling (Racine, 1972a). No careful survey of these transitory post-ictal changes has yet been made, but they certainly include the post-ictal inhibitory phenomena observed in the threshold rise (Sainsbury *et al.*, 1978; Freeman & Jarvis, 1981) and recycling (Engel & Ackermann, 1980) paradigms (for review, see Albertson, 1986). Conceivably, they also include processes related to the 'consolidation of the kindling trace'.

Binding changes

Only a few binding studies have been done at the 'ultra short' period of 30 minutes, but one of these was very extensive. Ashton *et al.* (1980) studied the binding of a number of ligands to homogenates prepared from the brains of male Wistar rats, amygdala-kindled on a twice-daily stimulation schedule to a criterion of 'at least two' (2–11, median 7) Stage 3 convulsions. Implanted and handled, non-stimulated, subjects served as controls. All subjects were sacrificed 30 min after the last convulsion, 'single-point' data being generated, rather than complete Scatchcard plots.

The results of this extensive study were totally negative. No significant difference between kindled and control subjects was found in any region of the brain. The various assays which contributed to this overall negative picture were as follows: (i) cholinergic system (muscarinic) – [^{3}H]dexetimide vs dexetimide in the frontal cortex and hippocampus; (ii) dopaminergic system – [^{3}H]haloperidol vs (+)-butaclamol in the striatum; (iii) GABA complex – [^{3}H]diazepam vs diazepam in the 'forebrain', [^{3}H]muscimol vs GABA in the cerebellum; (iv) noradrenergic system (alpha)-[^{3}H]WB-4101 vs noradrenaline in the 'forebrain'; (v) endorphinergic system – [^{3}H]naloxone vs dextromoramide in the 'forebrain'; (vi) serotonergic system-[^{3}H]spiperone vs (+)-butaclamol in the frontal cortex, nucleus accumbens/olfactory tubercle and hippocampus.

These negative findings are somewhat suprising. A number of the same systems show kindling-induced binding abnormalities at other post-kindling intervals, and some of the abnormalities are very long lasting (see below). Even if the effects of the most recent kindled seizure had not developed by 30 min, one would have expected Ashton *et al.* (1980) to observe the long-lasting changes caused by previous stimulations.

In considering these paradoxical data, it must be noted that the areas chosen for assay by Ashton *et al.* were sometimes over-inclusive (e.g. 'forebrain') and sometimes under-inclusive (e.g. cerebellum). Conceivably, some binding changes may have been overlooked. Alternately – as proposed by McIntyre & Roberts (1983) – it may be that the short-term biochemical effects of seizures obscure their long-term effects. This would be a biochemical parallel to the masking of long-term effects sometimes seen in electrophysiological studies (e.g. Racine, 1972a).

Recent studies by Schmutz *et al.* (1985) and by Tietz *et al.* (1985) seem to support this interpretation. Schmutz *et al.* amygdala-kindled male rats of the Tif:RAIf (SPF) strain on a daily schedule until Stage 4 convulsions had developed. Subjects were sacrificed 20 min after the last seizure and [^{3}H]flunitrazepam binding ('washed' homogenate, 'cold' ligand unspecified) was studied in the ipsilateral hippocampus – a site which shows clear B_{max} elevations at 24 h (Table 10.1). No changes were seen in either B_{max} or K_d at the 20-min interval. In similar experiments, Tietz *et al.* examined hippocampal benzodiazepine binding in animals amygdala-kindled to three Stage 5 convulsions and sacrificed either 'immediately' or 24 h after the last seizure (details in Table 10.1). Significant elevations in B_{max} were observed in the group sacrificed at 24 h but not in the group sacrificed immediately after kindling. Both of these studies suggest the existence of some factor in the immediate post-ictal period which masks long-term kindling-induced changes. In the noradrenergic system, this masking possibly lasts as long as 24 h (see Section 10.2.2). This question deserves further study.

10.2.2 *Short-term studies (30 min–1 day)*

By far the largest number of kindling/binding studies have been done 24 h post-kindling – or at intervals approaching 24 h. In the early kindling/binding studies, the need for longer post-seizure intervals was not appreciated. More recently, a 24 h group has usually been included – in addition to a 28-day group – for the sake of completeness.

Electrophysiological abnormalities

24 h after the last kindled seizure, the immediate sequelae of generalized seizure activity have disappeared (Mucha & Pinel, 1977; Sainsbury *et*

Table 10.1. *Receptor binding in kindled subjects: sacrifice 0–1 day post-ictal*[a]

Experimenters	Subjects	Assay	Results
		Cholinergic system Muscarinic receptors	
(Note: Nicotinic receptors have never been investigated at any time period.)			
McNamara (1978a) Duke University	Rats (m, Sprague–Dawley) amygdala kindled (hourly) to 1 Stage 5, 15 h to sacrifice	Filter, [^{3}H]QNB vs atropine	1 AMYG (ipsi) binding down (13–17%) 2 AMYG (contra) binding down (9%)
(Note: Subsequent Scatchard analysis showed changes in B_{max}, not K_d. Stimulation (without afterdischarge) or two ECS seizures had no effect.)			
Byrne, Gottlieb & McNamara (1980) Duke University	Rats (m, Sprague–Dawley), amygdala kindled (hourly) to 1 Stage 5, 15 h to sacrifice	Filter, [^{3}H]QNB vs atropine	1 AMYG (ipsi) binding down (12%) 2 AMYG (contra) unchanged 3 HPC (ipsi) binding down, (11%) 4 HPC (contra) binding down (19%) 5 CS (ipsi) unchanged 6 CX (contra) unchanged
(Note: Subsequent Scatchard analysis showed changes in B_{max}, not K_d. HPC changes were localized to FD, not CA. Pentylenetetrazol-induced spiking and seizures (1) did not cause similar changes.)			
Dasheiff & McNamara (1980) Duke University	Rats, (m, Sprague–Dawley), amygdala kindled (hourly) to 1 Stage 5, 19.6 h to sacrifice	Filter, [^{3}H]QNB vs atropine	1 FD (ipsi) binding down (13%) 2 FD (contra) binding down (14%) 3 CA (ipsi) binding down (14%) 4 CA (contra) binding down (9%)
(Note: Similar changes continued to occur after lesioning of major cholinergic input to the HPC. CAT was slightly decreased by kindling.)			
Dasheiff, Byrne, Patrone & McNamara (1981) Duke University	Rats, (m, Sprague–Dawley), amygdala kindled (hourly) to different stages: 2 Stage 2, 2 Stage 3, 2 Stage 4, 1 Stage 5. 18–24 h to sacrifice	Filter, [^{3}H]QNB vs atropine	1 AMYG (ipsi) binding down after Stage 4 (13%) and 5 (14%) 2 AMYG (contra) binding down after Stage 5 (20%) 3 FD (ipsi) binding down after Stage 4 (11%) and 5 (22%) 4 FD (contra) binding down after Stage 5 (20%)

Table 10.1. (*contd*)

Experimenters	Subjects	Assay	Results
			5 CA (ipsi) binding down after Stage 5 (14%) 6 CA (contra) unchanged (trend)
(Note: Subsequent Scatchard analysis showed changes in B_{max}, not K_d. Significant changes occurred only after development of Stage 4 and 5 seizures, Uptake, CAT, and AChE were unchanged.)			
Dasheiff, Savage & McNamara (1982) Duke University	Rats, (m, Sprague–Dawley), angular bundle kindled (twice daily) to 1 Stage 5, 24 h to sacrifice	Filter, [^{3}H]QNB vs atropine	1 FD (comb) binding down (13%) 2 CA (comb) binding down (14%) in both regio superior and inferior
(Note: Subsequent Scatchard analysis showed changes in B_{max}, not K_d. Similar changes were produced by 16 ECS seizures or by seizures induced via entorhinal lesions. Anticonvulsant drugs blocked the changes.)			
Savage & McNamara (1982) Duke University	Rats (m, Sprague–Dawley), amygdala kindled (90+ min) to 6 Stage 5, 24 h to sacrifice	Filter, [^{3}H]QNB vs atropine or carbechol	1 FD (comb) maximal binding down (22%) 2 CA (comb) maximal binding down (17%)
(Note: 'Maximal binding' was estimated from competition data. Analysis of assays involving carbachol showed the FD change was limited to the low-affinity site. CA changes occurred in both low- and high-affinity sites.)			
Savage, Dasheiff & McNamara (1983) Duke University	Rats (m, Sprague–Dawley), amygdala kindled (90+ min) to 3+ Stage 5, 24 h to sacrifice	Autoradiography, [^{3}H]QNB vs atropine	1 FD (ipsi) binding down (30%) 2 FD (contra) binding down (30%) 3 CA (ipsi) unchanged 4 CA (contra) unchanged
(Note: Changes in CA were uniformly distributed across the entire molecular and granule cell layers.)			
Dopaminergic/serotoninergic systems			
Gee, Hollinger, Bowyer & Killam (1979) University of California (Davis)	Rats (m, Sprague–Dawley), amygdala kindled (twice daily) to 4 stage 5, 24 h to sacrifice	Filter, [^{3}H]spiperone vs (+)-butaclamol	High-affinity sites: 1 AMYG (ipsi) B_{max} down (31%) 2 AMYG (contra) B_{max} down (25%) 3 CS (comb ?) unchanged 4 striatum (comb ?) unchanged

Table 10.1. (*contd*)

Experimenters	Subjects	Assay	Results
			Low Affinity Sites: 1 AMYG (ipsi) unchanged 2 AMYG (contra) unchanged 3 CX (comb ?) B_{max} up (45%) 4 striatum (comb ?) unchanged

(Note: Assay technique involved labelling of both dopaminergic and serotonergic receptors. Implanted controls received electrical stimulation (without after-discharge). The 'amygdala' sample contained some hippocampal tissue. K_d was decreased (affinity increased) in the high-affinity sites of both amygdalae. K_d was increased (affinity decreased) in the low-affinity sites of both amygdalae and in the high- and low-affinity sites of the striatum.)

GABA complex
$GABA_A$ receptors

(Note: $GABA_B$ receptors have not been investigated at any time period.)

Experimenters	Subjects	Assay	Results
Shin, Pedersen & McNamara (1985) Duke University	Rats (m, Sprague–Dawley), amygdala kindled (daily) to 3 Stage 4–5, 24 h to sacrifice	Autoradiography, $[^3H]$muscimol vs GABA	1 FD binding up (22%) 2 CAl unchanged 3 CX unchanged 4 SN unchanged

(Note: Analyses apparently involved both ipsi- and contralateral fascia dentata, but only *contralateral* cortex. Laterality of cornu ammonis and substantia nigra samples is not specified. Changes in FD were localized to the stratum granulosum (cell bodies) and stratum moleculare (dendritic trees). GABA receptor-mediated enhancement of benzodiazepine receptor binding was slightly attenuated.)

Benzodiazepine receptors; 'Central' receptors

(Note: 'Peripheral' receptors have not been studied at this time period.)

Experimenters	Subjects	Assay	Results
McNamara, Peper & Petrone (1980) Duke University	Rats, (m, Sprague–Dawley), amygdala kindled (daily) to 1+ Stage 5, 24 h to sacrifice	Filter, $[^3H]$diazepam vs diazepam ('washed' membranes)	1 AMYG (ipsi) unchanged (non-sig. 10% rise) 2 CX (ipsi) unchanged 3 CX (contra) unchanged 4 HPC (ipsi) binding up (35%) 5 HPC (contra) binding up (35%)

(Note: The contralateral amygdala was not assayed. Subsequent Scatchard analysis indicated that the HPC changes were in B_{max}, not K_d. Neither electrical stimulation (without aftercharge) nor 17 hypoxic episodes caused any change

Table 10.1. (*contd*)

Experimenters	Subjects	Assay	Results
in binding. A 19% increase in HPC binding did occur, however, after 17 (but not 7) daily ECS seizures.)			
Valdes, Dasheiff, Birmingham, Crutcher & McNamara (1982) Duke University, University of Utah	Rats (m, Sprague–Dawley), amygdala kindled (daily) to 1+ Stage 5, 24 h to sacrifice	Filter, [^{3}H]flunitrazepam vs diazepam ('washed' membranes)	1 FD(comb) binding up (41%) 2 CA (comb) unchanged (non-sig. 10% rise)
(Note: Right and left sides were combined after statistical analysis indicated no significant differences. Subsequent Scatchard analysis indicated the change was in B_{max}, not K_d. Subsequent autoradiography localized the change to granular (cell body) and moleculare (dendritic tree) areas of the FD. 19 daily ECS seizures increased FD binding by 33% (filter assay), without significantly affecting CA binding.)			
Fanelli & McNamara (1983) Duke University	Rats (m, Sprague–Dawley), amgydala kindled (daily) to 5–15 Stage 5, 24 h to sacrifice	Filter, [^{3}H]flunitrazepam vs diazepam ('washed' membranes)	1 FD (comb) B_{max} up (24%)
(Note: NaCl, pentobarbital and GABA all increased binding. NaCl and pentobarbitral were equally effective in kindled and control brains. GABA, however, was more effective in control than in kindled tissue.)			
Shin, Pedersen & McNamara (1985) Duke University	Rats, (m, Sprague–Dawley), amygdala kindled (daily) to 3 Stage 4–5, 24 h to sacrifice	Autoradiography, [^{3}H]flunitrazepam vs diazepam	1 FD binding up (38%) 2 CX unchanged 3 SN unchanged
(Note: Analyses apparently involved both ipsi- and contralateral fascia dentata, but only *contralateral* cortex. Laterality of substantia nigra samples is not specified. Changes in FD were localized to the stratum granulosum (cell bodies) and moleculare (dendritic tree). They took place in the Type 2 benzodiazepine receptor only. GABA-mediated enhancement of benzodiazepine receptor binding was slightly attenuated in the fascia dentata.)			

Table 10.1. (*contd*)

Experimenters	Subjects	Assay	Results
Tietz, Gomez & Berman (1985) Wayne State University	Rats (m, Long Evans), amygdala kindled (daily) to different levels: 1 afterdischarge, 1 Stage 3, or 3 Stage 5, 24 h to sacrifice	Filter, [^{3}H]diazepam vs diazepam ('washed' membranes)	1 AMYG (comb) unchanged (non-sig. 10% rise in B_{max} at all stages) 2 HPC (comb) B_{max} up (25% non-sig. rise after 1 discharge; 17% after Stage 3; 29% after 3 Stage 5)
(Note: Non-implanted animals were used as control subjects in this study. Changes were found in B_{max} only, not K_d.)			
Glutamate system			
Glutamate A and B receptors			
Savage, Werling, Nadler & McNamara (1984) Duke University (A preliminary report by the same authors appeared in 1982.)	Rats (m, Sprague–Dawley), angular bundle kindled (twice daily) to 3+ Stage 4, 24 h to sacrifice	Centrifugation, L-[^{3}H]glutamate vs quisqualate (glutamate A) or ibotenate (glutamate B)	1 HPC (comb) glutamate A binding up (38%) 2 glutamate B binding unchanged
(Note: Subsequent Scatchard analysis indicated a change in B_{max}, not K_d. Addition of Ca^{2+} increased binding, but decreased the kindling-induced elevation of binding.)			
Slevin & Ferrara (1985) University of Kentucky	Rats (m, Sprague–Dawley), entorhinal cortex kindled (daily) to 1, 8, 15, or 22 stimulations (22 = 2 Stage 5). Delay to sacrifice unspecified, but less than 24 h	Centrifugation? L-[^{3}H]glutamate vs L-glutamate (glutamate A)	1 HPC (ipsi) binding unchanged (non-sig. rise after 2 Stage 5) 2 HPC (contra) unchanged
(Note: Binding was measured both with and without Ca^{2+}. Pre-synaptic uptake of glutamate was also unchanged by kindling. ECS seizures (2) had no effect on either uptake or binding.)			

Table 10.1. (*contd*)

Experimenters	Subjects	Assay	Results
		Kainic acid receptors	
Savage, Nadler & McNamara (1984) Duke University	Rats, (m, Sprague–Dawley), amygdala or angular bundle kindled (90+ min) to 3+ Stage 4–5, 24 h to sacrifice	Autoradiography, [^{3}H]kainic acid vs kainic acid	1 FD (ipsi and contra) binding down (20–41%) 2 CA (ipsi and contra) binding down (47–61%)
(Note: Changes were seen only in the areas rich in kainic acid receptors – the stratum lucidum of CA3 and the molecular layer of the FD. Amygdala and angular bundle kindling produced equivalent results.)			
		Noradrenergic system	
(Note: α_1-receptors have not been studied at any time period.)			
		α_2-receptors	
Stanford & Jeffreys (1985) Oxford University	Rats (m, Sprague–Dawley) amygdala kindled (hourly) to 3 Stage 5. 24 h to sacrifice	Filter, [^{3}H]clonidine vs phentolamine	1 CX (comb) unchanged 2 'Olfactory' CX (comb) B_{max} down (25%)
(Note: 'Olfactory' cortex consisted of prepiriform, piriform and entorhinal cortices.)			
		β-receptors	
(Note: So far, β_1- and β_2-receptors have been studied in combination.)			
McNamara (1978a) Duke University	Rats (m, Sprague–Dawley), amygdala kindled (hourly) to 1 Stage 5, 15 h to sacrifice	Filter, [^{3}H]DHA vs (−)alprenolol	1 AMYG (ipsi) binding unchanged 2 AMYG (contra) binding unchanged
(Note: Stimulation (without afterdischarge) and two ECS seizures also produced no change.)			
Byrne, Gottlieb & McNamara (1980) Duke University	Rats (m, Sprague–Dawley), amygdala kindled (hourly) to 1 Stage 5, 15 h to sacrifice	Filter, [^{3}H]DHA vs (−)alprenolol	1 AMYG (ipsi) binding unchanged 2 AMYG (contra) binding unchanged 3 HPC (ipsi) binding unchanged 4 HPC (contra) binding unchanged 5 CX (ipsi) binding unchanged 6 CX (contra) binding unchanged

Table 10.1. (*contd*)

Experimenters	Subjects	Assay	Results
McIntyre & Roberts (1983) Carleton University	Rats (m, Wistar) amygdala kindled (daily) to 6 Stage 5, 24 h to sacrifice	Filter, $[^3H]$DHA vs (−)alprenolol	1 AMYG (ipsi) binding unchanged (non-sig. decrease) 2 AMYG (contra) binding unchanged 3 CX (comb) binding unchanged (non.sig. decrease)
(Note: Design involved a pause between the 5th and 6th Stage 5 seizures in order to match a 23-day group. (See Table 10.2.) Subsequent Scatchard analysis suggests a decrease in both B_{max} and K_d.)			
Stanford & Jefferys (1985) Oxford University	Rats (m, Sprague–Dawley), amygdala kindled (hourly) to 3 Stage 5, 24 h to sacrifice	Filter, $[^3H]$DHA vs (+/−)propranolol	1 CX (comb) B_{max} down (50%) 2 'Olfactory' CX (comb) B_{max} down (35%)
(Note: 'Olfactory' cortex consisted of the prepiriform, piriform and entorhinal cortices. A significantly lower K_d was seen in the 'olfactory' cortex.)			
Somatostatin receptors			
Never assayed at this time period.			

[a]Column 1 indicates names and affiliation of experimenters, plus the date of publication. Column 2 indicates species (and strain) of subjects, site, (inter-trial interval) and criterion of kindling, and delay to sacrifice. Column 3 indicates type of assay and labeled and unlabeled ligands. Column 4 indicates direction (and percentage) of changes relative to implanted but unstimulated control subjects. Abbreviations: AChE, acetylcholinesterase; AMYG, amygdala; B_{max}, maximal number of binding sites; CA, cornu ammonis; CAT, choline acetyltransferase; contra, contralateral (to stimulating electrode); comb, combined (ipsi- and contralateral sides pooled); DHA, dihydroalprenolol; ECS, electroconvulsive shock; FD, fascia dentata; HYPO, hypothalamus; GABA, γ-aminobutyric acid; ipsi, ipsilateral (to stimulating electrode); K_d, dissociation constant; m, male; QNB, quinuclidinyl benzilate; sig., significant; SN, substantia nigra; vs, versus.

al., 1978). A number of longer-lasting transitory changes are still present, however – in addition to the permanent changes produced by kindling. One of these is 'post-ictal resistance' to subsequent seizures, which may last more than a day (Sainsbury *et al.*, 1978), particularly if a massed-stimulation paradigm has been employed (Mucha & Pinel, 1977). Another – possibly related – phenomenon is the increased inhibition observed in fascia-dentata evoked potentials after kindling. This can be seen at one day (King *et al.*, 1985) and at two weeks (Tuff, Racine & Adamec, 1983), but not at one month after the last kindled seizure (King *et al.*, 1985). Another transient inhibitory phenomenon is the 'interference' effect, which has been reported to last up to two weeks (McIntyre & Goddard, 1973). An excitatory phenomenon, long-term potentiation, also lasts for several weeks (see Racine & Burnham, 1984).

Binding changes

Studies done at post-kindling intervals approximating 24 h have involved all of the well-known transmitter systems, plus a few of the systems that are not well-known (e.g. kainic acid). They are summarized in Table 10.1. As indicated, some sort of change has been reported in almost every system.

Cholinergic system The first system to receive serious attention was the cholinergic system, and, in particular, the muscarinic receptors. (Nicotinic binding has not been studied at any interval.) An initial report indicated that muscarinic binding was reduced in both the stimulated and the contralateral amygdalae 24 h after kindling (McNamara, 1978a). A subsequent study indicated that binding was also reduced in the ipsilateral and contralateral hippocampi, but not in the neocortex (Byrne *et al.*, 1980). Further studies then concentrated on locating the site of the hippocampal reductions. Some studies appeared to localize them to the fascia dentata, and especially to the granule and molecular layers (Byrne *et al.*, 1980; Savage *et al.*, 1983), while other studies found changes in both the fascia dentata and the cornu ammonis (Dasheiff & McNamara, 1980; Dasheiff *et al.*, 1981, 1982; Savage & McNamara, 1982). This question remains unresolved. Several other discrepancies have cropped up in this field. Early studies, for instance, suggested that binding changes were kindling-specific, i.e. that they could not be caused by electrical stimulation (without afterdischarge) or by the administration of generalized electroconvulsive shock seizures (McNamara, 1978a). A later study, however, indicated that a sufficient number of electroshock seizures (16) could cause similar changes (Dasheiff *et al.*, 1982). This finding – which had presumably been missed in the earlier study because of the smaller number (2) of seizures administered – seems consistent with the finding that the reductions only begin to occur after Stage 4 and 5 (generalized) kindled seizures have developed (Dasheiff *et al.*, 1981). A further discrepancy relates to a recent failure to find post-kindling muscarinic binding reductions in the amygdala (Savage *et al.*, 1983). The amygdala, of course, was the first site in which such binding changes were reported. This difference in results may relate to the different assays utilized (filter vs autoradiographic). It has also been suggested (Byrne *et al.*, 1980) that the 'amygdala' region assayed in the first studies was contaminated with hippocampal tissue. Binding changes in the amygdala have also been reported in certain of the later studies (e.g. Byrne *et al.*, 1980), however, which presumably utilized pure amygdala samples. This question requires further study.

In summary, then, it appears that generalized seizures, caused either by kindling or by the electroshock method, produce bilateral reductions in muscarinic binding in the fascia dentata, and perhaps the cornu ammonis and amygdala as well. It is interesting to note that these appear to relate to intense depolarization rather than to specific overstimulation via cholinergic afferents (Dasheiff & McNamara, 1980), and that they occur in the absence of changes in uptake or in the activity of the synthetic or degradative enzymes (Dasheiff *et al.*, 1981). Such changes might be expected to reduce the functional activity of the cholinergic system, and it has been suggested that they represent part of a down-regulation of excitatory systems which may contribute to post-ictal inhibitory events (Dasheiff *et al.*, 1981, 1982; Savage & McNamara, 1982).

Dopamine/serotonin systems A single study – described as a study of dopamine binding – has been done at 24 h (Gee *et al.*, 1979). The data are quite complex, with changes reported in both K_d and B_{max} for both 'high-affinity' and 'low-affinity' binding sites in both amygdalae and in the frontal cortex. (See Table 10.1 for detail.) Unfortunately this study was done early in the evolution of the dopamine binding assay, and it is probable – as the authors admit – that both dopamine and serotonin receptors were labeled. It is probably safest to conclude that dopamine and/or serotonin binding is changed at 24 h. Obviously, this study should be repeated with improved techniques.

GABA complex The second most studied system at the 24-h interval has been the GABA complex. The GABA complex consists of three separate subunits: (i) the GABA receptor, (ii) the benzodiazepine receptor, and (iii) the barbiturate (or picrotoxin) receptor (Olsen, 1981a). A single study – an autoradiographic assay by Shin *et al.* (1985) – has measured binding to the GABA receptor site itself at this time period.

This study found elevated GABA binding (B_{max}) in the fascia dentata at 24 h, but not in the cornu ammonis, cortex or substantia nigra. The changes in the fascia dentata could be localized to the stratum granulosum (cell bodies) and stratum moleculare (dendritic trees).

All of the other studies of the GABA complex at 24 h have investigated binding to the GABA-modulatory benzodiazepine site. 'Washed' membrane preparations have been used. (Crude homogenates have not been studied at 24 h.) The first report was by McNamara *et al.* (1980), who indicated that benzodiazepine binding (B_{max}) was bilaterally elevated in the hippocampus at 24 h, but not in the amygdala or the cortex. Neither electrical stimulation (without kindling) nor repeated hypoxic episodes produced these changes. Similar changes could be produced, however, by 17 (but not 7) generalized ECS seizures (see also Valdes *et al.*, 1982). Later studies from the same group indicated that the hippocampal elevations occurred in the fascia dentata but not the cornu ammonis (Valdes *et al.*, 1982), and that they could be localized to the stratum granulosum and stratum moleculare (Shin *et al.*, 1985). A recent study by Shin *et al.* (1985) suggests that the changes take place in the Type 2 (but not Type 1) 'central' receptor. (The 'peripheral' benzodiazepine site has not been assayed at this time period.) Another recent study by Tietz *et al.* (1985) appears to suggest that such changes are seen only after the development of Stage 3–5 kindled seizures. This report – implying that the changes result from generalized seizure activity – seems consistent with the previous report that they can be caused by repeated ECS seizures (McNamara *et al.*, 1980). Careful inspection of Tietz' data, however, indicates that binding changes just as large as those seen after Stage 3–5 seizures were seen after one discharge. These failed to attain significance because of the larger variance in the data at this earlier time period. Thus, the question of when hippocampal benzodiazepine binding abnormalities develop is one which could benefit from further study.

In summary, bilateral elevations in B_{max} are seen in both GABA and benzodiazepine binding 24 h after the last kindled seizure. They have been reported, so far, only in the hippocampus, where they are localized to the fascia dentata, strata granulosum and moleculare. (As noted above, abnormalities in muscarinic binding are also seen in this locus.) It has been suggested that they are caused by generalized seizure activity rather than by 'kindling *per se*', but this is a question which requires further study (see discussion below). If these changes indicate an up-regulation of the GABA system – and this has yet to be proven – they may relate to the post-ictal inhibitory phenomena seen at 24 h (see Shin *et al.*, 1985). Binding to the third unit of the complex, the barbiturate receptor, has not yet been studied at any time period.

Before leaving the GABA complex, receptor interactions must be discussed. It is known that binding to each of the subunits of the GABA complex increases binding to the others (Olsen, 1981a). Fanelli & McNamara (1983), working at 24 h in the fascia dentata, found that the ability of GABA to enhance benzodiazepine binding was reduced after kindling. Shin *et al.* (1985) have reported a similar (though slight) attenuation. This interesting observation suggests that at 24 h there may be some 'uncoupling' between the GABA and benzodiazepine receptors. The enhancing effects of sodium chloride and pentobarbital on benzodiazepine binding are unchanged (Fanelli & McNamara, 1983).

Glutamate system Studies of the effect of kindling on both the glutamate A (quisqualate sensitive) and glutamate B (ibotenate sensitive) sites have been done at 24 h. There is some confusion about the results. Savage, Werling *et al.* (1984) report that glutamate B sites are unchanged in kindled rats at this time period, but that the B_{max} for glutamate A binding in the hippocampus is increased by about 40%. They suggest that this change – the only elevation in excitatory receptors reported so far – may relate to the long-term potentiation which occurs during kindling. Slevin & Ferrara (1985), however, have also studied glutamate A binding in the hippocampus at 24 h and failed to find any significant change caused by kindling – although there was a slight (non-significant) elevation in the ipsilateral hippocampus. Comparing their results to those of Savage, Werling *et al.*, Slevin and Ferrara argue that the discrepancy cannot be explained by differences in placement (entorhinal cortex vs angular bundle) or in the unlabeled ligand (L-glutamate vs quisqualate). They finally conclude that the Savage *et al.* may have observed an apparent change in glutamate A binding due to the accidental labeling of a certain number of kainic acid receptors. A recent study indicating that kainic acid binding is *reduced* at 24 h (see below) casts doubt on this explanation. This question remains unresolved.

Kainic acid receptors Kainic acid binds to a possible subclass of glutamate receptors. A single experiment has been done on kainic acid binding at 24 h. Large, bilateral binding reductions have been found in both the cornu ammonis and the dentate gyrus (Savage *et al.*, 1984). The reduction in the cornu ammonis (47–61%) is one of the largest binding changes ever reported after kindling. Unfortunately – as noted below – this interesting observation has never been followed up by experiments at later time periods.

Noradrenergic system Studies of both α_2- and β-noradrenergic binding have been done at 24 h. (The α_1-receptor has never been studied at any time period.) The α_2-receptor has been the object of a single study (Stanford & Jefferys, 1985), which suggests that binding is reduced in 'olfactory' cortex, but not in neocortex at 24 h. ('Olfactory' cortex combines the prepiriform, piriform and entorhinal areas.) Several studies of β-adrenergic binding have been done, and these have produced apparently contradictory results. McNamara reported that β-binding was unchanged in the amygdalae at this interval (McNamara, 1978a). Later he extended his findings to indicate that β-binding was unchanged in the bilateral amygdalae, hippocampi and cortices (Byrne *et al.*, 1980). McIntyre & Roberts (1983) confirmed that there were no significant differences at this time interval – although trends toward reduction were seen in the ipsilateral amygdala and cortex – but argued that reductions were really there, masked by the short-term effects of the last seizure. Stanford & Jefferys (1985) have recently reported large reductions (30–50%) at 24 h in the 'olfactory' cortex – not assayed by other investigators – and in the neocortex – where previous investigators found no change. The major conflict in these studies concerns the neocortex – where McNamara's group and McIntyre & Roberts reported no change, but Stanford & Jefferys reported a large reduction. A careful examination of the data offers a possible solution. McNamara's data and most of McIntyre's data were derived from 'single point' experiments – experiments done with a single concentration of radioactive ligand. Single point experiments cannot discriminate changes in B_{max} and K_d. A Scatchard analysis in McIntyre's experiment shows a drop in B_{max} at 24 h which looks just as large as the drop he observed at 23 days. It is counterbalanced, however, by a rise in affinity (drop in K_d) which gave the overall impression, in the single-point data, that there was no change. Something similar may have occurred in McNamara's single-point experiments. In Stanford & Jefferys' 'olfactory' cortex data the same effect is seen – reduced B_{max}, increased affinity – but there is no confusion since all the data were subjected to Scatchard analysis. Thus, it appears that the B_{max} for β-adrenergic binding may be reduced at 24 h, but that it may be obscured in single-point experiments by a rise in affinity.

In passing, it should be noted that significant K_d shifts have been reported at 24 h in both noradrenaline binding and dopamine binding experiments (see below), although they seem to be rare in other systems. It may be unwise to do single-point experiments when dealing with a catecholaminergic system.

Summary and discussion: short-term studies Thus, at the 24-h interval B_{max} changes have been reported in a large number of systems. Elevations have been reported in the $GABA_A$, benzodiazepine (washed homogenate), and glutamate A systems, and reductions have been reported in the cholinergic, kainic acid, and α- and β-adrenergic systems. The dopamine and/or serotonin systems may be changed as well, but the data are ambiguous due to the technique employed. K_d changes have been reported much less often, being limited to the noradrenergic and (possibly) dopamine/serotonin systems. Most of the binding changes which have been observed seem to have occurred either in the hippocampus or the amygdala – but this may have been primarily due to the fact that these have been the areas most often chosen for assay. (Multiple-area studies have been rare at 24 h.) Conflicting data exist in several different areas, suggesting a need for further experimentation.

Before concluding this discussion of the 24-h data, it may be worth discussing one further question: What aspect of the kindling procedure causes binding changes? Is it electrical stimulation, kindling *per se* or generalized seizure activity? This question – which has been addressed in several of the studies done at 24 h – contains certain inherent conceptual problems. The first part of the question is clear, and allows of an unequivocal answer. Repeated electrical stimulation at frequencies which do not cause motor seizure development (e.g. 1 Hz) does not seem to cause binding changes. This has been demonstrated in both the cholinergic system (McNamara, 1978a) and the benzodiazepine system (McNamara *et al.*, 1980). The second part of the question, however, which attempts to distinguish 'kindling' from the effects of repeated generalized seizure activity, is somewhat confused. The problem is, of course, that repeated generalized seizures cause permanent epileptogenic brain changes (i.e. 'kindle') just as focal seizures do (Ramer & Pinel, 1976; Pinel & Van Oot, 1977). Thus, both focal and generalized seizures 'kindle', and both are equally likely to be associated with long-lasting biochemical changes. The earlier binding studies, which appeared to differentiate 'kindling' from repeated ECS seizures (e.g. McNamara, 1978a), usually used small numbers of ECS seizures. Recent work, which has employed larger numbers of ECS seizures, has generally found their effects to be similar to those of traditional kindling (McNamara *et al.*, 1980; Dasheiff *et al.*, 1982).

10.2.3 *Intermediate-term studies (2–27 days)*

After 24 h, the number of binding/kindling studies drops off sharply. A moderate amount of work has been done in the period from 2–27 days, however, and some interesting results have been obtained. Studies done from 2–27 days allow us to classify some abnormalities as 'transient', while others may be recognized as candidates for long-term study.

Electrophysiological abnormalities
During the period from 2–27 days, the temporary electrophysiological changes resulting from kindling tend to disappear. Their decline is gradual, however, rather than rapid. Post-seizure resistance, for instance, may last for several days after massed stimulations (Ramer & Pinel, 1976; Pinel & Van Oot, 1977), while the 'interference' effect lasts over a week (McIntyre & Goddard). Enhanced inhibition in the hippocampus lasts over three weeks (R. J. Racine, personal communication), as does long-term potentiation (Racine & Burnham, 1984). Interictal spiking gradually dies down to a low level during this period, although an enhanced *tendency* toward interictal spiking seems to be a permanent feature of kindling (R. J. Racine, personal communcation). Thus, during this period a number of transitory changes gradually fade, while the permanent changes resulting from kindling remain.

Binding changes
Table 10.2 presents the 2–27 day binding data currently available. Systems assayed include the cholinergic system, the dopamine system, the GABA complex, and the noradrenergic and somatostatin systems. The glutamate, kainic acid and serotonin systems have not been studied at this time period.

Cholinergic system The hippocampal reductions observed in muscarinic cholinergic binding appear to be transitory. They are observed at 24 h and at three days post-ictal, but they disappear before a week is up (Dasheiff & McNamara, 1980).

Dopamine binding Data on the persistence of dopamine binding changes in electrically kindled animals are not available. Csernansky *et al.* (1985), however, report that bilateral elevations in the dopamine 2 receptor, induced in the amygdalae by lidocaine kindling, last for at least three days.

GABA complex The hippocampal elevations in GABA A binding, observed at 24 h (Shin *et al.*, 1985), have disappeared by two weeks (Tuff, Racine & Mishra, 1983). The bilateral elevations in hippocampal benzodiazepine binding seen at 24 h ('washed' homogenate), however, continue to be seen at two weeks, as do bilateral elevations in the amygdalae (Tuff, Racine & Mishra, 1983; Niznik *et al.*, 1984). Recent work has shown that these are seen *only* in washed homogenates, not in crude homogenates (Niznik *et al.*, 1984). Bilateral reductions in the striatum ('washed' homogenate) have also been reported at this time period by

Table 10.2. *Receptor binding in kindled subjects: sacrifice 1–27 days post-ictal*[a]

Experimenters	Subjects	Assay	Results
		Cholinergic system Muscarinic receptors	
McNamara (1978b) Duke University	Rats (m, Sprague–Dawley) amygdala kindled (hourly) to 1 Stage 5, 3 days to sacrifice	Filter, [^{3}H]QNB vs atropine	1 AMYG (ipsi) binding unchanged 2 AMYG (contra) binding unchanged
(Note: The 'amygdala' samples contained a certain amount of hippocampal tissue. Binding was also unchanged in two large blocks of extra-focal tissue, designated as 'central' and 'hemispheric'.)			
Dasheiff & McNamara (1981) Duke University	Rats (m, Sprague–Dawley), amygdala kindled (hourly) to 1 Stage 5, 3 or 7 days to sacrifice	Filter, [^{3}H]QNB vs atropine	1 AMYG (ipsi) binding unchanged 2 AMYG (contra) binding unchanged 3 FD (ipsi) binding unchanged 4 FD (contra) binding down at 3 days (11%), not at 5 5 CA (ipsi) binding unchanged 6 CA (contra) binding unchanged
(Note: Subsequent Scatchard analysis showed a change in B_{max}, not K_d.)			
		Dopaminergic system Dopamine$_2$ receptors	
(Note: Dopamine$_1$ receptors have never been investigated at any time period.)			
Csernansky, Csernansky, Glick & Hollister (1985) Stanford University	Rats (m, Sprague–Dawley), lidocaine kindled (daily) to Stage 4–5 (45 days), 3 days to sacrifice	Centrifugation, [^{3}H]spiperone vs sulpiride	1 AMYG (comb) B_{max} up (approx 20%) 2 ACC (comb) unchanged (non-sig. up) 3 Striatum (comb) unchanged
(Note: The receptor change correlated with a rise in stereotypic behavior after apomorphine injection.)			

Table 10.2. (*contd*)

Experi-menters	Subjects	Assay	Results
		GABA complex	
		$GABA_A$ receptors	
Tuff, Racine & Mishra (1983) McMaster University	Rats (m, Royal Victoria hooded), amygdala kindled (daily) to 6 Stage 5, 2 weeks to sacrifice	Centrifugation, [^{3}H]GABA vs GABA, and filtration, [^{3}H]muscimol vs GABA	1 AMYG (ipsi) no change 2 AMYG (contra) no change 3 HPC (ipsi) no change 4 HPC (contra) no change 5 CX (ipsi) no change 6 CX (contra) no change 7 Striatum (ipsi) no change 8 Striatum (contra) no change
(Note: The ventral forebrain, hypothalamus, midbrain, cerebellum and brain stem also showed no change.)			
		Benzodiazepine site; 'Central' receptors	
(Note: Peripheral receptors were also investigated in some studies. See notes.)			
Tuff, Racine & Mishra (1983) McMaster University	Rats (m, Royal Victoria hooded), amygdala kindled (daily) to 6 Stage 5, 2 weeks to sacrifice	Filter, [^{3}H]flunitrazepam vs diazepam ('washed' membranes)	1 AMYG (ipsi) binding up (15%) 2 AMYG (contra) binding up (14%) 3 HPC (ipsi) unchanged (trend up) 4 HPC (contra) unchanged 5 CX (ipsi) unchanged 6 CX (contra) unchanged 7 Striatum (ipsi) binding down (13%) 8 Striatum (contra) binding down (11%)
(Note: The ventral forebrain, hypothalamus, midbrain, cerebellum and brain stem showed no significant changes. Subsequent Scatchard analysis indicated that the observed changes were in B_{max}, not K_d. Further kindling of the FD in 6 subjects (after amygdala kindling) produced significant elevations of binding in the HPC (16%).)			

Table 10.2. (*contd*)

Experimenters	Subjects	Assay	Results
Niznik, Kish & Burnham (1983) University of Toronto	Rats (m, Royal Victoria hooded), amygdala kindled (daily) to 6 Stage 5, 2 weeks to sacrifice	Filter, [^{3}H]flunitrazepam vs diazepam (crude homogenate)	1 AMYG (ipsi) unchanged 2 AMYG (contra) unchanged 3 HPC (ipsi) unchanged 4 HPC (contra) unchanged 5 CX (ipsi) B_{max} down (20%) 6 CX (contra) unchanged 7 Striatum (ipsi) unchanged 8 Striatum (contra) unchanged 9 HYPO (comb) B_{max} down (20%)
Niznik, Burnham & Kish (1984) University of Toronto	Rats (m, Royal Victoria hooded), amygdala kindled (daily) to 6 Stage 5, 15 days to sacrifice	Filter, [^{3}H]flunitrazepam vs clonazepam	Crude homogenate preparation: 1 AMYG (ipsi) unchanged 2 AMYG (contra) unchanged 3 HPC (contra) unchanged 4 HPC (contra) unchanged 5 CX (ipsi) binding down (23%) 6 CX (contra) unchanged 7 HYPO (comb) binding down (20%) 'Washed' membrane preparation: 1 AMYG (ipsi) B_{max} up (20%) 2 AMYG (contra) B_{max} up (21%) 3 HPC (ipsi) B_{max} up (18%) 4 HPC (contra) B_{max} up (18%) 5 CX (ipsi) unchanged 6 CX (contra) unchanged 7 HYPO (comb) unchanged

Table 10.2. (*contd*)

Experi-menters	Subjects	Assay	Results
(Note: Binding was also unchanged in the ipsilateral and contralateral striata and in the cerebellum (comb). This was true for both homogenate preparations. Similar results were obtained when diazepam was used as the unlabeled ligand. When 100 μM GABA was added to the 'washed' assay, binding was increased, but there was essentially no change in the results. GABA enhancement of benzodiazepine binding appeared to be normal in the kindled tissue. Further assays utilizing [^{3}H]R05-4864 and unlabeled R05-4864 showed no abnormalities in 'peripheral' binding in any area or in either homogenate.)			
Rondouin, Chicheportiche, Lerner-Natoli, Ben Attia, Privat & Baldy-Moulinier (1986) Ecole Natinale Supérieure de Chemie	Rats (m? Sprague–Dawley), olfactory bundle kindled (once or twice daily) to unspecified criterion. 1 week to sacrifice	Filter, [^{3}H]diazepam vs diazepam (preparation unspecified)	1 AMYG (comb?) B_{max} up (23–26%) 2 Olfactory bulb (comb?) B_{max} up (23–26%) 3 HPC (comb?) B_{max} unchanged
(Note: A 20–30% decrease in K_d was observed in the kindled olfactory bulb (and amygdala?). Parallel assays showed no change in GABA levels, or GABA synthetic or degradative enzymes. GABA uptake, however, was increased in kindled brains.)			
		Glutamate system	
		Glutamate A and glutamate B receptors	
Slevin & Ferarra (1985) University of Kentucky	Rats (m, Sprague–Dawley), entorhinal cortex kindled (daily) to 2 Stage 5, 3 days to sacrifice	Centrifugation? L-[^{3}H]glutamate vs L-glutamate (glutamate A)	1 HPC (ipsi) unchanged (non-sig. rise, about 15%) 2 HPC (contra) unchanged
(Note: Binding was measured both with and without Ca^{2+}. Pre-synaptic uptake of glutamate was also unchanged by kindling. ECS seizures (2) had no effect on either uptake or binding.)			
		Kainic acid receptors	
Never assayed at this time period.			
		Noradrenergic system	
		α_2-receptors	
Stanford & Jefferys (1985) Oxford University	Rats (m, Sprague–Dawley), amygdala kindled (hourly) to 3 Stage 5, 21 days to sacrifice	Filter, [^{3}H]clonidine vs phentolamine	1 CX (comb) unchanged (non'sig. 18% down)

Table 10.2. (*contd*)

Experimenters	Subjects	Assay	Results
(Note: 'Olfactory' cortex was not statistically evaluated at 21 days due to a loss of subjects. 'Limited data' suggested that the difference observed at 24 h had disappeared.)			
		β-receptors	
McNamara (1978b) Duke University	Rats (m, Sprague–Dawley), amygdala kindled (hourly) to 1 Stage 5, 3 days to sacrifice	Filter, [^{3}H]DHA vs (−)alprenolol	1 AMYG (ipsi) binding down (11%) 2 AMYG (contra) binding down (12%)
(Note: The 'amygdala' samples contained a certain amount of hippocampal tissue. Subsequent Scatchard analysis indicated a change primarily in B_{max}, not K_d. Beta binding was unchanged in two large extrafocal blocks of tissue, designated as 'central' and 'hemispheric'. Electrical stimulation (without afterdischarge) caused no change.)			
McIntyre & Roberts (1983) Carleton University	Rats (m, Wistar) amygdala kindled (daily) to 6 Stage 5, 23 days to sacrifice	Filter, [^{3}H]DHA vs (−)alprenolol	1 AMYG (ipsi) binding down (approx. 50%) 2 AMYG (contra) binding unchanged (non-sig. decrease) 3 CX (comb) binding down (approx. 20%)
(Note: Subsequent Scatchard analysis indicated a change in B_{max}, not K_d.)			
Stanford & Jefferys (1985) Oxford University	Rats (m, Sprague–Dawley), amygdala kindled (hourly) to 3 Stage 5, 21 days to sacrifice	Filter, [^{3}H]DHA vs (+/−)propranolol	1 CX (comb) unchanged (non-sig. decrease of 28%)
(Note: Cortical binding was significantly lower than unhandled controls in both B_{max} and K_d, but not significantly lower than handled controls. 'Olfactory' cortex was not statistically evaluated at 21 days due to a loss of subjects. 'Limited data' suggested that the difference observed at 24 h had disappeared.)			
		Somatostatin receptors	
Higuchi, Kokubu, Sikand, Wada & Friesen (1984) University of Manitoba	Rats (m, Royal Victoria hooded), amygdala kindled (daily), kindling criterion unspecified, 2 weeks to sacrifice	Centrifugation, ^{125}I (D Tyr 8) SRIF vs SRIF	1 TEMPORAL CX (comb) unchanged 2 CX (comb) B_{max} up (8%) 3 HPC (comb) B_{max} down (21%)
(Note: 'Temporal CX' includes amygdala, entorhinal cortex and piriform cortex. Preliminary studies indicated significant declines in B_{max} in all three areas assayed, but it was concluded that these were artifactual in the temporal cortex and cortex, reflecting elevated levels of endogenous SRIF.)			

[a]Presentation of data and abbreviations as in Table 10.1. New Abbreviation: SRIF, somatostatin.

Tuff, Racine & Mishra (1983). Niznik *et al.* (1984) report a smaller (non-significant) trend in the same direction. In *crude* homogenates, *reductions* in ipsilateral cortical and in hypothalamic benzodiazepine binding have been reported at the two-week time period (Niznik *et al.*, 1983, 1984). These are seen *only* in crude homogenates, not in washed homogenates (Niznik *et al.*, 1984). The fact that binding changes in this system are homogenate-dependent suggests that the actual changes involved may not take place in receptor number, but in receptor state or in endogenous modulators (see Niznik *et al.*, 1984, for discussion).

Studies of GABA enhancement of benzodiazepine binding suggest that this has returned to normal by two weeks post-kindling (Tuff, Racine & Mishra, 1983; Niznik *et al.*, 1984). The 'uncoupling' seen at 24 hours seems to be transient.

A recent study by Randouin *et al.* (1986) provides an interesting footnote to the benzodiazepine area. Working in homogenates derived from subjects sacrificed one week after olfactory bulb kindling, Randouin *et al.* found an elevated B_{max} in the amygdala and the olfactory bulb, but not in the hippocampus. Since Randouin's homogenate preparation is not specified, it is hard to make exact comparisons with previous studies. It is interesting to note, however, that olfactory bundle kindling seems to produce a pattern of changes different from *either* pattern reported after amygdala kindling. This study underlines the fact that most of our studies on kindling biochemistry so far are studies on the biochemistry of amygdala/entorhinal kindling.

Glutamate binding The intermediate-term data concerning the persistence of glutamate binding are somewhat ambiguous. Slevin & Ferrara (1985) studied glutamate A binding in the hippocampus at three days post-ictal and failed to find any change. The same investigators, however, had also failed to find elevated binding at 24 h – when Savage *et al.* reported a 38% increase. Slevin & Ferrara do report a non-significant trend toward increased binding at both time periods. Perhaps a replication of this study is in order.

Noradrenergic binding The decreased α_2-noradrenergic binding in 'olfactory' cortex, observed at 24 h, *may* have dissipated by three weeks (Stanford & Jefferys, 1985). This is not entirely clear, however, since a number of animals were lost in Stanford & Jefferys' three-week group, and the remaining data were not subjected to statistical analysis. With regard to beta binding, McIntyre & Roberts (1983) have reported decreased β-noradrenergic binding in the ipsilateral (stimulated) amygdala and in the neocortex at 23 days. Stanford & Jefferys, who also examined beta binding in neocortex and 'olfactory' cortex at 21 days, again report ambiguous data. In the 'olfactory' cortex – reduced at 24 h – they feel that the reduction may have disappeared. This is a non-statistical impression, however, based on limited data. In the neocortex, they report a reduction of 28% when kindled subjects are compared to implanted controls. This 'trend' – which is actually larger than the reduction reported by McIntyre & Roberts – was not significant, however, perhaps due to the variability of the data. (Significance *was* found when the kindled subjects were compared to a group of *non-implanted* controls.)

Since changes of some sort were found by both McIntyre & Roberts and by Stanford & Jefferys, it seems safe to conclude that beta binding is reduced for at least three weeks in both the amygdala and the neocortex. Although these studies do not quite meet our 28-day criterion, the period involved is relatively long, and it seems quite possible that the changes are permanent. McIntyre & Roberts interpret these data as supporting the hypothesis that kindling results from a post-synaptic down regulation of noradrenergic receptors. The data on α_2-binding and on β-binding in the 'olfactory' cortex are less satisfactory. These studies should be repeated.

Somatostatin binding Higuchi *et al.* (1984) have reported small elevations in cortical somatostatin binding at two weeks, and larger reductions in hippocampal somatostatin binding at the same time. Somatostatin binding in 'temporal' cortex (amygdala plus associated juxtallocortex) is unchanged. (Note: preliminary studies had suggested significant reductions in somatostatin binding in cortex, hippocampus and 'temporal' cortex. It was later concluded that the apparent reductions in the cortex and 'temporal' cortex were artefacts caused by kindling-induced changes in the levels of endogenous somatostatin.)

Summary: intermediate-term studies In summary, the intermediate-term data suggest that the abnormalities reported in muscarinic cholinergic and $GABA_A$ binding are transient, whereas the changes reported in α-adrenergic and glutamate A binding *may* be transient. Certain other changes – including the changes observed in benzodiazepine binding, β-adrenergic binding and somatostatin binding – last throughout the medium range, and are candidates for study at later intervals. As indicated below, some of the desired long-interval studies have been done, while others have not.

10.2.4 *Long-term studies: changes possibly permanent (28+ days)*

At 28+ days post-kindling, the crucial interval for identifying long-term changes, only four studies have been done. All of these have been published quite recently. The paucity of long-interval data is, at present, the most serious problem in the kindling/binding field.

Electrophysiological abnormalities

The transitory electrophysiological changes caused by kindling – threshold rise, interference, etc. – have either disappeared or fallen to near-baseline levels by 28 days. The basic electrophysiological changes involved in the kindling process, on the other hand – threshold drop at the focus, enhanced seizure spread to extra-focal sites, etc. – are permanent and may easily be observed at this time period. Assays conducted at 28+ days, therefore, provide biochemical information relevant to the long-lasting changes which constitute the physiological essence of the kindling phenomenon.

Because of the importance of long-term data in locating permanent abnormalities, most recent studies have tended to include a 28-day group. Actually, it might be wise to use an even longer interval. Certain transient changes are very long lasting (e.g. long-term potentiation) and may still be present at 28 days (R. J. Racine, personal communication). The maintenance of kindled animals for these long periods, however, is both difficult and expensive. For practical reasons, 28 days seems to have been accepted as a criterion of 'permanence'.

Binding changes

Table 10.3 presents the data from experiments in which subjects were sacrificed 28 or more days after the last kindled seizure. Only the GABA complex ($GABA_A$ and central benzodiazepine receptors) and the glutamate system have been investigated so far. All of the other systems – including the cholinergic, dopaminergic, noradrenergic, serotonergic, kainic acid and somatostatin systems – still await investigation.

GABA complex Shin *et al.* (1985), working with an autoradiographic assay, have found $GABA_A$ binding to be normal in the fascia dentata at 28 days. Tuff, Racine & Mishra (1983), of course, had already reported it to be normal in the hippocampus at the shorter interval of two weeks. Thus, the study of Shin *et al.* helps to confirm that the hippocampal elevations, observed at one day, are transient. With regard to benzodiazepine binding, the elevations observed in 'washed' homogenates at one day (McNamara *et al.*, 1980, etc.) and at two weeks (Tuff, Racine & Mishra, 1983) seem to be transitory. They are not seen at 28 days (Shin *et al.*, 1985). The reductions observed in crude homogenate at two weeks, however, seem to be very long lasting. Similar decreases have been reported in the ipsilateral cortex and hypothalamus of animals sacrificed two months after the last seizure (Burnham *et al.*, 1983).

Glutamate system The elevations in glutamate A receptor binding, observed in the hippocampus at one day (Savage, Werling *et al.*, 1984), but apparently not at three days (Slevin & Ferrara, 1985), are definitely gone by 28 days – as reported by the researchers who found the 24-h change (Savage, Werling *et al.*, 1984).

Summary and Discussion: long-term studies Thus, the changes observed earlier in benzodiazepine binding (crude homogenate) seem to be very long lasting, while the changes observed in $GABA_A$ binding, washed-homogenate benzodiazepine binding and glutamate binding appear to be transient.

While definite data are lacking for other systems at 28 days, certain tentative statements may be made. It is probably safe to assume, that the cholinergic system, which had normalized by three days (McNamara, 1978; Dasheiff & McNamara, 1981) and the α-adrenergic system, which had probably normalized by 21 days (Stanford & Jeffries, 1985), remain normal at 28+ days post-ictal. With regard to the β-adrenergic, somatostatin, and dopamine 2 systems – changed in 'intermediate' studies but not assayed at later periods – we can only conclude that they *may* show long-term changes. Further data will be needed to confirm this possibility.

10.3 Conclusions and prospective

Sections 10.1 and 10.2 of this review have discussed the basic rationale for kindling/binding studies, and the kindling/binding data which are currently available. Section 10.3 will consider the conclusions which can be drawn from the present data, and the future data which will be needed to clarify the picture.

10.3.1 *Conclusions from the present data*

Section 10.1 suggested that an initial goal of kindling/binding studies is to locate neurotransmitter systems changed by kindling. A first and obvious conclusion to be drawn from the present data is that the assay works very well for this purpose. A post-kindling change of some sort has been reported in virtually every system studied. Thus, the binding technique has proved to be a sensitive index of kindling-induced transmitter abnormalities. It is a technique which holds considerable promise for future studies.

Section 10.1 also indicated that the long-range goal of kindling/assay studies is to relate biochemical data to behavioral and electrophysiological data in hopes of establishing (or disproving) causal relationships.

Table 10.3. *Receptor binding in kindled subjects: sacrifice 28 or more days post-ictal*[a]

Experimenters	Subjects	Assay	Results
Cholinergic system			
Never assayed at this time period.			
Dopaminergic system			
Never assayed at this time period.			
GABA complex			
$GABA_A$ receptors			
Shin, Pedersen & McNamara (1985) Duke University	Rats (m, Sprague–Dawley) amygdala kindled (daily) to 3 Stage 4–5, 28 days to sacrifice	Autoradiography, $[^3H]$muscimol vs GABA	1 FD unchanged 2 CA1 unchanged 3 CX unchanged 4 SN unchanged
(Note: Analyses apparently involved both ipsi- and contralateral FD, but only *contralateral* cortex. Laterality of cornu ammonis and substantia nigra samples is not specified.)			
Benzodiazepine receptors; 'Central' receptors			
(Note: Peripheral receptors were also investigated in some studies. See notes.)			
Burnham, Niznik, Okazaki & Kish (1983) University of Toronto	Rats (m, Royal Victoria Hooded), amygdala kindled (daily) to 6 Stage 4–5, 60 days to sacrifice	Filter, $[^3H]$flunitrazepam vs diazepam (crude homogenate)	1 AMYG (ipsi) unchanged 2 AMYG (contra) unchanged 3 HPC (ipsi) unchanged 4 HPC (contra) unchanged 5 CX (ipsi) B_{max} down (15%) 6 CX (contra) unchanged 7 Striatum (ipsi) unchanged 8 Striatum (contra) unchanged 9 HYPO (comb) B_{max} down (19%)
(Note: No changes were seen in the thalamus, cerebellum, or pons–medulla. Binding to the 'peripheral' site was also studied in filter assays which involved $[^3H]$R05-4864 vs R05-4864. No change was found in any area.)			
Shin, Pedersen & McNamara (1985) Duke University	Rats (m, Sprague–Dawley), amygdala kindled (daily) to 3 Stage 4–5, 28 days to sacrifice	Autoradiography, $[^3H]$flunitrazepam vs diazepam	1 FD (comb) unchanged 2 CX unchanged 3 SN unchanged

Table 10.3. (*contd*)

Experi-menters	Subjects	Assay	Results
(Note: Analyses apparently involved both ipsi- and contralateral fascia dentata, but only *contralateral* cortex. Laterality of substantia nigra samples is not specified.			
	Glutamate system		
	Glutamate A and B receptors		
Savage, Werling, Nadler & McNamara (1984) Duke University (A preliminary report by the same authors appeared in 1982.)	Rats (m, Sprague–Dawley), angular bundle kindled (twice daily) to 3+ Stage 4, 28 days to sacrifice	Centrifugation, L-[^{3}H]glutamate vs quisqualate (glutamate A) or ibotenate (glutamate B)	1 HPC (comb) glutamate A unchanged glutamate B unchanged
	Kainic acid receptors		
Never assayed at this time period.			
	Noradrenergic system		
Never assayed at this time period.			
	Somatostatin receptors		
Never assayed at this time period.			

[a]Presentation of data and abbreviations as in Table 10.1.

Can the present data help us toward that second goal? Certainly, some initial steps can be taken. Although far from complete, the present data allow a crude sorting of the observed changes in terms of duration, and such a categorization has important functional implications.

It is clear, for instance, that most kindling-induced binding abnormalities are transient in nature. They disappear within a few days or weeks after the last seizure. Transient changes of this sort cannot be *directly* related to permanent aspects of the kindling phenomenon. They may, perhaps, be involved in 'laying down the kindling trace'. Alternately, they may represent non-specific effects of ictal excitation or attempts by the brain to suppress further seizure activity. Among the transient abnormalities which have been observed are the changes in muscarinic cholinergic binding, $GABA_A$ binding, central benzodiazepine binding (washed homogenate), and glutamate A binding.

There are also a few systems which show long-term, possibly permanent binding changes. These changes are indicative of abnormalities which are perhaps as long-lasting as the kindling effect itself. One example is the homogenate-dependent decrease in benzodiazepine binding (crude homogenate) which has been observed after a delay of two months (Burnham *et al.*, 1983). Reductions in beta-adrenergic binding have also been reported as long as 23 days after the last seizure (McIntyre & Roberts, 1983). (While these do not meet the 28-day criterion, they are quite long-lasting and may be permanent.) Thus, both the GABA complex and the noradrenergic systems show prolonged abnormalities after kindling. The present data are not sufficient to tell us whether these changes are *causally* related to the persistence of kindling. They do, however, indicate that the GABA complex and the noradrenergic system are good candidates for further study.

In certain other systems, the data are unclear. Kindling-induced abnormalities have been observed for as long as anyone has bothered to look, and it is possible that they are permanent. In these systems, however, the crucial long-term data are lacking. These ambiguous cases include the changes seen in dopamine binding (longest interval: three days), kainic acid binding (longest interval: 24 h) and somatostatin binding (longest interval: two weeks). Further binding research on these systems is badly needed – as is research on those systems which have not as yet been studied (e.g. the serotonin system).

Thus, the present data indicate that kindling causes transitory changes in many systems, long-lasting changes in the GABA complex and noradrenergic systems, and changes of unknown duration in several other systems. Is it possible to go farther, and relate the shorter and longer lasting biochemical changes to the short- and long-term electrophysiological changes which occur after kindling? A number of such hypotheses have been framed, and noted above in Section 10.2. Briefly summarized, the transitory increases in inhibitory binding (e.g. $GABA_A$ receptors) and decreases in excitatory binding (e.g. muscarinic receptors) have been hypothesized to relate to increased post-ictal inhibition (e.g. Dasheiff *et al.*, 1981; Shin *et al.*, 1985), whereas the one instance of temporarily increased binding in an excitatory system (glutamate A receptors) has been linked to long-term potentiation (Savage, Werling *et al.*, 1984). The long-lasting decrease in binding in an inhibitory system (β-noradrenergic receptors) has been seen as consistent with the noradrenergic theory of kindling (McIntyre & Roberts, 1983).

While such hypotheses are stimulating – and consistent with the available data – extended discussion of them would be premature. The present data are so incomplete, and incomplete in so many different ways, that critical analysis is impossible. At the present time, for instance, we have complete time-course data for only one system (muscarinic binding) and complete spatial distribution data for none. In only one system (muscarinic binding) do we have sufficient biochemical data to indicate whether the observed binding abnormality is related to hypo- or hyperactivity. At the present time, therefore, extensive theoretical discussion can hardly be profitable. What we obviously require is more data.

10.3.2 *Future perspectives*

What future studies will be needed to clarify this picture? As indicated by the above discussion, a great many data are missing – particularly data from long-term studies. Rather than compiling a list of all of the missing information, it may be more fruitful to consider the larger question, 'How may we establish that a biochemical brain change is *causally* related to the persistence of the kindling phenomenon'. This is a question which has never been fully considered in the literature. Its answer should provide some general guidance for future studies in the binding/kindling field. Similar strategies, of course, can be evolved to relate transitory biochemical abnormalities to short- and intermediate-term electrophysiological changes.

To establish that a kindling-related biochemical change is *causally* related to the persistence of kindled seizures, three different types of data are needed:

(i) *Biochemical data* The first step, of course, is to ascertain that a biochemical change occurs. This has already been done for a number of systems. Beyond that, however, we must also have a clear idea of where the change occurs (spatial distribution) and of how long it lasts (time course). Likewise, it is important to know how the change relates to other parameters in the system, so that its functional significance can be assessed. The *causal* changes related to the persistence of kindling will probably have a net excitatory effect.

(ii) *Electrophysiological data* Once the time course and spatial distribution of an abnormality are known, they can be compared to the time course and spatial distribution of the electrophysiological abnormalities induced by the kindling process – threshold drop, interictal spiking, enhanced evoked potentials and so on. Biochemical changes *causally* related to the persistence of kindling should show a good temporal and spatial correlation to one of these persistent electrophysiological abnormalities.

(iii) *Pharmacological data* Conceivably, a biochemical abnormality might show good temporal and spatial correlations without being causally related to the kindling process. It might, for instance, represent an attempt by the brain to antagonize the abnormalities related to kindling. This problem can be met by the use of pharmacological techniques. If a biochemical change is *causally* related to kindling, then pharmacological induction of the change in normal subjects should induce a kindling-like state, and pharmacological reversal of the change in kindled subjects should return them to normal.

In summary, three sorts of interrelated data are necessary to establish a causal relationship between a biochemical abnormality and the persistence, of kindling – each of them necessary, and none of them sufficient. How should future researchers proceed to gather such data? One logical sequence would be the following: (i) *Initial binding studies* should be done to indicate whether a kindling-induced biochemical abnormality exists and whether it is long lasting. Assays might be done at 24 h and 28 days. A relatively small number of sites could be assayed, including those particularly relevant to the ligand, or those particularly susceptible to kindling-induced abnormalities (e.g. the hippocampus). (ii) *Further biochemical studies* might then be carried out to ascertain whether the binding abnormality related to hyper- or hypo-function in the system. These need not include a survey of all possible parameters – a single downstream parameter might be sufficient to indicate the functional state of the entire system (e.g. receptor-related ion flux). (iii) *Anatomical distribution studies* could then be done to determine the spatial distribution of the abnormality. The autoradiographic binding technique, introduced into the kindling field by McNamara's group, would be particularly useful for this sort of study. The distribution of binding changes would be compared to the distribution of kindling-induced electrophysiological abnormalities. (If the spatial distribution of electrophysiological changes is unknown, electrophysiological mapping will be necessary.) (iv) *Time-course studies* could then be done to indicate the duration of the biochemical changes in the various different loci. The standard binding assay would be appropriate for this sort of study. These data would be compared to the time courses of the relevant electrophysiological changes. (If the duration of the electrophysiological changes is unknown, electrophysiological time-course studies will be necessary.) (v) *Pharmacological studies* could finally be done to indicate whether the pharmacological induction/normalization of the biochemical abnormality induces/antagonizes kindling.

The above program involves a great deal of work – certainly a great deal more than is common in the kindling/biochemistry field. These steps are all necessary, however, to answer the question, 'What causes kindling?' and to provide eventual clues to the much more important question, 'What causes epilepsy?'

References

Albertson, T. E. (1986). Amygdala-kindled postictal inhibition: Effect of intertrial intervals on repeated days. *Experimental Neurology*, **92,** 197–206.

Ashton, D., Leysen, J. E. & Wauquier, A. (1980). Neurotransmitters and receptor binding in amygdaloid kindled rats: Serotonergic and noradrenergic modulatory effects. *Life Sciences*, **27,** 1547–56.

Burnham, W. M., Niznik, H. B., Okazaki, M. M. & Kish, S. J. (1983). Binding of ^{3}H-flunitrazepam and ^{3}H-R05-4864 to crude homogenates of amygdala kindled rat brain: two months post-seizure. *Brain Research*, **279,** 259–62.

Byrne, M. C., Gottlieb, R. & McNamara, J. O. (1980). Amygdala kindling induces muscarinic cholinergic receptor declines in a highly specific distribution within the limbic system. *Experimental Neurology*, **69,** 85–98.

Csernansky, J. G., Csernansky, C. A., Glick, S. A. & Hollister, L. E. (1985). Lidocaine kindling is accompanied by an increase in apomorphine stereotypy and mesolimbic dopamine D_2 receptor density. *Psychopharmacology Bulletin*, **21,** 707–11.

Dasheiff, R. M., Byrne, M. C., Patrone, V. & McNamara, J. O. (1981). Biochemical evidence of decreased muscarinic cholinergic neuronal communication following amygdala-kindled seizures. *Brain Research*, **206,** 233–8.

Dasheiff, R. M. & McNamara, J. O. (1980). Evidence for an agonist independent down regulation of hippocampal muscarinic receptors in kindling. *Brain Research*, **195,** 345–53.

Dasheiff, R. M., Savage, D. D. & McNamara, J. O. (1982). Seizures down-regulate muscarinic cholinergic receptors in hippocampal formation. *Brain Research*, **235,** 327–34.

Engel, J. & Ackermann, R. F. (1980). Interictal EEG spikes correlate with decreased, rather than increased, epileptogenicity in amygdaloid kindled rats. *Brain Research*, **190,** 543–8.

Fanelli, R. J. & McNamara, J. O. (1983). Kindled seizures result in decreased responsiveness of benzodiazepine receptors to GABA. *Journal of Pharmacology and Experimental Therapeutics*, **226,** 147–50.

Freeman, F. G. & Jarvis, M. F. (1981). The effect of interstimulation interval on the assessment and stability of kindled seizure thresholds. *Brain Research Bulletin*, **7,** 629–33.

Gee, K. W., Hollinger, M. A., Bowyer, J. F. & Killam, E. K. (1979). Modification of dopaminergic receptor sensitivity in rat brain after amygdaloid kindling. *Experimental Neurology*, **66,** 771–7.

Goddard, G. V. (1983). The kindling model of epilepsy. *Trends in Neuroscience*, **6,** 275–9.

Goddard, G. V., McIntyre, D. & Leech, C. (1969). A permanent change in brain function resulting from daily electrical stimulation. *Experimental Neurology*, **25,** 295–330.

Higuchi, T., Kokubu, T., Sikand, G. S., Wada, J. A. & Friesen, H. G. (1984). A study of somatostatin receptors in amygdaloid-kindled rat brain. *Journal of Neurochemistry*, **43,** 1271–6.

Kairiss, E. W., Racine, R. J. & Smith, E. K. (1984). The development of interictal spike during kindling in the rat. *Brain Research*, **322,** 101–10.

Kalichman, M. W. (1982a). Pharmacological investigation of convulsant gamma-aminobutyric acid (GABA) antagonists in amygdala-kindled rats. *Epilepsia*, **16,** 163–71.

Kalichman, M. W. (1982b). Neurochemical correlates of the kindling model of epilepsy. *Neuroscience and Neurobehavioural Review*, **6,** 165–81.

Kalichman, M. W. & Burnham, W. M. (1980). Locomotor and convulsive responses to picrotoxin in amygdala-kindled rats. *Experimental Neurology*, **70,** 167–72.

King, G. L., Dingledine, R., Giacchino, J. L. & McNamara, J. O. (1985). Abnormal neuronal excitability in hippocampal slices from kindled rats. *Journal of Neurophysiology*, **54,** 1295–304.

Lefkowitz, R. J., Caron, M. G. & Stiles, G. L. (1984). Mechanisms of membrane-receptor regulation. *The New England Journal of Medicine*, **310,** 1570–9.

Lloyd, K. G., Munari, C., Worms, P., Bossi, L., Bancaud, J., Talairach, J. & Morselli, P. L. (1981). The role of GABA mediated neurotransmission in convulsive states. In *GABA and Benzodiazepine Receptors*, ed. E. Costa, G. Di Chiara & G. L. Gessa, pp. 199–206. New York: Raven Press.

Marsden, C. D. (1976). Neurology. In *A Textbook of Epilepsy*, ed. J. Laidlaw & A. Richens, pp. 15–55. Edinburgh: Churchill Livingstone.

Mathieson, G. (1975). Pathology of temporal lobe foci. In *Complex Partial Seizures and Their Treatment*, ed. J. K. Penry & D. D. Daly, pp. 163–85. New York: Raven Press.

McIntyre, D. C. & Goddard, G. V. (1973). Transfer, interference and spontaneous recovery of convulsions kindled from the rat amygdala. *Electroencephalography and Clinical Neurophysiology*, **35,** 533–43.

McIntyre, D. C. & Roberts, D. C. S. (1983). Long-term reduction in beta-adrenergic receptor binding after amygdala kindling in rats. *Experimental Neurology*, **82,** 17–24.

McNamara, J. O. (1978a). Muscarinic cholinergic receptors participate in the kindling model of epilepsy. *Brain Research*, **154,** 415–20.

McNamara, J. O. (1978b). Selective alterations of regional beta-adrenergic receptor binding in the kindling model of epilepsy. *Experimental Neurology*, **61,** 582–91.

McNamara, J. O. (1984). Role of neurotransmitters in seizure mechanisms in the kindling model of epilepsy. *Federation Proceedings*, **43,** 2516–22.

McNamara, J. O., Byrne, M. C., Dasheiff, R. M. & Fitz, J. G. (1980). The kindling model of epilepsy: a review. In *Progress in Neurobiology*, vol. 15, ed. J. W. Phillis & G. Kerkut, pp. 139–59. Oxford: Pergamon Press.

McNamara, J. O., Peper, A. M. & Patrone, V. (1980). Repeated seizures induce long-term increase in hippocampal benzodiazepine receptors. *Proceedings of the National Academy of Science, USA*, **77,** 3029–32.

Meldrum, B. S. (1975). Epilepsy and gamma-aminobutyric acid-mediated inhibition. *International Review of Neurobiology*, **17,** 1–36.

Mucha, R. F. & Pinel, J. P. (1977). Postseizure inhibition of kindled seizures. *Experimental Neurology*, **54**, 266–82.

Niznik, H. B., Burnham, W. M. & Kish, S. J. (1984). Benzodiazepine receptor binding following amygdala-kindled convulsions: differing results in washed and unwashed brain membranes. *Journal of Neurochemistry*, **43**, 1732–6.

Niznik, H. B., Kish, S. J. & Burnham, W. M. (1983). Decreased benzodiazepine receptor binding in amygdala kindled rat brains. *Life Sciences*, **33**, 425–30.

Olsen, R. W. (1981a). GABA-benzodiazepine-barbiturate receptor interactions. *Journal of Neurochemistry*, **37**, 1–13.

Olsen, R. W. (1981b). The GABA postsynaptic membrane receptor-ionophore complex. Site of action of convulsant and anticonvulsant drugs. *Molecular and Cellular Biochemistry*, **39**, 261–79.

Peterson, S. L. & Albertson, T.E. (1982). Neurotransmitter and neuromodulator function in the kindled seizure and state. *Progress in Neurobiology*, **19**, 237–70.

Pinel, J. P. J. & Van Oot, P. H. (1977). Intensification of the alcohol withdrawal syndrome following periodic electroconvulsive shocks. *Biological Psychiatry*, **12**, 749–86.

Racine, R. J. (1972a). Modification of seizure activity by electrical stimulation: I. Afterdischarge threshold. *Electroencephalography and Clinical Neurophysiology*, **32**, 269–79.

Racine, R. J. (1972b). Modification of seizure activity by electrical stimulation: II. motor seizure. *Electroencephalography and Clinical Neurophysiology*, **32**, 281–94.

Racine, R. J. (1978). Kindling: The first decade. *Neurosurgery*, **3**, 234–52.

Racine, R. J. & Burnham, W. M. (1984). The kindling model. In *The Electrophysiology of Epilepsy*, ed. P. Schwartzkroin & H. Wheal, pp. 153–71. London: Academic Press.

Racine, R. J., Gartner, J. G. & Burnham, W. M. (1972). Epileptiform activity and neural plasticity in limbic structures. *Brain Research*, **47**, 262–8.

Ramer, D. & Pinel, J. P. J. (1976). Progressive intensification of motor seizures produced by periodic electroconvulsive shock. *Experimental Neurology*, **51**, 421–33.

Rondouin, G., Chichêportiche, M., Lerner-Natoli, M., Ben Attia, M., Privat, A. & Baldy-Moulinier, M. (1986). Inhibitory processes in limbic kindling. In *Kindling*, vol. 3, ed. J. A. Wada, pp. 361–71. New York: Raven Press.

Sainsbury, R. S., Bland, B. H. & Buchan, D. H. (1978). Electrically induced seizure activity in the hippocampus: Time course for postseizure inhibition of kindled seizures. *Behavioral Biology*, **22**, 479–88.

Savage, D. D. & McNamara, J. O. (1982). Kindled seizures selectively reduce a subpopulation of (^{3}H)-quinuclidinyl benzilate binding sites in rat dentate gyrus. *Journal of Pharmacology and Experimental Therapeutics*, **222**, 670–3.

Savage, D. D., Dasheiff, R. M. & McNamara, J. O. (1983). Kindled seizure-induced reduction of muscarinic cholinergic receptors in rat hippocampal formation: evidence for localization to dentate granule cells. *Journal of Comparative Neurology*, **221**, 106–12.

Savage, D. D., Nadler, J. V. & McNamara, J. O. (1984). Reduced kainic acid binding in rat hippocampal formation after limbic kindling. *Brain Research*, **323**, 128–31.

Savage, D. D., Werling, L. L., Nadler, J. V. & McNamara, J. O. (1982). Selective increase in L-^{3}H-glutamate binding to a quisqualate-sensitive site

on hippocampal synaptic membranes after angular bundle kindling. *European Journal of Pharmacology*, **85,** 255–6.
Savage, D. D, Werling, L. L., Nadler, J. V. & McNamara, J. O. (1984). Selective and reversible increase in the number of quisqualate-sensitive glutamate binding sites on hippocampal synaptic membranes after angular bundle kindling. *Brain Research*, **307,** 332–5.
Schmutz, M., Klein, M., Klebs, K., Bernasconi, R., Bittiger, H. & Baltzer, V. (1985). Pharmacological and neurochemical aspects of kindling. *Journal of Neural Transmission*, **63,** 143–55.
Shin, C., Pedersen, H. B. & McNamara, J. O. (1985). Gamma-aminobutyric acid and benzodiazepine receptors in the kindling model of epilepsy: A quantitative radiohistochemical study. *Journal of Neuroscience*, **5,** 2696–701.
Slevin, J. T. & Ferrara, L. P. (1985). Lack of effect of entorhinal kindling on L-(^{3}H)-glutamic acid presynaptic uptake and postsynaptic binding in hippocampus. *Experimental Neurology*, **89,** 48–58.
Stanford, S. C. & Jefferys, S. R. (1985). Down-regulation of alpha-2 and beta-adrenoceptor binding sites in rat cortex caused by amygdalar kindling. *Experimental Neurology*, **90,** 108–17.
Tietz, E. I., Gomez, F. & Berman, R. F. (1985). Amygdala kindled seizure stage is related to altered benzodiazepine binding site density. *Life Science*, **36,** 183–90.
Tower, D. B. (1976). GABA and seizures: Clinical correlates in man. In *GABA in Nervous System Function*, ed. E. Roberts, T. N. Chase & D. B. Tower, pp. 461–78. New York: Raven Press.
Tuff, L. P., Racine, R. J. & Adamec, R. (1983). The effects of kindling on GABA-mediated inhibition in the dentate gyrus of the rat: I. Paired-pulse depression. *Brain Research*, **277,** 79–90.
Tuff, L. P., Racine, R. J. & Mishra, R. K. (1983). The effects of kindling on GABA-mediated inhibition in the dentate gyrus of the rat: II. Receptor binding. *Brain Research*, **277,** 91–8.
Valdes, F., Dashieff, R. M., Birmingham, F., Crutcher, K. A. & McNamara, J. O. (1982). Benzodiazepine receptor increases after repeated seizures. Evidence for localization to dentate granule cells. *Proceedings of the National Academy of Science, USA*, **79,** 193–7.

11

Imaging of regional cerebral metabolism and blood flow in epilepsy

George J. Siegel, Bassel Abou-Khalil and
J. Chris Sackellares

11.1 Clinical features and classification of epilepsy

Epilepsy is defined as a condition of recurrent seizures. An epileptic seizure represents an abrupt and transient disturbance of central nervous system function resulting from a paroxysmal excessive discharge of a group of cortical neurons. The location and number of these cells and the pattern of spread of the discharges within the brain vary remarkably in different types of epilepsy. Therefore, the clinical manifestations of seizures include a variety of motor, sensory, affective, autonomic, psychic, or cognitive phenomena. Consciousness may be impaired in certain types of seizures.

Epileptic seizures are divided into three categories (i) Partial seizures; (ii) Generalized seizures; (iii) Unclassified seizures. Partial seizures are those in which the first clinical and electroencephalographic (EEG) changes indicate initial activation of a system of neurons limited to a part of one cerebral hemisphere. Partial seizures can be further divided into simple partial and complex partial seizures depending on whether consciousness is preserved or impaired. In generalized seizures, the first clinical and EEG changes indicate bilateral involvement of both hemispheres from the outset. Epileptic syndromes, each with its own constellation of these seizure types and characteristic clinical features, are classified separately (Commission on Classification, 1981, 1985).

11.2 Electrophysiology

11.2.1 *Partial seizures*

Current models for the cellular pathophysiology of seizures envisage three processes in focal epileptogenesis: intrinsic burst activity, disinhibition, and excitatory synaptic coupling (Prince & Connors, 1984).

Both histopathologic (Engel *et al.*, 1982a) and physiologic studies (Schwartzkroin & Knowles, 1984) on resected temporal lobes of patients with complex partial seizures suggest that the mesial temporal cortex is most often the site of the epileptogenic focus. The clinical EEG abnormality most specific to epilepsy consists of spikes and sharp waves. In patients with partial seizures the spikes are often focal, arising frequently from one temporal lobe and recorded optimally with mesiobasal electrodes. However, the spikes may be widespread in one or both hemispheres. Not uncommonly, spikes are not detected at all in patients suspected of having partial seizures. Detection of spikes depends on adequate sampling and the position of recording electrodes with regard to distance from the spike locus and the orientation relative to the electrical dipole (Pedley, 1984).

Localization of an epileptogenic focus is one of the most important concerns in evaluating patients with refractory complex partial seizures for epilepsy surgery (Ajmone-Marsan, 1984; Engel, 1984a) and for research into metabolic and blood flow correlates. The epileptogenic focus is defined as the site in the brain where the seizure discharge is initiated. The location of the interictal spike activity recorded from surface electrodes (including scalp, nasopharyngeal, and sphenoidal electrodes) is a useful guide to the location of the epileptogenic focus, but it provides inaccurate or incomplete localization in a significant proportion of patients (Ajmone-Marsan, 1984). Ictal scalp EEG recordings improve accuracy, but interobservor disagreement may be as high as 40% with regard to lateralization (Spencer *et al.*, 1985). Interictal data from depth electrodes often show bilateral abnormalities. Using ictal recordings from depth EEG for localization of the epileptogenic focus results in the best prediction of success following surgical resection (Spencer *et al.*, 1982). Use of implanted electrodes, however, is limited by significant risks, and depth recording also may be inconclusive because the electrodes may not be optimally located for detecting the initial focal electrical events prior to their spread. Thus, an infallible standard does not exist for determining the location of the epileptogenic focus. Nevertheless, when available, focal ictal onset on depth recording provides the most reliable localization of that focus (Spencer *et al.*, 1985).

11.2.2 *Generalized seizures*

The electrophysiology of generalized epilepsy in humans has been more difficult to study. The typical interictal EEG abnormality in generalized epilepsies is the diffuse spike and wave discharge synchronous in both hemispheres. The mechanism of its generation has been the subject of controversy, but the most favored hypothesis, the corticoreticular hypothesis proposed by Gloor (1984), stresses the importance of the interaction between an abnormal diffusely hyperexcitable cortex and the thalamus and midbrain reticular formation. The mechanism of that interaction remains unknown. Also, the striking differences in clinical manifestations among the types of generalized epilepsies are not explained.

11.3 Histologic features

Most pathologic studies in epilepsy have been performed on resected temporal lobe tissue from patients having undergone surgical therapy for complex partial seizures. Where *en bloc* anterior temporal lobectomies were done, significant abnormalities were found in 75–97% of patients, the most common lesion being mesial temporal sclerosis (46–52% of cases). Other atrophic lesions, tumors, and vascular malformations were seen in 34–45% (Green & Scheetz, 1964; Falconer & Taylor, 1968; Falconer, 1974; Turner & Wyler, 1981). Mesial temporal sclerosis is characterized microscopically by neuronal loss and gliosis in the hippocampus. These changes sometimes extend into neighboring structures. Hippocampal pyramidal and granule cells show simplification of their dendrites. The causal factors of these histopathologic changes are unknown. It has been hypothesized both that local hypoxia or ischemia *in utero* or in early life is a causal factor in the sclerosis and that the seizures produce pathology through excessive metabolism and a relative ischemia (see Corsellis & Meldrum, 1976). The role of mesial temporal sclerosis in epileptogenesis (Babb *et al.*, 1984a,b; Schwartzkroin & Knowles, 1984) and the possible mechanisms of epileptogenesis have been discussed elsewhere (Delgado-Escueta *et al.*, 1986).

11.4 Brain metabolism and blood flow

J. Hughlings Jackson in the 1870s postulated that in epilepsy '... there occasionally occur excessive liberations of energy' associated with 'paroxysmal excessive discharges' in portions of grey matter that have 'high tension' and 'unstable equilibrium' (Taylor, 1958). It remained for later generations of scientists from various disciplines to elucidate the physiologic and biochemical relationships between neuronal activity and metabolism. Neuronal resting and action potentials depend on the flux of Na^+ and K^+ down their concentration gradients through special channels located in the membrane (Hille, 1981). The concentration gradients, in turn, are continuously restored and maintained through active transport catalyzed by the membrane-bound enzyme, $(Na^+ + K^+)$-stimulated adenosinetriphosphatase (Skou, 1957). In this reaction, ATP is hydrolyzed to $ADP+P_i$ and the chemical bond energy in ~P is converted to the work of ion transport. The concentration gradients for Na^+ and K^+ represent the energy reservoir for the membrane electrical potentials and it is estimated that at least 30–50% of oxygen utilization or of ATP turnover in brain serves the maintenance of these gradients (Siegel *et al.*, 1981). In isolated nerve and ganglia, a linear relationship could be shown clearly between oxygen utilization and neuronal stimulation (Sokoloff, 1981). Through the influence of $[ATP]/[ADP][P_i]$ ratios on the regulation of glycolysis and mitochondrial oxidative phosphorylation, cation transport related to electrical activity is the major determinant of metabolic rate in brain (Siegel *et al.*, 1981; Sokoloff, 1981).

The development of the nitrous oxide technique by Kety & Schmidt (1948) for the measurement of cerebral blood flow opened the way for research into whole brain metabolism *in vivo*. Under most physiologic conditions, blood flow and metabolism were found to be coupled so that the oxygen extraction ratio was relatively constant. Metabolic rate was found to be reduced in humans in association with confusion or coma due to various causes and in anesthesia (Sokoloff, 1981). During experimental generalized seizures in animals, increases of metabolic rate by 1.5 to 5 times were observed with perfusion being proportional to or greater than metabolic rate (Duffy & Plum, 1981). Blood flow is believed to be regulated to serve brain metabolic needs (autoregulation) but the range and mechanism of the coupling of perfusion to metabolism regionally is a subject for research (Duffy & Plum, 1981; Sokoloff, 1981, 1984).

The nitrous oxide method, being invasive, was not suitable for human studies. Since only mean hemispheric values could be obtained, interesting changes in heterogeneous regions of brain related to particular functions could not be detected.

Another method, based on the clearance of a tracer, xenon-133, is capable of showing regional cortical blood flow. The earliest studies of human epilepsy with this technique showed focal hyperemia in relation to epileptic discharges and focal reductions in blood flow interictally (Ingvar, 1975). These results showed the necessity for studying both interictal and ictal states in epilepsy. The ^{133}Xe clearance method, however, is limited in spatial resolution and in its showing only lateral cortex and not deep structures.

A signal advance in the study of brain metabolism was the development of the $[^{14}C]$2-deoxyglucose (2-DG) autoradiographic method by Sokoloff *et al.* (1977) for measuring regional glucose metabolism in animals. This discovery enabled the measurement of metabolic rates three-dimensionally in discrete brain regions and the study of metabolic correlations with specific brain functions (for references, see Sokoloff, 1981, 1984). This model takes advantage of the fact that 2-DG competes with glucose for hexokinase and forms 2-deoxyglucose 6-phosphate (2-DG 6-P) which, unlike glucose 6-phosphate, remains in brain for relatively long periods. The amount of 2-DG 6-P accumulated in the steady state during 40 minutes after injection of the tracer can be used to calculate the rate of glucose metabolism. The power of this method was soon demonstrated in the study of experimental focal seizures in animals. Increased glucose metabolism was observed at the epileptogenic foci and through the anatomic projections of the seizure discharges (Collins *et al.*, 1976, 1983).

Development of computer assisted tomography and the positron camera permitted the use of a host of tracers labeled with short-lived positron-emitting radionuclides (^{18}F, ^{15}O, ^{11}C, ^{13}N) in producing three-dimensional images of the brain (Ter-Pogossian *et al.*, 1970, 1975). With the appropriate tracer and compartmental model, quantitative images could be derived non-invasively in humans from metabolic, blood flow, receptor binding, and various other properties in brain (Phelps & Mazziotta, 1985). Reivich (1977) and Phelps (1979) and their colleagues developed the steady-state 2-DG model of Sokoloff (1977) with the use of [^{18}F]2-fluoro-2-deoxyglucose (FDG) and PET scanning (FDG PET) to measure local cerebral metabolic rate for glucose (LCMRG) in humans. Inhalation of oxygen-15 labeled CO_2 and O_2 were applied by Jones and colleagues to measure steady-state regional blood flow and oxygen metabolism (Frackowiak *et al.*, 1980, 1984). Dynamic methods based on bolus intravenous $H_2{}^{15}O$ and a single inhalation of $^{15}O_2$ were developed to measure blood flow and oxygen metabolism in brief intervals (Raichle *et al.*, 1984; Mintun *et al.*, 1984).

The strength of these imaging methods is that changes in metabolism or blood flow accurately identify regions in which there are structural and/or physiologic changes relative to a defined state. In brain, physiologic energy consuming changes are related to excitatory and inhibitory neuronal events (Ackermann *et al.*, 1984). The weakness is that, since the metabolic or perfusion rates are the net results of multiple processes, the final value is not necessarily proportional to any single variable. The absence of a net regional change under some given condition does not eliminate the possibility of some signficant structural or physiologic changes in that region.

The methods, theories, and applications for these imaging procedures have been extensively described in recent books and symposia (Walker, 1984; Phelps *et al.*, 1985; Reivich & Alavi, 1985). This chapter discusses only the clinical observations made with these methods in epilepsy. Since most of the available information in epilepsy consists of data on LCMRG obtained from FDG PET scans, these are discussed separately.

11.5 LCMRG in partial seizures

11.5.1 *Interictal studies*

The first study of local cerebral glucose metabolism in patients with epilepsy comprised a group of 50 sequential patients with partial seizure disorders investigated by Kuhl (1980a) and Engel (1982d) and their co-workers. These patients, in the main refractory to medical therapy, were under evaluation for surgical resection of an epileptogenic focus. While all had surface electrode EEG recordings, about half had depth electrodes as well and half underwent temporal lobe resection after identification of an epileptogenic focus. All the patients had PET scans with FDG interictally. This group provides the first and largest array of available data correlating surface EEG, depth electrode EEG, surgical treatment outcome, and tissue pathology with regional brain metabolism in patients with partial complex seizures.

The most remarkable single observation was that in about two-thirds of the patients the interictal scans showed local or widespread reductions in LCMRG ipsilateral to a well-lateralized EEG focus (Engel *et al.*, 1982d). This result was consistent with earlier reports of interictal reductions in cerebral cortical blood flow as measured by the intracarotid ^{133}Xe method (Ingvar, 1975; Lavy *et al.*, 1976).

Similar hypometabolic regions were found in the three other studies with FDG PET scans performed (Theodore *et al.*, 1983; Theodore, 1984; Gloor *et al.*, 1984; Yamamoto *et al.*, 1984; Abou-Khalil *et al.*, 1986). An example is shown in Fig. 11.1. In our experience with 32 patients with partial seizures, 24 have well-lateralized EEG foci. Among the latter group, 18 patients demonstrate ipsilateral and three show contralateral hypometabolism while three others have no significant metabolic asymmetry. Among the eight patients with non-lateralized EEG, three exhibit focal hypometabolism, and five show no asymmetry. There are 24 instances of focal metabolic asymmetry of which 21 are in patients with well-lateralized EEGs. 75% of patients with unilateral or one dominant EEG focus had one ipsilateral hypometabolic zone. As noted, the hypometabolic and EEG foci were in opposite hemispheres in three instances but these EEG foci were not verified with depth electrodes (Abou-Khalil *et al.*, 1986).

In some instances in which FDG scans could be repeated in the same patient, no obvious changes in the LCMRG pattern were noted (Kuhl *et al.*, 1980a). On the other hand, postictal scans repeated soon after seizures have shown widening and intensification of a hypometabolic region or the new appearance of focal hypometabolism as compared to the interictal scan (Abou-Khalil *et al.*, 1986).

While the criteria for defining EEG foci and for evaluating hypometabolism are not necessarily uniform in all reported studies, the following general conclusions can be drawn regarding interictal FDG PET scans and EEG foci:

(i) There is a high correlation between scans showing a unilateral focal reduction in LCMRG and the finding of well-lateralized EEG abnormalities in the ipsilateral hemisphere.

(ii) There are poor correlations between LCMRG and EEG abnormalities when either (a) the PET scans show either no focal reductions or bilateral reductions in LCMRG; or (b) the EEG abnormalities are bilateral without a predominant lateralized focus.

(iii) Normal PET scans are more often found with non-lateralized EEG findings and vice versa.

The finding of focal interictal hypometabolism is surprising since it is not expected from Jackson's postulation (Taylor, 1958) upon which models of focal epilepsy have been largely based for over a century.

Fig. 11.1. Interictal FDG scan: Left lateral temporal hypometabolism in a patient with a left mesial temporal epileptogenic focus. The graph represents the average LCMRG in eight-pixel columns between the two horizontal lines, from left to right.

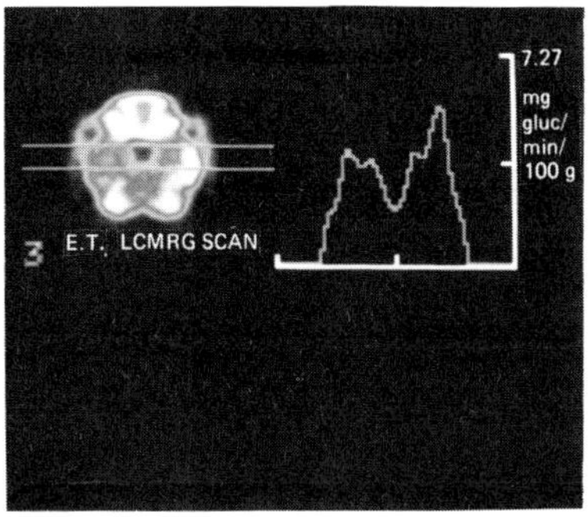

The concept expressed by Jackson does not indicate a qualitative but rather a quantitative difference between interictal and ictal states. However, the metabolic studies have revealed a fundamentally different physiologic process interictally that leads to a net reduced 'tension' and 'instability', in Jackson's terms, in certain neuronal networks. The relation to ictal states which are associated with increased metabolic rate is discussed later.

11.5.2 *Ictal studies in partial seizures*

The first human seizures studied with PET scans were reported by Kuhl *et al.* (1980a) and, including these, FDG PET scans have been reported on at least 13 patients during partial seizures of various types (Engel *et al.*, 1982b, 1983; Theodore *et al.*, 1983). In these studies, the seizures occurred during the 40 minute period after injection of FDG.

The principal observation in common among these cases is that the interictal hypometabolic region becomes hypermetabolic during the seizure (Fig. 11.2). The changes may be several-fold relative to the opposite cortex or may be seen only as reductions in the interictal asymmetry. In some patients the hypermetabolism extends to contiguous and projection regions, notably temporal and frontal, in the same and contralateral hemisphere and the change in adjacent regions is not necessarily constant in different seizures in the same patient (Engel *et al.*, 1983). The regional patterns of changes vary considerably among the subjects studied. There

Fig. 11.2. (*A*) Interictal FDG scan: Although a complex partial seizure occured 11 minutes after FDG injection, this scan can be considered mainly interictal because of weighting of the first minutes after FDG injection (*B*) Ictal FDG scan: FDG was injected immediately after the onset of a complex partial seizure. This scan represents a combination of ictal and postictal LCMRG. Note the increased LCMRG in the left temporal lobe which was slightly hypometabolic in scan A, and the decreased LCMRG in the remainder of the brain.

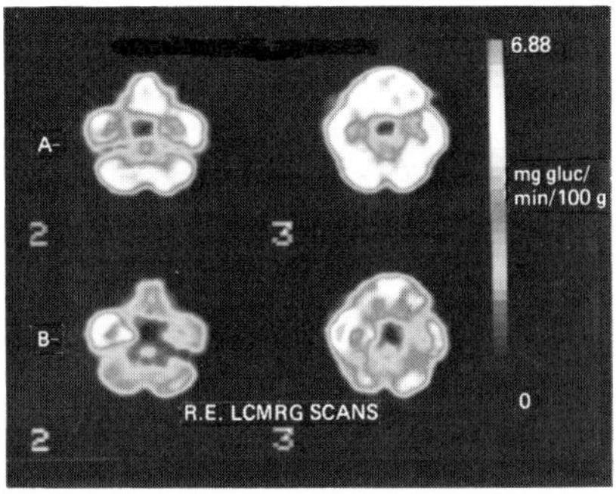

is a paucity of data regarding changes in mesiobasal or deep structures and in cerebellum in humans although hypermetabolism in the thalamus was noted in at least one patient (Engel *et al.*, 1983, pt. 3).

Reductions in metabolism bilaterally outside the hypermetabolic zone seem to occur when consciousness is lost during the seizure (Engel *et al.*, 1983; Theodore *et al.*, 1983). These reductions are postulated to be the results of postictal depression.

The hypermetabolism of the epileptogenic focus spreading to include contiguous cortex and projection regions during seizures confirms Jackson's concepts of the 'paroxysmal excessive discharge' associated with 'energy liberation' (Taylor, 1958). We have already noted that the interictal hypometabolism is a qualitatively different process. It follows that the interictal process, perhaps one leading to stabilization, is overcome or switched off at the onset of the seizure. It has been said by Jackson that the cortical abnormality in epilepsy is permanent with a varying state (see Taylor, 1958, p. 95) which description conforms precisely to the overall metabolic observations.

The FDG scans are not suitable for studying the regional or temporal sequence of changes through interictal, ictal, and postictal states. Since the FDG uptake period is about 40 minutes, while seizures rarely exceed five minutes in duration, the scans are the time average of variable combinations of ictal and postictal events spreading or receding through the brain. The brain state is changing during this period so that quantitative correlations from such averages are precluded. Resolution of ictal and postictal events and of epileptogenic foci from their projection regions will depend on application of dynamic methods with tracer substances such as oxygen-15 that permit multiple scans in short time periods (Sackellares *et al.*, 1986).

11.5.3 *Pathology related to hypometabolism*

The pathologic significance of the focal hypometabolism could be partially evaluated together with the efficacy of surgery therapy in the series of patients reported by Engel *et al.*, (1982a). In this series, complete metabolic and pathologic data were available for 25 patients who underwent *en bloc* resection of an anterior temporal lobe. Operations were performed only on temporal lobes believed to evince well-lateralized epileptogenic foci by EEG criteria. Among these 25 well-studied patients, 18 had PET scans exhibiting single hypometabolic regions ipsilateral to the EEG focus, three had normal scans, two had contralateral hypometabolic foci (possibly related to damage produced by depth electrodes, according to the authors), and two had bilateral hypometabolic foci. Gross or microscopic pathology was found in 19 of the temporal lobe surgical specimens. Preoperatively, all of these 19 subjects demonstrated a hypometabolic region in the tissue later resected. Regarding the six patients with histologically normal resected tissue, the preoperative PET scans were normal in three and showed contralateral hypometabolism in the two with possible depth electrode damage. Only one patient with normal tissue had a distinct ipsilateral hypometabolic region preoperatively.

These data prove a high positive correlation between a visually identified hypometabolic region on an FDG PET scan and structural pathology in the ipsilateral anterior temporal lobe (Engel *et al.*, 1982a). Similar results were obtained in later studies (Theodore *et al.*, 1983, 1984). However, this conclusion may be applied only to patients with well-lateralized epileptogenic foci by EEG criteria. Operations usually are not performed on patients whose EEGs do not show well-lateralized foci. Therefore, the pathologic significance of the presence or absence of hypometabolism cannot be investigated in the absence of an associated EEG focus.

11.5.4 *Prediction of treatment results*

The treatment outcome of temporal lobe resection was defined by the frequency of seizures postoperatively (Engel *et al.*, 1982a). All but one of the 25 were improved. Most experienced only rare or no seizures postoperatively. This is so although five did not have hypometabolism in the resected lobe and six of the resections showed no pathology. The individual who did not improve was one who had had hypometabolism on the preoperative PET scan which was contralateral to the EEG focus. However, the second patient with contralateral hypometabolism was free of seizures after surgery (Engel *et al.*, 1982a). In another group, a single patient in whom depth electrode discharges were contralateral to focal metabolism had no improvement after resection of the temporal lobe indicated by the EEG (Theodore *et al.*, 1983). While the numbers are small, the outcome of surgical treatment seems not predictable from the absence or presence of hypometabolism or of finding structural pathology by conventional means in the resected tissue in these studies.

11.5.5 *Correlations with clinical features*

In none of the reported studies was there any evidence for correlation of hypometabolism with frequency of EEG epileptiform discharges during the scan, seizure frequency, duration of seizure disorder, types of complex partial seizures, or age of onset. Hypometabolism has been observed in all instances in which CT or MRI scans show focal abnormalities (Abou-Khalil *et al.*, 1986; Theodore *et al.*, 1986b; Latack *et al.*, 1986). However, it is known from studies of neoplasms and infarctions that hypometabolism is produced by structural lesions that are not necessarily epileptogenic (Kuhl *et al.*, 1980b; Newmark *et al.*, 1983).

The available data regarding anticonvulsant drug effects in humans indicate that phenobarbital withdrawal leads to generally increased LCMRG with no changes in the relative hypometabolism where it is found and other drugs seem not to have an effect (Theodore *et al.*, 1986a). There have been no reports of FDG PET scans performed before and after chronic treatment with anticonvulsant drugs. Whether the result after phenobarbital withdrawal reflects prior chronic metabolic suppression by barbiturate or a rebound effect is an interesting topic for research.

11.5.6 *Theories of hypometabolism*

The histologic characteristics associated with focal hypometabolism are of considerable interest. In 15 of the 19 temporal lobe specimens showing lesions, the pathology consisted of mesial temporal sclerosis involving the hippocampal pes, dentate gyrus, and subiculum, to various degrees. The remaining four lesions consisted of tumor, heterotopia, or angioma (Engel *et al.*, 1982a).

Within the resected portions of temporal lobes, the pathological finding in the cases with mesial temporal sclerosis was neuron loss ranging from 'more or less complete neuron loss in different regions of the hippocampal pes and dentate gyrus to only mild and random cell loss in hippocampus and subiculum'. In the most severe case, the amygdala also showed neuron loss. The severity of neuron loss was graded and correlated with the percentage decrease in LCMRG. However, the zone of hypometabolism often involved most of the temporal lobe and was considerably larger than the extent of the structural lesion demonstrated by pathological examination (Engel *et al.*, 1982a). Similar results were reported by Theodore (1983, 1984).

In a more recent study of patients with demonstrable mesial temporal lobe epileptogenic foci, LCMRG was analyzed separately in mesial and lateral temporal lobe cortex (Abou-Khalil *et al.*, 1985). These data show that the relative hypometabolism is of a much greater degree in the lateral than in the mesial cortex although the epileptiform EEG activity is greatest or present only in the mesial leads (Fig. 11.1). These observations suggest that functional neuronal connections exist between mesial and broad regions of lateral temporal cortex in man. The lesser degree of hypometabolism observed mesially despite the expected neuronal loss in the same location suggests that the surviving cells have increased ion flux or firing rates. This might represent the site of permanent cortical instability supposed by Hughlings Jackson (Taylor, 1958). Hypometabolism in the lateral cortex may be due to deafferentation from mesial neuronal loss or from possible inhibitory influences of mesial cortex activity (Abou-Khalil *et al.*, 1985). The apparent correlation of neuron dropout in mesial temporal lobe structures with reductions in LCMRG which involve most of the temporal lobe, may be additional evidence for more widespread hippocampal–lateral neocortical pathways than have been demonstrated earlier by anatomic methods (Jones & Powell, 1970; Rosene & Van Hoesen, 1977; Engel *et al.*, 1978; Watson *et al.*, 1983; Ackermann *et al.*, 1984).

Possible causes of the temporal lobe hypometabolism are: local structural loss or damage not yet appreciated by conventional histologic methods, reduced activation or increased inhibition of neuronal activity, or variation in vascular perfusion, as discussed by Engel *et al.*, (1982c). The net asymmetry in metabolic rate may be the resultant of multiple physiologic and structural factors locally or of activity in remote ipsilateral or contralateral pathways. Whatever structural or physiologic changes may be found in the lateral temporal neocortex, a satisfactory hypothesis will have to account for the relationship of changes in the lateral neocortex to the neuron loss and epileptiform activity in the mesial cortex.

11.6 Clinical use of the FDG PET scan in diagnosis of partial seizures

The available PET studies with FDG in epilepsy show that a locally hypometabolic scan represents additional confirmation of an epileptogenic region when it coincides with a clear EEG focus. While the FDG PET scan cannot yet be used independently, it is stated that the FDG PET scan may help identify epileptogenic lesions (Engel *et al.*, 1982c; Engel, 1984b). It is necessary to define explicitly the types of cases in which the PET scan is useful diagnostically. Estimating the incidence of falsely negative or positive scans depends on selecting a standard for comparison. Based on the experience of Engel and colleagues (1982c), which represents the most comprehensive EEG data available, about one-third of normal PET scans in patients with refractory partial epilepsy (5/15) are associated with well-lateralized EEG foci and may be considered falsely negative while 10% of focally abnormal scans (4/35) are associated with non-localizing EEG data from depth and/or surface electrodes. In the latter type of cases, surgery is usually not performed and, therefore, verification will be lacking. These proportions are similar to those found by inspection of the data in the other reports (Theodore, 1984; Gloor *et al.*, 1984; Abou-Khalil *et al.*, 1986). Therefore, the FDG PET scan cannot be used presently to decide for or against surgery.

The finding of regional hypometabolism on the FDG PET scan may be very useful, on the other hand, to indicate when additional information is needed. In the experience of Engel's group, 13 patients in whom ictal onset was recorded from depth electrodes and who underwent surgery were among those whose resected temporal lobes showed pathology. Detection of the side of ictal onset from depth electrodes in these patients disagreed in only one instance with the PET scan. In contrast, each of interictal depth and scalp and even ictal scalp recordings showed multiple disagreements (Engel *et al.*, 1982c, Table 4). Thus, from inspection of these data, the laterality of focal reductions in LCMRG, when present in patients with partial seizures, is strongly correlated with ictal recordings from depth electrodes. Several investigators have shown that ictal onset data recorded from depth electrodes are the most reliable in predicting surgical outcome and are in disagreement with surface ictal data in at least 40% of cases (Engel *et al.*, 1981; Spencer *et al.*, 1982; 1985). Therefore, if the PET scan shows hypometabolism conflicting with surface EEG data, this would indicate the need for depth electrode recordings to localize the epileptogenic focus.

If regional hypometabolism coincides with well-lateralized surface EEG data, the need for depth electrode implantation may be relieved (Engel *et al.*, 1982c). This consideration may depend also on whether the focus is in the temporal lobe in which localization from surface leads is more accurate than elsewhere (Spencer *et al.*, 1985). Currently, however, the PET scan does not help in lateralizing the epileptogenic focus where the surface EEG discharges are bilateral or shifting since in these cases, the PET scan is often normal (Abou-Khalil *et al.*, 1986). Additional data are needed to determine the significance of an abnormal PET scan in the presence of bilateral EEG foci. Possibly, dynamic ictal studies with oxygen-15 will be more powerful than FDG scans in localizing ictal sites (Sackellares *et al.*, 1986).

11.7 Primary generalized seizures

The types of generalized seizures so far studied with PET scans are absence seizures, ECT induced tonic–clonic seizures, and the Lennox–Gastaut syndrome.

11.7.1 *Absence*

Patients with absence seizures associated with 3 Hz generalized spike-and-slow-wave complexes in the EEG were studied by Engel *et al.*, (1985). Hyperventilation was performed by the patients for 10 min after injection of the FDG in the initial (ictal) scan and in a repeat (control) scan several months after abolition of seizures with anticonvulsant drug treatment. EEG monitoring during the FDG uptake period indicated the number of seizures.

In three of the four patients studied, the EEGs during the ictal scans showed frequent generalized 3 Hz spike-and-slow-wave complexes associated with clinical absences. Both the ictal and control PET scans exhibited no focal asymmetries or unusual patterns of LCMRG but the global LCMRG rates in the ictal scans were 2.5 to 3.5 times greater than in the control hyperventilation studies in which no seizures occurred. The global LCMRG values in the ictal scans were higher than those in patients with partial seizures or generalized seizures after electroconvulsive therapy possibly because the absences are not followed by postictal depression as are other types of seizures (Engle *et al.*, 1985).

Another group of nine patients, of whom seven had both absence and generalized tonic–clonic seizures, one had absence seizures only, and one had tonic-clonic seizures only, was studied by Theodore *et al.*, (1985). The interictal EEGs showed no epileptiform discharges despite hyperventilation and the interictal PET scans showed normal metabolic rates and no asymmetry to focal hypometabolism

Three of these patients also had scans during seizures. Two of these patients had hyperventilation-induced generalized spike and wave discharges, one with blinking and one without obvious behavioral changes Metabolic rates were diffusely increased and no focal changes were noted in their ictal scans. These findings are similar to those of Engel *et al.*, (1985) in absence seizures.

11.7.2 *Absence status*

One patient reported by Theodore and colleagues (1985) had a prolonged absence status, then repetitive episodes of unresponsiveness interspersed with confusion. The EEG showed generalized 5 Hz repetitive sharp waves leading into 2.5 – 3 Hz spike-and-slow-wave complexes. Confusion was accompanied by 4–6 Hz irregular slowing on the EEG. This ictal scan showed 20–39% decreases in LCMRG in many cortical and subcortical regions bilaterally. No focal changes were observed. The EEG activity and postictal confusion episodes suggested that these were atypical absences. The decreased metabolism may be correlated with the presence of postictal confusion and EEG slowing as seen after partial or secondarily generalized seizures, or after generalized tonic–clonic seizures and contrasts with results in classical absence with 3 Hz spike-and-slow-wave complexes (Engel *et al.*, 1985).

11.7.3 *Tonic-clonic seizures*

The effect of electroconvulsive therapy on LCMRG was studied in several patients. A PET scan was obtained after FDG was injected at the time of electroshock therapy (ictal) and another scan was performed after FDG injection at the onset of EEG depression at a later treatment session (postictal). An interictal scan was performed in between treatments. The ictal scan revealed globally increased metabolic rates while the postictal scan exhibited globally decreased rates compared to the interictal scan (Engel *et al.*, 1982b).

It is remarkable that generalized absence seizures are similar to ECT seizures in showing diffuse increases in metabolic rate, presumably in all of the brain. Yet, absence seizures are quite different in showing no postictal depression, either metabolically, on EEG, or behaviorally. The measurement of metabolic rate apparently does not discriminate between inhibitory and excitatory neuronal activity. The increases were greater during absence seizures than during ECT, presumably because of the prolonged postictal depression in the latter which is included in the FDG uptake period.

11.7.4 *Lennox–Gastaut syndrome*

Lennox–Gastaut syndrome is a severe form of epilepsy manifesting various types of generalized seizures associated with slow spike-and-slow-wave complexes in the EEG, often frontally but also diffusely with shifting patterns. The neurologic examination and intellect are often abnormal. Congenital or hereditary factors are frequently encountered. Two such patients exhibited hypometabolism in the left temporal lobes, by 55% and 59%, compared to the right sides (Gur *et al.*, 1982). In another series of 10 patients, either bilateral frontal cortex hypometabolism or no metabolic changes were noted (W. H. Theodore, personal communication).

11.8 Oxygen-15 PET scan studies

PET scan methods were developed with the use of oxygen-15 labeled O_2 and CO_2 to measure steady state regional oxygen metabolic rate (rCMRO), blood flow (rCBF) and oxygen extraction ratio (rOER)

(Frackowiak *et al.*, 1980). A scan is first performed to measure blood flow during inhalation of $C^{15}O_2$ which transfers the label to $H_2{}^{15}O$ in the lungs through the catalytic action of carbonic anhydrase. Then a scan is performed during inhalation of $^{15}O_2$ to measure rOER. The product of rOER and rCBF yields the oxygen metabolic rate.

Bernardi *et al.* (1983) and Depresseux *et al.* (1983) found that in the interictal state many patients showed focal reductions in rCMRO and rCBF in regions containing the epileptogenic focus. In addition, Bernardi *et al.* (1983) described decreases, although smaller, in the contralateral hemisphere and in both cerebellar hemispheres in epileptic patients. Ictal activity, when studied, was accompanied by focally, multifocally, or generally increased rCBF and rCMRO up to 2.4 times the normal (Depresseux *et al.*, 1983). Zones of reduced rCBF and rCMRO were reported to be similar to but more diffuse than those with FDG (Gloor *et al.*, 1984; Yamamota *et al.*, 1984).

An important question is whether blood flow and metabolic rate are coupled in epileptic brain and during seizures. In one study (Depresseux *et al.*, 1983), coupling between perfusion and oxygen metabolism was reported to be normal in all cases so that rOER was not significantly changed. In contrast, Bernardi *et al.* (1983) observed a significant increase in the rOER on interictal scans in the temporal lobe ipsilateral to the EEG focus. It has been proposed from studies of cerebrovascular disease that an increase in rOER indicates the presence of relative ischemia or failure of blood flow to satisfy metabolic demands (see Frackowiak *et al.*, 1984, for references). Ischemia has been postulated as both a cause and an effect of temporal lobe mesial sclerosis and seizures (Corsellis & Meldrum, 1976). Therefore, the analysis of rOER is of considerable importance in the study of the pathology and physiology of epilepsy. The few results so far obtained with the use of oxygen-15 in partial seizures are conflicting.

Dynamic methods for the measurement of oxygen metabolism with a single whiff of $^{15}O_2$ and of blood flow with an intravenous bolus of oxygen-15 labeled water (Raichle *et al.*, 1984) will permit more rapid and repeated imaging. So far, there are very few data with the use of these dynamic methods in the study of seizures. rCBF was measured with the intravenous $H_2{}^{15}O$ method of Raichle in a small number of patients with partial seizures. Interictally, a focal reduction in rCBF corresponding to a reduction in LCMRG and an EEG focus was found in one patient. Ictal scans in two patients showed increases in rCBF corresponding to the EEG foci (Sackellares *et al.*, 1986). Figure 11.3 shows an example of focal interictal hypoperfusion. The same region demonstrated hyperperfusion during a partial seizure induced by hyperventilation. Hyperventilation itself may produce a 30–50% generalized reduction in cerebral blood flow (Fig. 11.4). There have been no reports of the effect of hyperventilation on metabolism. Considerably more research into the coupling of oxygen metabolism and blood flow to brain functions is required with the use of these methods.

Fig. 11.3. H_2O[O-15] scan: Effect of a complex partial seizure on blood flow in the same patient as in Fig. 2. (*A*) Preictal rCBF. (*B*) Ictal rCBF; a complex partial seizure was precipitated by hyperventilating for one minute. Note the marked hyperemia in the left temporal lobe corresponding to the epileptogenic focus. (*C*) rCBF 10 minutes after the seizure. Note the slight persistent hyperemia in the left temporal lobe.

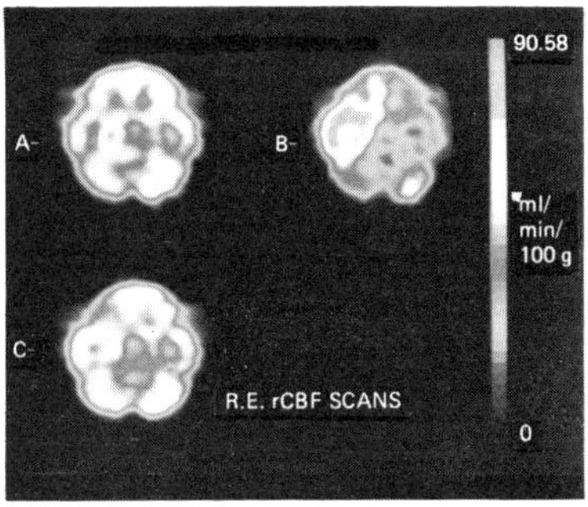

Fig. 11.4. H_2O[O–15] scan: Effect of hyperventilation on blood flow. (*A*) rCBF interictally. Note the reduced blood flow in the left temporal lobe corresponding to the site of focal epileptiform activity on EEG.(*B*) rCBF during hyperventilation. The left temporal reduction in blood flow is still noted. Cerebral blood flow is 35% lower than in A.(*C*) rCBF 10 minutes after hyperventilation. A rebound increase in blood flow is seen. (*D*) rCBF 22 minutes after hyperventilation approaches baseline values.

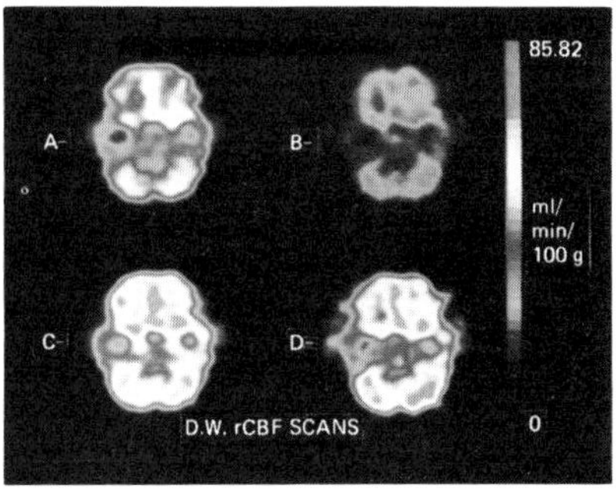

11.9 Other blood flow studies

Most of the xenon-133 studies of rCBF are consistent with the FDG studies in showing interictal reductions of perfusion in partial seizures (Ingvar, 1975; Lavy *et al.*, 1976; Bonte *et al.*, 1983; Rosadini *et al.*, 1983, 1984) and no interictal reductions or asymmetries in patients with primary generalized seizures (Sakai *et al.*, 1978; Rosadini *et al.*, 1983, 1984; Touchon *et al.*, 1986). Patients with asynchronous bilateral EEG abnormalities showed no asymmetries or reductions in rCBF (Baldy-Moulinier *et al.*, 1985; Touchon *et al.*, 1986). Also, in patients studied during *petit mal* seizures, blood flow was found to be increased diffusely in grey and white matter (Sakai *et al.*, 1978), in accord with PET scan results. However the patterns of interictal hypoperfusion found in partial seizures with ^{133}Xe methods are much more varied than those of LCMRG observed in the FDG scans. In addition, some observations of interictal hyperperfusion have been reported (Hougaard *et al.*, 1976; Sakai *et al.*, 1978). Whether these differences between results with FDG PET and ^{133}Xe studies are related to the differences in methodology or to the pathophysiology of blood flow as compared to that of glucose metabolism is not yet clear. As yet, there are few PET studies of blood flow in epilepsy.

Research into other methods for measuring cerebral blood flow in epilepsy includes the use of [^{123}I]isopropyl-iodo-amphetamine with single photon emission computed tomography (Magistretti *et al.*, 1983; Sanabria *et al.*, 1983). This is a new and relatively untried tool which may prove useful, particularly for cortical blood flow measurements. It has an advantage over PET scans in not requiring a cyclotron and in being much less costly and labor-intensive.

11.10 Conclusions

The metabolic and blood flow studies are concordant in showing relative interictal reductions in glucose and oxygen metabolic rates and perfusion in regions of the hemisphere ipsilateral to lateralized EEG foci in many but not all patients with partial seizures. The patterns with blood flow, however, seem less consistently correlated than those with FDG. During partial seizures, the epileptogenic focus and the distribution of seizure discharge are occupied by hypermetabolism and hyperperfusion. In patients with primary generalized seizures, on the other hand, no focal asymmetries or reductions in metabolism or blood flow interictally are found. During generalized seizures, the cerebrum demonstrates bilateral diffuse increases in metabolism and blood flow.

Considerably more data, together with development of standardized methods for accurate analysis of landscapes of blood flow and metabolism, are required to recognize both the range of normal variations under various conditions and the deviations that can be related to abnormal function. Standardization is required also for comparison of data from different studies.

Research is needed in the dynamic study of regional blood flow and metabolism with methods for rapid and repeated imaging to assess autoregulation, the possible presence of relative ischemia, and the temporal and regional sequence of changes from interictal to ictal to postictal states.

The authors' work was supported by NIH grant NS15655. The authors are grateful for the technical assistance of R. Marshall, J. Rothley, and A. Tournow in the performance of PET and EEG studies.

References

Abou-Khalil, B. W., Sackellares, J. C., Hichwa, R. D., Weinberger, L. M., & Siegel, G. J. (1987). Local cerebral metabolic rate for glucose (LCMRG) in patients with chronic refractory partial seizures. *Advances in Epileptology: sixteenth Epilepsy International Symposium*, p. 143. New York: Raven Press.

Abou-Khalil, B. W., Siegel, G. J., Hichwa, R. D., Sackellares, J. C. & Gilman, S. (1985). Topography of glucose hypometabolism in epilepsy of mesial temporal origin, *Ann. Neurol.*, **18,** 151.

Ackermann, R. F., Finch, D. M., Babb, T. L. & Engel, J., Jr (1984). Increased glucose metabolism during long-duration recurrent inhibition of hippocampal pyramidal cells. *Neuroscience*, **4,** 251–64.

Ajmone-Marsan, C. (1984). Electroencephalographic studies in seizure disorders: additional considerations. *Clin. Neurophysiol.*, **1,** 143–57.

Babb, T. L., Brown, W. J., Pretorius, J., Davenport, C., Lieb, J. P. & Crandall, P. H. (1984a). Temporal lobe volumetric cell densities in temporal lobe epilepsy. *Epilepsia*, **25,** 729–40.

Babb, T. L., Lieb, J. P., Brown, W. J., Pretorius, J. & Crandall, P. H. (1984b). Distribution of pyramidal cell density and hyperexcitability in the epileptic human hippocampal formation. *Epilepsia*, **25,** 721–8.

Baldy-Moulinier, M., Valmier, J., Touchon, J., Billiard, M., Besset, A. & Cadilhac, J. (1985). Débits cérébraux régionaux diminués en periode intercritique dans l'épilepsie du lobe temporal. *Rev. Neurol.*, **141,** 18–27.

Bernardi, S., Trimble, M. R., Frackowiak, R. S. J., Wise, R. J. S. & Jones, T. (1983). An interictal study of partial epilepsy using positron emission tomography and the oxygen-15 inhalation technique. *Neurol. Neurosurg. Psychiatry*, **46,** 473–7.

Bonte, F. J., Stokely, E. M., Devous, M. D. & Homan, R. W. (1983). Single-photon tomographic study of regional cerebral blood flow in epilepsy. A preliminary report. *Arch. Neurol.*, **40,** 267–70.

Collins, R. C., Kennedy, C., Sokoloff, L. & Plum, F. (1976). Metabolic anatomy of focal motor seizures. *Arch. Neurol.*, **33,** 536–42.

Collins, R. C., Tearse, R. G. & Lathman, E. W. (1983). Functional anatomy of limbic seizures: focal discharges from medial entorhinal cortex in rat. *Brain Res.*, **280,** 25–40.

Commission on Classification and Terminology of the International League Against Epilepsy (1981). Proposal for revised clinical and electroencephalographic classification of epileptic seizures. *Epilepsia*, **22,** 489–501.

Commission on Classification and Terminology of the International League Against Epilepsy (1985). Proposal for classification of epilepsies and epileptic syndromes. *Epilepsia*, **26,** 268–78.

Corsellis, J. A. N. & Meldrum, B. S. (1976). Epilepsy. In *Greenfield's Neuropathology*, ed. W. Blackwood & J. A. N. Corsellis, pp. 771–95. London: Edward Arnold.

Delgado-Escueta, A. V., Ward, A. A., Jr, Woodbury, D. M. & Porter, R. J. (1986). *Basic Mechanisms of the Epilepsies*. New York: Raven Press.

Depresseux, J. C., Frank, G. & Sadzot, B. (1983). Regional cerebral blood flow and oxygen uptake rate in human focal epilepsy. In *Cerebral Blood Flow, Metabolism and Epilepsy*, ed. M. Baldy-Moulinier, D. H. Ingvar and B. S. Meldrum, pp. 76–81. London: John Libbey.

Duffy, T. E. & Plum, F. (1981). Seizures, coma, and major metabolic encephalopathies. In *Basic Neurochemistry*, 3rd edn, ed. G. J. Siegel, R. W. Albers, B. W. Agranoff & R. Katzman, pp. 693–718. Boston: Little, Brown & Co.

Engel, J., Jr (1984a). A practical guide for routine EEG studies in epilepsy. *Clin. Neurophysiol.*, **1,** 109–42.

Engel, J. (1984b). The use of positron emission tomographic scanning in epilepsy. *Ann. Neurol.* **15,** *(suppl)*, S180–91.

Engel, J. Jr, Brown, W. J., Kuhl, D. E., Phelps, M. E., Mazziotta, J. C. & Crandall, P. H. (1982a). Pathological findings underlying focal temporal lobe hypometabolism in partial epilepsy. *Ann. Neurol.*, **12,** 518–28.

Engel, J. Jr, Kuhl, D. E. & Phelps, M. E. (1982b). Patterns of human local cerebral glucose metabolism during epileptic seizures. *Science*, **218,** 64–6.

Engel, J. Jr, Kuhl, D. E., Phelps, M. E. & Crandall, P. H. (1982c). Comparative localization of epileptic foci in partial epilepsy by PCT and EEG. *Ann. Neurol.*, **12,** 529–37.

Engel, J. Jr, Kuhl, D. E., Phelps, M. E. & Mazziotta J. C. (1982d). Interictal cerebral glucose metabolism in partial epilepsy and its relation to EEG changes. *Ann. Neurol.*, **12,** 510–7.

Engel, J. Jr, Kuhl, D. E., Phelps, M. E., Rausch, R. & Nuwer, M. (1983). Local cerebral metabolism during partial seizures. *Neurology*, **33,** 400–13.

Engel, J. Jr, Lubens, P., Kuhl, D. E. & Phelps, M. E. (1985). Local cerebral metabolic rate for glucose during petit mal absences. *Ann. Neurol.*, **17,** 121–8.

Engel, J. Jr, Rausch, R., Lieb, J. P., Kuhl, D. & Crandall, P. H. (1981). Correlation of criteria used for localizing epileptic foci in patients considered for surgical therapy of epilepsy. *Ann. Neurol.*, **9,** 215–24.

Engel, J. Jr, Wolfson, L. & Brown, L. (1978). Anatomical correlates of electrical and behavioral events related to amygdaloid kindling. *Ann. Neurol.*, **3,** 538–44.

Falconer, M. A. (1974). Mesial temporal (Ammon's horn) sclerosis as a common cause of epilepsy. Aetiology, treatment, and prevention. *Lancet*, II, 767–70.

Falconer, M. A. & Taylor, D. C. (1968). Surgical treatment of drug-resistant epilepsy due to mesial temporal sclerosis. Etiology and significance. *Arch. Neurol.*, **19,** 353–61.

Frackowiak, R. S. J., Lenzi, G. L., Jones, T. & Heather, J. D. (1980). Quantitative measurement of regional cerebral blood flow and oxygen metabolism in man using ^{15}O and positron emission tomography: theory, procedure and normal values. *J. Comput. Assist. Tomogr.*, **4,** 727–36.

Frackowiak, R. S. J., Wise, R. J. S., Gibbs, J. M., Jones, T. (1984). Positron emission tomographic studies in aging and cerebrovascular disease at Hammersmith Hospital, *Ann. Neurol.*, **15** *(suppl)*, S112–18.

Gloor, P. (1984). Electrophysiology of generalized epilepsy. In *Electrophysiology of Epilepsy*, ed. P. A. Schwartzkroin & H. V. Wheal, pp. 107–36. London: Academic Press Inc.

Gloor, P., Yamamoto, L., Ochs, R., Feindel, W., Gotman, J., Quesney, L. F., Meyer, E. & Thompson, C. (1984). Regional cerebral metabolism measured by positron emission tomography in patients with partial epilepsy: correlation with EEG findings. In *Advances in Epileptology: fifteenth Epilepsy International Symposium,* ed. R. J. Porter *et al.*, New York: Raven Press. pp. 99–103.

Green, J. R. & Scheetz, D. G. (1964). Surgery of epileptogenic lesions of the temporal lobe. *Arch. Neurol.*, **10,** 135–48.

Gur, R. C., Sussman, N. M., Alavi, A., Gur, R. E., Rosen, A. D., O'Connor, M., Goldberg, H. I., Greenberg, J. H. & Reivich, M. (1982). Positron emission tomography in two cases of childhood epileptic encephalopathy (Lennox-Gastaut Syndrome). *Neurology,* **32,** 1191–4.

Hille, B. (1981) Excitability and ionic channels. In *Basic Neurochemistry*, 3rd edn, ed. G. J. Siegel, R. W. Albers, B. W. Agranoff & R. Katzman, pp. 95–105. Boston: Little, Brown & Co.

Hougaard, K., Oikawa, T., Sveinsdottir, E., Skinhoj, E., Ingvar, D. H. & Lassen, N. A. (1976). Regional cerebral blood flow in focal cortical epilepsy. *Arch. Neurol.*, **33,** 527–35.

Ingvar, D. H. (1975). rCBF in focal cortical epilepsy. In *Cerebral Circulation and Metabolism*, ed. T. W. Langfitt *et al.*, pp. 361–4. Berlin: Springer Verlag.

Jones, E. G. & Powell, T. P. S. (1970). An anatomical study of converging sensory pathways within the cerebral cortex of the monkey, *Brain*, **93,** 793–820.

Kety, S. S. & Schmidt, C. F. (1948). The nitrous oxide method for quantitative determination of cerebral blood flow in man: theory, procedure and normal values. *J. Clin. Invest.*, **27,** 476–83.

Kuhl, D. E., Engel, J. Jr, Phelps, M. E. & Selin, C. (1980a). Epileptic patterns of local cerebral metabolism and perfusion in humans determined by emission computed tomography of ^{18}FDG and $^{13}NH_3$. *Ann. Neurol.*, **8,** 348–60.

Kuhl, D. E., Phelps, M. E., Kowell, A. P., Metter, E. J., Selin, C. & Winter, J. (1980b). Effects of stroke on local cerebral metabolism and perfusion: mapping by emission computed tomography of ^{18}FDG and $^{13}NH_3$, *Ann. Neurol.*, **8,** 47–60.

Latack, J. T., Abou-Khalil, B. W., Siegel, G. J., Sackellares, J. C., Gabrielson, T. O. & Aisen, A. M. (1986). Magnetic resonance imaging, computed tomography, and positron emission tomography in patients with partial seizures. *Radiology*, **159,** 159–63.

Lavy, S., Melamed, E., Portnoy, Z. & Carmon, A. (1976). Interictal regional cerebral blood flow in patients with partial seizures. *Neurology*, **26,** 418–22.

Magistretti, P., Uren, R., Shomer, D., Blume, H., Holman, B. & Hill, T. (1983). Emission tomographic scans of cerebral blood flow using I^{123} iodoamphetamine in epilepsy. In *Nuclear Medicine and Biological Advances*, ed. C. Raynaud, pp. 139–43. Paris: Pergamon Press.

Mintum, M. A., Raichle, M. E., Martin, W. R. W. & Herscovitch, P. (1984). Brain oxygen utilization measured with ^{15}O radiotracers and positron emission tomography. *J. Nucl. Med.* **25,** 177–87.

Newmark, M. E., Theodore, W. H., Sato, S., De La Paz, R., Patronas, N., Brooks, R., Jabbari, B. & Di Chiro, G. (1983). EEG, transmission computed tomography, and positron emission tomography with fluorodeoxyglucose ^{18}F. *Arch. Neurol.*, **40,** 607–10.

Pedley, T. A. (1984). Epilepsy and the human electroencephalogram. In *Electrophysiology of Epilepsy*, ed. P. A. Schwartzkroin & H. V. Wheals, pp. 1–30. London: Academic Press Inc.

Phelps, M. E., Huang, S. C., Hoffman, E. J., Selin, C. S., Sokoloff, L. & Kuhl, D. E. (1979). Tomographic measurement of local cerebral glucose metabolic rate in humans with (F-18)2-fluoro-2-deoxy-D-glucose: validation of method. *Ann. Neurol.*, **6,** 371–88.

Phelps, M. E. & Mazziotta, J. C. (1985). Positron emission tomography: human brain function and biochemistry. *Science*, **228,** 799–809.

Phelps, M. E., Mazziotta, J. & Schelbert, H. R. (1985). *Positron Emission Tomography and Autoradiography*. New York: Raven Press.

Prince, D. A. & Connors, B. W. (1984). Mechanisms of epileptogenesis in cortical structures. *Ann. Neurol.*, **16** *(suppl)*, S59–64.

Raichle, M. E., Herscovitch, P., Mintun, M. A., Martin, W. R. W. & Powers, W. (1984). Dynamic measurements of local blood flow and metabolism in the study of higher cortical function in humans with positron emission tomography. *Ann. Neurol.,* **15** *(suppl.)*, S48–9.

Reivich, M. & Alavi, A. (ed.) (1985). *Positron Emission Tomography*. New York: Alan R. Liss, Inc.

Reivich, M., Kuhl, D., Wolf, A., Greenberg, J., Phelps, M., Ido, T., Casella, V. Fowler, J., Gallagher, B., Hoffman, E., Alavi, A. & Sokoloff, L. (1977). Measurement of local cerebral glucose metabolism in man with 18-F-2-fluoro-2-deoxy-glucose. *Acta Neurol. Scand.*, **56,** (suppl. 64), 190–1.

Rosadini, G., Arvigo, F., Ferrillo, F., Gris, A., Rodriguez, G., Sannita, W. G., Romano, P. & Sandini, G. (1984). Flussimetria ematica cerebrale regionale nello studio delle lateralizzazioni emisferiche in soggetti con epilessia. *Boll. Lega. It. Epil.*, *45/6*, 205–7.

Rosadini, G., Ferrillo, F., Rodriguez, G., Sannita, W. G. & Arvigo, F. (1983). rCBF and quantitative EEG correlations in epileptic patients. In *Cerebral Blood Flow, Metabolism and Epilepsy*, ed. M. Baldy-Moulinier, D. H. Ingvar & B. S. Meldrum, pp. 26–32. London: John Libbey.

Rosene, D. L., & Van Hoesen, G. W. (1977). Hippocampal efferents reach widespread areas of cerebral cortex and amygdala in the Rhesus monkey. *Science,* **198,** 315–7.

Sackellares, J. C., Abou-Khalil, B. W., Siegel, G. J., Gilman, S., Hichwa, R. D., Hutchins, G. & Berent, S. (1986). Interictal, ictal and postictal measures of local cerebral blood flow in temporal lobe epilepsy. *Neurol.*, **36,** (Suppl. 1), 338.

Sakai, F., Meyer, J. S., Naritomi, H. & Hsu, M. C. (1978). Regional cerebral blood flow and EEG in patients with epilepsy. *Arch. Neurol.*, **35,** 648–57.

Sanabria, E., Chauvel, P., Askienazy, S., Vignal, J. P., Trottier, S., Chodkiewicz, J. P. & Bancaud, J. (1983). Single photon emission computed tomography (SPECT) using ^{123}I-isopropyl-iodo-amphetamine (IAMP) in partial epilepsy. In *Cerebral Blood Flow, Metabolism and Epilepsy*, ed. M. Baldy-Moulinier, D. H. Ingvar & B. S. Meldrum, pp. 82–7. London: John Libbey.

Schwartzkroin, P. A. & Knowles, W. D. (1984). Intracellular study of human epileptic cortex: in vitro maintenance of epileptiform activity? *Science*, **223,** 709–12.

Skou, J. C. (1957). The influence of some cations on an adenosinetriphosphatase from peripheral nerve, *Biochim. Biophys. Acta*, **23,** 394–401.

Siegel, G. J., Stahl, W. L. & Swanson, P. D. (1981). Ion transport. In *Basic Neurochemistry*, 3rd edn, ed. G. J. Siegel, R. W. Albers, B. W. Agranoff & R. Katzman, pp. 107–43. Boston: Little, Brown & Co.

Sokoloff, L. (1981). Circulation and energy metabolism of the brain. In *Basic Neurochemistry*, 3rd edn, ed. G. J. Siegel, R. W. Albers, B. W. Agranoff & R. Katzman, pp. 471–95. Boston: Little, Brown & Co.

Sokoloff, L. (1984). Modeling metabolic processes in the brain in vivo. *Ann. Neurol.*, **15** *(suppl.)*, S1–11.

Sokoloff, L., Reivich, M., Kennedy, C., Des Rosiers, M. H., Patlak, C. S., Pettigrew, K. D., Sakurada, O. & Shinohara, M. (1977). The [^{14}C]deoxyglucose method for the measurement of local cerebral glucose utilization: theory, procedure, and normal values in the conscious and anesthetized albino rat. *J. Neurochem.*, **28,** 897–916.

Spencer, S. S., Spencer, D. D., Williamson, P. D. & Mattson, R. H. (1982). The localizing value of depth electroencephalography in 32 patients with refractory epilepsy. *Ann. Neurol.*, **12,** 248–53.

Spencer, S. S., Williamson, P. D., Bridges, S. L., Mattson, R. H., Ciccheti, D. V. & Spencer, D. D. (1985). Reliability and accuracy of localization by scalp ictal EEG. *Neurology*, **35,** 1567–75.

Taylor, J., ed. (1958). *Selected Writings of John Hughlings Jackson*, vol. I, pp. 94–6, 100, 279. New York: Basic Books, Inc.

Ter-Pogossian, M. M., Eichling, J. O., Davis, D. O. & Welch, M. J. (1970). The measure in vivo of regional cerebral oxygen utilization by means of oxyhemoglobin labeled with radioactive oxygen-15. *J. Clin. Invest.*, **49,** 381–91.

Ter-Pogossian, M. M., Phelps, M. E., Hoffman, E. J. & Mullani, N. A. (1975). A positron-emission transaxial tomograph for nuclear medicine imaging (PETT), *Radiology*, **114,** 89–98.

Theodore, W. H. (1984). Positron emission tomography in partial seizure disorders. In *Advances in Epileptology: fifteenth Epilepsy International Symposium*, ed. R. J. Porter *et al.*, pp. 87–91. New York: Raven Press.

Theodore, W. H., Brooks, R., Margolin, R., Patronas, N., Sato, S., Porter, R. J., Mansi, L., Bairamian, D. & DiChiro, G. (1985). Positron emission tomography in generalized seizures. *Neurology*, **35,** 684–90.

Theodore, W. H., DiChiro, G., Margolin, R., Fishbein, D., Porter, R. J. & Brooks, R. A. (1986a). Barbiturates reduce human cerebral glucose metabolism. *Neurology*, **36,** 60–4.

Theodore, W. H., Dorwart, R., Holmes, M., Porter, R. J. & DiChiro, G. (1986b). Neuroimaging in epilepsy: comparison of positron emission tomography (PET), magnetic resonance imaging (MRI), and computed tomography (CT). *Advances in Epileptology: sixteenth Epilepsy International Symposium*. New York: Raven Press. (In press.)

Theodore, W. H., Newmark, M. E., Sato, S., Brooks, R., Patronas, N. La Paz, R., DiChiro, G., Kessler, R. M., Margolin, R., Manning, R. G., Channing, M. & Porter, R. J. (1983). [^{18}F]Fluorodeoxyglucose positron emission tomography in refractory complex partial seizures. *Ann. Neurol.*, **14,** 429–37.

Touchon, J., Valmier, J. & Baldy-Moulinier, M. (1986). Regional cerebral blood flow during interictal state: differences between temporal lobe epilepsy and primary generalized epilepsy. *Eur. Neurol.*, **25,** 43–52.

Turner, D. A. & Wyler, A. R. (1981) Temporal lobectomy for epilepsy: mesial temporal herniation as an operative and prognostic finding. *Epilepsia*, **22,** 623–9.

Walker, M. D. (Conference Chairman) (1984). Research issues in positron emission tomography, *Ann. Neurol.*, **15** *(suppl.)*, S1–204.

Watson, R. E., Edinger, H. M. & Siegel, A. (1983). A [^{14}C]2-deoxyglucose analysis of the functional neural pathways of the limbic forebrain in the rat. III. The hippocampal formation, *Brain Res. Rev.*, **5,** 133–76.

Yamamoto, Y. L., Ochs, R., Ammann, W., Meyer, E., Evans, A. C., Cooke, B., Izawa, M., Kato, A., Gloor, P., Feindel, W. H., Diksic, M. & Thompson, C. J. (1984). Changes of energy metabolism and regional cerebral blood flow studied by positron emission tomography in the interictal phase of partial epilepsy. *Acta Neurochir*, **33,** 35–46.

12

A review of the attentional deficit disorder of childhood

Lisa A. Raskin, Sally E. Shaywitz, Bennett A. Shaywitz, George M. Anderson, James F. Leckman and Donald J. Cohen

12.1 Introduction

An abundance of research has focused on the etiology, neurochemical basis and treatment of the attention deficit disorder of childhood (ADD) (Shaywitz & Shaywitz, 1983). Much of the concern about ADD stems from its growing prevalence in the school-age population; studies estimate that anywhere between 3% and 20% of school-age children show symptoms of the disorder. Symptoms are also much more likely to occur in boys than in girls (Whalen & Henker, 1976).

Although research in the area of ADD has been considerable, much of it is difficult to interpret. Clinicians, researchers, and physicians often have different understandings of the diagnosis which makes comparisons between studies difficult. In the most recent publication of the Diagnostic and Statistical Manual (DSM III) of the American Psychiatric Association (1980) a multiaxial system is suggested for the diagnoses of ADD, which takes into account the child's behavioral profile, neurological assessments, as well as the severity of psychosocial stressors in the child's life (American Psychiatric Association, 1980; Camp & Winsberg, 1984). With the advent of new diagnostic criteria, research in the area of ADD will no doubt be enhanced by more consistent diagnoses of subject populations.

According to the DSM III the cardinal signs of ADD are impulsivity, distractability, an inability to sustain attention over time, all of which may lead to learning disorders. When these behaviors occur simultaneously with age-inappropriate hyperactivity, the diagnosis of ADD+H (hyperactivity) is suggested. In fact, ADD+H is undoubtedly the more prevalent diagnosis among younger populations. While the symptoms of ADD+H are typically diagnosed before the child is seven, problems with activity tend to diminish by the junior high school years while problems with attention can persist into adulthood (American Psychiatric Association, 1980; Shaywitz & Shaywitz, 1984).

To date, no single etiology has been identified for ADD or ADD+H. Suggestions have been made that factors such as a child's inherited predisposition, pre- and perinatal complications, or early lead poisoning may all contribute to the emergence of the disorder. None of these single factors, however, can by itself, reliably predict ADD or ADD+H (see Rapoport & Ferguson, 1981; Shaywitz & Shaywitz, 1983; Camp & Winsberg, 1984, for review). In the past it was believed that children who suffered from attention and/or motor deficits had organic brain dysfunction and hence the diagnosis for such children was 'Minimal Brain Damage or Dysfunction' (MBD). However, the inability to identify gross differences in the brains of these children no doubt contributed to the change in nosology from 'brain damage' to a more descriptive term of 'attention deficit disorder' (Shaywitz & Shaywitz, 1984). Although researchers have been unable to identify gross alterations in the brains of MBD or ADD children, recent advances in the field of biological psychiatry have turned investigators towards determining if abnormalities exist in the brain chemistry of ADD children. In particular, investigators have focused on whether the monoamine systems, i.e. serotonin (5-HT), norepinephrine (NE), and dopamine (DA) are aberrant in ADD children.

Early speculations which implicated the catecholamines in ADD emerged in part because of the successful treatment of the disorder with stimulant medication. Psychomotor stimulants, such as dextroamphetamine (Dexedrine) have long been used to treat the impulsivity, inattentiveness and hyperactivity displayed by ADD children (Bradley, 1937; Whalen & Henker, 1980). The ability of stimulants to produce an apparent decrease in motor activity led to the proposal that the effect of amphetamine was 'paradoxical' in ADD children and that this paradoxical drug effect perhaps reflected an anomaly in brain chemistry (Snyder, 1973; Wender, 1971). Given that dextroamphetamine acts to increase catecholamines at the synapse, and that it apparently reversed the symptoms of ADD, it was further suggested that these ADD symptoms resulted from a catecholamine deficiency (Wender, 1971). However, it should be noted that although a drug improves symptoms of a disorder, the disorder need not stem from a lack of endogenous levels of the drug. For example, although aspirin alleviates symptoms of rheumatic fever, rheumatic fever does not stem from an aspirin deficiency (Shaywitz & Shaywitz, 1983). In addition, about 20% of children diagnosed as ADD or ADD+H show no improvement following stimulant medication

(Shaywitz & Shaywitz, 1984). Thus, early speculations implicating a role for catecholamines in ADD needed to be assessed by more direct, systematic measures.

The two main approaches taken by recent investigators have been (i) to analyze the levels of monoamine precursors or metabolites in the cerebrospinal fluid (CSF), blood and/or urine of ADD children, and (ii) to develop animal models which parallel the symptoms of ADD children with the hope of understanding the neurochemical basis of such symptoms and how they respond to treatment (Shaywitz, Yager & Klopper, 1976). The present chapter will review the clinical studies performed with ADD children, including the pharmacotherapy utilized and then present an animal model which may have clinical utility for understanding this behavioral syndrome.

12.2 Clinical studies

When evaluating clinical studies which have investigated the neurochemical basis of ADD it must be kept in mind that most studies performed to date have not utilized the new diagnostic criteria proposed by the DSM III. Future studies which adhere to the DSM III guidelines will allow for more systematic comparison across clinical populations. Another problem which is inherent in the data assessing the neurochemistry of ADD is that the techniques available cannot directly assess central nervous system (CNS) function. Given that the CNS is not easily accessible in humans, researchers turn to measuring neurotransmitter metabolite levels in the cerebrospinal fluid (CSF), blood and urine, as a 'window' to the CNS. However, these techniques are not ideal, and therefore the data which are generated from such studies must be interpreted with caution. Perhaps with the introduction of nuclear magnetic resonance (NMR) or positron emission tomography (PET) into clinical medicine a more accurate measurement of neurochemical correlates of behavior disorders will soon be available. Thus, the following sections will review the research performed on the neurochemistry of ADD with considerations of the limitations of existing research techniques.

12.2.1 *Basal levels of monoamine metabolites in ADD*

Clinical studies which assess central serotonergic (5-HT) function in ADD children have used the following measures: levels of whole blood 5-HT, free and total levels of the amino acid precursor, tryptophan, in plasma, (Ferguson *et al.*, 1981) platelet levels of serotonin,

(Rapoport *et al.*, 1974c) and the levels of major metabolite 5-hydroxy-indoleacetic acid (5-HIAA) in the CSF (Shaywitz, Cohen & Bowers, 1977), blood (Coleman, 1971) and urine (Wender *et al.*, 1971). Studies which use peripheral measures of 5-HT to reflect CNS function are particularly problematic, given that 5-HT is found predominantly in the gastrointestinal tract and blood platelets. Only about 2% of the body's 5-HT is in the CNS (Cooper, Bloom & Roth, 1982) making it difficult to determine the contribution of central 5-HT to peripheral measures of 5-HT function. Perhaps a more accurate measurement of central 5-HT function can be found in assessing the levels of 5-HIAA in lumbar CSF. It has been estimated that about 50% of lumbar CSF originates rostral to the spinal cord and would therefore reflect brain function (Garelis *et al.*, 1974). The use of probenecid, a technique which blocks the egress of metabolites from the CSF, may increase the measure of central 5-HIAA from lumbar CSF (Bowers, 1978). More recently however, it has been proposed that probenecid loading may not lead to more stable measures of monoamine metabolites. Probenecid may have a differential effect on clinical vs nonclinical populations thus complicating the comparisons of metabolite levels between groups (see Camp & Winsberg, 1984). However, with or without probenecid, the best available measure of central 5-HT function appears to be measurements of 5-HIAA in lumbar CSF. That measurement, while perhaps the most accurate, must still be considered carefully given that about 50% of the 5-HIAA may represent spinal cord 5-HT function (Garelis *et al.*, 1974).

To date, only two studies have actually analyzed the levels of 5-HIAA in the CSF of ADD children. Shetty & Chase (1976) compared the basal levels of 5-HIAA in CSF of 23 children diagnosed as 'hyperactive' with those of six children in a control group, and found no differences between the groups. Shaywitz *et al.*, (1977) measured the levels of CSF 5-HIAA in a group of boys who were clinically homogeneous and would meet the current criteria for ADD+H. Their 5-HIAA levels were compared with a control group who suffered from minor neurological difficulties, although none of the difficulties were in attention or activity. Using the probenecid technique, no differences were found in CSF 5-HIAA levels between the ADD+H children and the control group. Thus, both studies which utilized the most effective technique currently available for analyzing CNS 5-HT metabolite levels suggest that 5-HT levels were not significantly altered in ADD (Shetty & Chase, 1976; Shaywitz *et al.*, 1977).

The studies which have measured peripheral levels of 5-HT in ADD children are not only difficult to interpret but have sometimes yielded inconsistent results. For example, although Bhagauan, Coleman & Coursin (1975) reported a decrease in blood platelet levels of 5-HT in hyperactives as compared with controls, Rapoport *et al.* (1974) were unable to replicate those findings. In addition, although Coleman (1971) reported a decrease in 5-HIAA levels in whole blood of hyperactive children, a more recent study showed that whole blood levels of 5-HT were not different between hyperactive and control groups (Ferguson *et al.*, 1981). This latter study showed that levels of free and total tryptophan were also not different in their clinically diagnosed population (Ferguson *et al.*, 1981). Measurement of urinary 5-HIAA levels in children diagnosed as MBD have also been shown to be similar to control values (Wender *et al.*, 1971). In sum, the measures of peripheral levels of 5-HT function do not reveal any consistent alteration in 5-HT function in ADD children (Coleman, 1971; Rapoport *et al.*, 1974) and this is confirmed by CSF studies which more accurately reflect CNS 5-HT function (Shetty & Chase, 1976; Shaywitz *et al.*, 1977).

Research investigating levels of catecholamine (CA) function in ADD children has more consistently suggested that these neurotransmitter systems may be aberrant in clinical populations. Measurement of norepinephrine (NE) function has been attempted by measuring the level of dopamine betahydroxylase (DBH), the enzyme which converts DA to NE, in plasma (Rapoport, Quinn & Lambrecht, 1974), and by measuring the principal metabolite of CNS norepinephrine, 3-methoxy-4-hydroxyphenylglycol (MHPG) in the urine (Shekim, Dekirmenjian & Chapel, 1977, 1979). Rapoport *et al.* (1974) reported no significant levels of DBH in the plasma of hyperactive vs normal children. A difference in DBH levels between the two groups of children may not have been observed in this study, however, because levels of DBH tend to be extremely variable in normal groups of children (Shaywitz & Shaywitz, 1983). MHPG levels can be measured in the CSF but, unlike that which is reported for the 5-HT system, this is not the best reflection of brain NE function. Apparently most of the MHPG measured in lumbar CSF is derived from NE in the spinal cord and not the brain (Garelis *et al.*, 1974).

A more accurate measure of brain NE function comes from assessing MHPG levels in urine given that, in man, about 60% of MHPG found in urine originates in the brain (Maas *et al.*, 1979). Although there was an early report showing no differences in MHPG levels in the urine of MBD versus normal chidren (Wender *et al.*, 1971), more recent studies have reported differences between hyperactive and normal children (Shekim *et al.*, 1977, 1979). This work is complicated by the fact that the direction of the differences has varied across studies. Shekim and his associates have reported in two studies that basal levels of urinary MHPG were significantly lower in hyperactive children. Urinary levels of the peripheral NE metabolites normetanephrine and metanephrine were also significantly lower in the hyperactive group (Shekim *et al.*, 1977, 1979). Interestingly, Kahn & Dekirmenjian (1981) reported that urinary MHPG levels in hyperactive children were significantly different from controls; however, in this case the MHPG values of the hyperactive children were significantly higher than their control counterparts.

Although the findings of both lower and higher MHPG levels in hyperactive children are inconsistent, several explanations can be offered for these data. First, Camp & Winsberg (1984) have pointed out that the control values of MHPG in the study reported by Khan & Dekirmenjian were significantly lower than control values usually reported in other studies, whereas the MHPG levels in the hyperactive children were comparable to that which other investigators report. According to Camp & Winsberg (1984) MHPG values of the hyperactive children in Kahn & Dekirmenjian's study may in fact have been lower than control values if a different control population had been chosen. This speculation is interesting although troublesome because there is no reason to suspect that this particular group would represent a different population from controls used in other studies. This finding rather sheds light on the possible variability of MHPG levels in normal children. Camp & Winsberg (1984) also suggest that discrepancies in MHPG levels between studies may reflect error in the urine-sampling procedures utilized.

Another way of looking at the findings of both an excess and a deficit of MHPG in ADD children has been previously proposed by Raskin *et al.* (1984b). Following the suggestion of Maas (1979) for the understanding of noradrenergic mediation of affective disorders, it has been proposed that attempting to determine whether there is 'too much or too little' of a neurotransmitter level is perhaps not as helpful as determining whether or not specific transmitters function properly within certain boundaries (Maas, 1979; Raskin *et al.*, 1984b). If one accepts the findings of the work performed on NE metabolite levels in ADD, it appears that these children may suffer from some aberration in NE; whether it is too much or too little is as yet unknown. A confirmation of this proposal must await studies which utilize similar urine-sampling procedures, similar diagnostic criteria for the clinical population, and similar methods for choosing control groups.

Clinical studies in which dopamine (DA) function is assessed have relied upon measurement of one of the main DA metabolites, homovanillic acid (HVA) which can be measured in CSF, blood and urine. Although it is feasible to measure the other main DA metabolite, DOPAC, the procedure is difficult and therefore has not been utilized very much clinically (Bowers, 1978; Cooper *et al.*, 1982). Measures of HVA in urine reflect both central and peripheral levels of DA function and are therefore difficult to interpret. Wender *et al.* (1971) have reported no difference in urinary HVA levels between hyperactive and normal children; however, it is possible that levels of HVA from peripheral DA were masking differences in central HVA in this measure. Perhaps a more accurate reflection of CNS DA comes from HVA which is measured in lumbar CSF. It has, in fact, been suggested that the HVA which is measured in lumbar CSF comes from areas located around the lateral ventricles, such as the caudate, which contains the majority of CNS DA (Garelis *et al.*, 1974).

Two studies have measured CSF HVA levels in ADD children and have compared them with control populations. In the study in which Shetty & Chase (1976) measured CSF 5-HT metabolites and found no differences in hyperactive children, similar results were reported for the levels of the CSF DA metabolite, HVA. However, as also previously noted, the procedures of this experiment did not include probenecid loading which, by blocking egress of the metabolites from CSF, may allow for a more accurate reflection of central neurotransmitter function (Bowers, 1978). The results of this study are further complicated by the fact that only six control subjects were used. The importance of a randomly sampled and sufficiently large control group for comparison cannot be over-emphasized. In the study in which 5-HT metabolites were measured in lumbar CSF by Shaywitz *et al.* (1977) lumbar HVA levels were also measured following probenecid loading. As previously noted, the advantage of this study was that the group of boys was clinically homogeneous and although then diagnosed as MBD, would fit the current DSM III classification of ADD+H.

MBD boys were compared with a control group of children who suffered from problems such as urinary incontinence or emotional difficulties; however, no control subjects exhibited disorders of activity or attention. MBD boys had no history of seizures and had not received any medication for at least two weeks prior to the study. Results of the study showed that the concentration of HVA per unit probenecid was significantly lower in MBD boys than in the control group. That 5-HT metabolites were not significantly different between the groups and DA metabolites were, suggests that this technique was sensitive enough to detect a selective deficit in MBD boys. Further confirmation of these results is warranted, however, because although the control group was large, only six MBD boys were tested in this study.

Support for the role of DA in attention deficits may also come from a preliminary report which assessed the behavioral effects of exogeneous human growth hormone (hGH) in young boys. Results of this double-blind study suggested that hGH may be involved in enhancing attention (Smith *et al.*, 1985). Connections linking GH and DA function (Bansal, Lee & Woolf, 1981) make this an interesting line of research to pursue.

The possibility that disorders of attention in childhood may involve aberrations in DA is consistent with the vast literature which links disorders of attention and DA dysfunction in adult schizophrenia (Snyder *et al.*, 1974). Given the converging lines of evidence which implicated DA dysfunction in ADD children, Shaywitz and his colleagues have designed an animal model which shows that neonatal DA depletion leads to behaviors which are similar to those exhibited by ADD+H children. That animal model will be discussed in detail later in this chapter. The value of an animal model is that it may have clinical utility in determining the contribution that each of the catecholamines play in attention and activity disorders in childhood.

12.2.2 *Pharmacotherapy*

Although a variety of drugs, i.e. antipsychotics, antidepressants, have been used in the treatment of ADD, the most effective results have been reported following the use of stimulant medication (Shaywitz & Shaywitz, 1984). Stimulants such as dextroamphetamine (Dexedrine), methylphenidate (Ritalin), and magnesium pemoline (Cylert) reportedly enhance performance on tests which require response inhibition vigilance and selective attention (Whalen & Henker, 1976, 1980). Although clear improvements have been observed in about 70–80% of treated children during laboratory tests, it has not yet been established whether this enhanced performance will translate into improvement in academic performance over the long term (Rapoport, 1983).

Much of the earlier research which assessed the effect of stimulant medication for ADD children utilized dextroamphetamine; however, more recently researchers have suggested that due to fewer side effects methylphenidate should be the preferred medication (Shaywitz & Shaywitz, 1984). An additional problem of treatment with dextroamphetamine is the fact that the peak in behavioral performance following medication does not correlate with the peak of drug levels in plasma (Rapoport, 1983). In a recent study, S. E. Shaywitz *et al.* (1982) reported that within the range of 0.3–0.8 mg/kg of methylphenidate, there is a dose-related correlation between plasma levels of drug and an increase in performance on cognitive tests. This positive correlation has not been observed, however, in higher doses (1.0 mg/kg) of the drug (Sprague & Sleator, 1977). The finding that there is a relationship between blood methylphenidate levels and behavioral performance should expedite future research attempting to determine the changes in neurochemistry which correlate with enhanced performance to medication.

Although the use of stimulant medication has been shown to be effective in attenuating ADD symptomatology, it has been difficult to determine the neurochemical basis for such improvements. The early proposal that stimulants improve performance because they increase levels of catecholamines, which may be deficient in ADD children, has been difficult to substantiate. Surprisingly, most studies which measure post-medication metabolite levels in ADD children show that a *decrease* in CA metabolite levels is correlated with an *increase* in behavioral performance. For example, Shekim and his associates (1977, 1979) have shown that following two weeks of daily 0.5 mg/kg dextroamphetamine administration, hyperactive boys had MHPG levels which were significantly lower than their baseline MHPG levels. This finding was later confirmed by Brown, Hunt & Rapoport (1981). Furthermore, Shekim *et al.*, reported that a decrease in MHPG from baseline levels was seen only in children who displayed enhanced performance on medication and was not observed in non-responders. A decrease in lumbar CSF levels of HVA was also observed following dextroamphetamine treatment in hyperactive children (Shetty & Chase, 1976) although no change has been observed in urinary levels of the DA metabolite following amphetamine (Shetty & Chase, 1976; Brown *et al.*, 1981).

One or more possible phenomena may explain why treatment with a drug which increases CA leads to a decrease in CA metabolites in ADD children. On the one hand it has been argued that, at the neuronal level, an increase in the amount of either NE or DA at the synapse would, through feedback inhibition (Bunney & Aghajanian, 1975, 1976), lead to a decrease of neurotransmitter release and hence fewer metabolites (Shekim *et al.*, 1977). Although reasonable, this postulation does not address the question of why children with a purported deficit in certain neurotransmitter functions show a reversal of their symptoms when that neurotransmitter is further decreased. In other words, if ADD children show low levels of MHPG why would amphetamine, which enhances their performance, further decrease levels of MHPG?

Another possible explanation for a decrease in metabolites following amphetamine administration may be found in the time course used during the urine-sampling procedure. Pharmacokinetic studies have shown that amphetamine exerts its greatest behavioral effect during the absorption phase of the drug rather than during the peak in plasma levels of drug concentration (Rapoport, 1983). Yet there is no indication in the studies previously cited (Shetty & Chase, 1976; Shekim *et al.*, 1977, 1979; Brown *et al.*, 1981) of the relationship between metabolite levels, plasma levels of amphetamine and medication-induced behavioral improvement. Perhaps metabolite levels actually increase during the absorption phase of the drug but are decreased by the time clinical measures are taken. An increase in excretion in phenethylamine (PEA), an endogenous chemical which is structurally similar to the catecholamines and amphetamine, has been reported following amphetamine treatment in ADD children (Zametkin *et al.*, 1984). Since it has been determined by Shaywitz and her colleagues that an increase in behavioral performance is correlated with peak levels of methylphenidate in plasma (S.E. Shaywitz *et al.*, 1982) it would be interesting to determine how levels of MHPG and HVA change during the peak of efficacy in methylphenidate administration.

Although the stimulants have been shown to be effective in 70–80% of children diagnosed with ADD or ADD+H, there remain children who are non-responders to such medication. In a recent study, Gastfried, Biederman & Jellinek (1984) report that treatment with the antidepressant Desipramine had a beneficial effect on a small group of children who had previously not responded to stimulants. Although other antidepressants have previously been used in the treatment of ADD they have reportedly not been as effective as stimulants (Rapoport, *et al.*, 1974a). However, following desipramine treatment there was an increase in behavioral performance which was augmented by the fact that drug side effects, although present initially, appeared to be mild with extended treatment (Gastfried *et al.*, 1984). The discovery of new and safe medication for the treatment of ADD is not only critical clinically, but can hopefully shed more light on the neurochemical basis of pharamcotherapy.

12.3 An animal model

Based on results showing that a catecholamine deficiency may be present in ADD children, Shaywitz and his colleagues (Shaywitz *et al.*, 1976) have proposed an animal model for this clinical disorder. The advantages of an animal model are many: neurotransmitter levels can be directly altered and measured, behavior can be systematically

Bhagauan, H. N., Coleman, M. & Coursin, D. B. (1975). The effect of pyridoxine hydrochloride on blood serotonin and pyridoxal phosphate contents in hyperactive children. *Pediatrics*, **55,** 437–41.

Bowers, M. B. (1978). CSF acid monoamine metabolites in psychotic syndromes: what might they signify? *Biological Psychiatry,* **13,** 375–83.

Bradley, C. (1937). The behavior of children receiving benzedrine. *American Journal of Psychiatry*, **94,** 557–85.

Brown, G. L., Ebert, M. H., Hunt, R. D. & Rapoport, J. (1981). Urinary 3-methoxy-4-hydroxyphenylglycol and homovanillic acid response to d-amphetamine in hyperactive children. *Biological Psychiatry*, **16,** 779–87.

Bunney, B. S. & Aghajanian, G. K. (1975). Evidence for drug actions in both pre- and postsynaptic catecholamine receptors in the CNS. In *Pre and Post-synaptic Receptors*, ed. E. Usden & W. E. Bunney. New York: Marcel Dekker.

Bunney, B. S. & Aghajanian, G. K. (1976). d-amphetamine induced inhibition of central dopaminergic neurons: mediation by a striato-nigral feedback pathway. *Science*, **192,** 391–3.

Camp, J. A. & Winsberg, G. G. (1984). Clinical utility of animal models of childhood hyperkinesis. *Clinical Neuropharmacology* , **7,** 185–221.

Coleman, M. (1971). Serotonin concentration in whole blood of hyperactive children. *Journal of Pediatrics*, **78,** 985–90.

Cooper, J. R., Bloom, F. E. & Roth, R. H. (1982). *The Biochemical Basis of Neuropharmacology*. New York: Oxford University Press.

Ferguson, H. B., Pappas, B. A., Trites, R. L., Peters, D. A. V. & Taub, H. (1981). Plasma free and total syndrome: no evidence for the serotonin deficiency hypothesis. *Biological Psychiatry,* **16,** 231–8.

Garelis, E., Young, S. N., Lal, S. & Sourkes, T. L. (1974). Monoamine metabolites in lumbar CSF. The question of their origin in relation to clinical studies. *Brain Research*, **79,** 1–8.

Gastfriend, D. R., Biederman, J. & Jellinek, M. S. (1984). Desipramine in the treatment of adolescents with attention deficit disorder. *American Journal of Psychiatry*, **141,** 906–8.

Heffner, T. G. & Seiden, L. S. (1982). Possible involvement of serotoninergic neurons in the reduction of locomotor hyperactivity caused by amphetamine in neonatal rats depleted of brain dopamine. *Brain Research*, **224,** 81–90.

Khan, A. U. & Dekirmenjian, H. (1981). Urinary excretion of catecholamine metabolites in hyperkinetic child syndrome. *American Journal of Psychiatry*, **138,** 108–10.

Lipton, S. V., McGrough, J. P. & Shaywitz, B. A. (1980). Effects of apomorphine on escape performance and activity in developing rat pups treated with 6-hydroxydopamine. *Pharmacology, Biochemistry and Behavior*, **13,** 371–7.

Maas, J. W. (1979). Neurotransmitters and depression: too much, too little, or too unstable? *Trends in Neuroscience*, December, 306–8.

Maas, J. W., Greene, N. M., Hattox, S. E. & Landis, D. H. (1979). Neurotransmitter metabolite production by human brain. In *Catecholamines: Basic and Clinical Frontiers,* ed. E. Usdin, I. J. Kopin & J. Barchas. New York: Pergamon Press.

McLean, J. H., Kostrzewa, R. M. & May, J. G. (1976). Behavioral and biochemical effects of neonatal treatment of rats with 6-hydroxydopa. *Pharmacology, Biochemistry and Behavior*, **4,** 601–7.

Miller, F. E., Heffner, T. G., Kotake, C. & Seiden, L. S. (1981). Magnitude and duration of hyperactivity following neonatal 6-hydroxydopamine is related to the extent of brain dopamine depletion. *Brain Research*, **229,** 123–32.

Morgan, D. N., McLean, J. H. & Kostrzewa, R. M. (1979). Effects of 6-hydroxydopamine and 6-hydroxydopa or development of behavior. *Pharmacology, Biochemistry and Behavior*, **11,** 309–12.

Olton, D. S. & Samuelson, R. J. (1976). Remembrance of places past: spatial memory in rats. *Journal of Experimental Psychology, Animal Behavior Processes,* **2,** 97–116.

Pappas, B. A. & Sobrian, S. K. (1972). Neonatal sympathectomy for 6-hydroxydopamine in the rat: no effects on behavior but changes in endogenous brain norepinephrine. *Life Sciences,* **11,** 653–9.

Pearson, D. E., Raskin, L. A., Shaywitz, B. A., Anderson, G. M. & Cohen, D. J. (1984) Radial arm maze performance in rats following neonatal dopamine depletion. *Developmental Psychobiology*, **17,** 505–17.

Pearson, D. E., Teicher, M. H., Shaywitz, B. A., Cohen, D. J., Young, J. G. & Anderson, G. M. (1980). Environmental influences on body weight and behavior in developing rats after neonatal 6-hydroxydopamine. *Science*, **209,** 715–7.

Rapoport, J. L. (1983). Stimulant drug treatment of hyperactivity: an update. In *Childhood Psychopathology and Development,* ed. S. Guze, F. Earls & J. Barrett. New York: Raven Press.

Rapoport, J. L. & Ferguson, H. B. (1981). Biological validation of the hyperkinetic syndrome. *Developmental Medical Child Neurology*, **23,** 667–82.

Rapoport, J. L., Quinn, P. O., Bradbard, G., Riddle, K. D. & Brooks, E. (1974a) Imipramine and methylphenidate treatment of hyperactive boys. *Archives of General Psychiatry*, **30,** 789–93.

Rapoport, J. L., Quinn, P. O. & Lamprecht, F. (1974b). Minor physical anomalies and plasma dopamine-beta-hydroxylase activity in hyperactive boys. *American Journal of Psychiatry*, **131,** 386–90.

Rapoport, J. L., Quinn, P. O., Scribnau, N. & Murphy, D. (1974)c). Platelet serotonin of hyperactive school-age boys. *British Journal of Psychiatry*, **125,** 138–40.

Rapoport, J. L. Zametkin, A. (1980). Attention deficit disorder. *Psychiatric Clinics of North America*, **3,** 425–40.

Raskin, L. A., Shaywitz, B. A., Anderson, G. M., Cohen, D. J., Teicher, M. H. & Linakis, M. (1983). Differential effects of selective dopamine, norepinephrine or catecholamine depletion on activity and learning in the developing rat. *Pharmacology, Biochemistry & Behavior*, **19,** 743–9.

Raskin, L. A., Shaywitz, B. A., Shaywitz, S. A. Cohen, D. J. & Anderson, G. M. (1984a). Early brain damage and attentional deficit disorder: an animal model. In *Early Brain Damage*, vol. 1, C. R. Almli & S. Finger. pp. 111–23. New York: Academic Press.

Raskin, L. A., Shaywitz, S. E., Shaywitz, B. A., Anderson, G. M. & Cohen, D. J. (1984b). Neurochemical correlates of Attention Deficit Disorder. *Pediatric Clinics of North America*, **31,** 387–96.

Shaywitz, B. A., Cohen, D. J. & Bowers, M. B. (1977a). CSF monoamine metabolites in children with minimal brain dysfunction: evidence fior alteration of brain dopamine. *Journal of Pediatrics*, **90,** 67–71.

Shaywitz, B. A., Gordon, J. W., Klopper, J. H. & Zelterman, D. A. (1977b). The effect of 6-hydroxydopamine on habituation of activity in the developing rat pup. *Pharmacology, Biochemistry and Behavior*, **6,** 391–6.

Shaywitz, B. A., Klopper, J. H. & Gordon, J. W. (1978). Methylphenidate in 6-hydroxydopamine-treated developing rat pups. *Archives of Neurology*, **35,** 463–9.
Shaywitz, B. A., Teicher, M. H., Cohen, D. J., Anderson, G. M., Young, T. G. & Levitt, P. (1984). Dopaminergic but not noradrenergic mediation of hyperactivity and performance deficits in the developing rat pup. *Psychopharmacology*, **82,** 73–7.
Shaywitz, B. A., Yager, R. D. & Klopper, J. H. (1976a). Selective brain dopamine depletion in developing rats: an experimental model of minimal brain dysfunction. *Science*, **191,** 305–8.
Shaywitz, B. A., Yager, R. D., Klopper, J. H. & Gordon, J. W. (1976b). Paradoxical response to amphetamine in developing rats treated with 6-hydroxydopamine. *Nature*, **261,** 153–5.
Shaywitz, S. E. & McGraw, K. (1982). Gifted and learning disabled: shared behavior characteristics of gifted and learning disabled children. *Pediatric Research,* **16,** 93.
Shaywitz, S. E., Sebrects, M. & Jatlow, M., Anderson, G. M., Young, J. G., Cohen, D. J. & Shaywitz, B. A. (1982). Plasma methylphenidate levels predict attention and activity: results in a double-blind placebo study. *Pediatric Research*, **16,** 93.
Shaywitz, S. E. & Shaywitz, B. A. (1983). Biological influences in attentional disorders. In *Developmental Behavioral Pediatrics*, ed. M. D. Levine *et al.* Philadelphia: W. B. Saunders.
Shaywitz, S. E. & Shaywitz, B. A. (1984). Diagnosis and management of attention deficit disorder: a pediatric perspective. *Pediatric Clinics of North America*, **31,** 429–57.
Shekim, W. O., Dekirmenjian, H. & Chapel, J. L. (1977) Urinary catecholamine metabolites in hyperkinetic boys treated with d-amphetamine. *American Journal of Psychiatry*, **134,** 1276–9.
Shekim, W. O., Dekirmenjian, H. Chapel, J. L. (1979). Urinary MHPG excretion in minimal brain dysfunction and its modification by d-amphetamine. *American Journal of Psychiatry*, **136,** 667–71.
Shetty, T. & Chase, T. N. (1976). Central monoamines and hyperactivity of childhood. *Neurology*, **26,** 1000–2.
Smith, M. O., Shaywitz, S. E., Shaywitz, B. A., Gertner, J., Raskin, L. A. & Gelwan, E. M. (1985). Exogenous growth hormone levels predict attentional performance: a preliminary report. *Developmental and Behavioral Pediatrics*, **6,** 273–8.
Sorenson, C. A., Vayer, J. S. & Goldberg, C. S. (1977). Amphetamine reduction of motor activity in rats after neonatal administration of 6-hydroxydopamine. *Biological Psychiatry*, **12,** 133–7.
Sprague, R. L. & Sleator, E. K. (1977). Methylphenidate in hyperkinetic children: differences in dose effects on learning and social behavior. *Science*, **198,** 1274–6.
Snyder, S. H. (1973). How amphetamine acts in minimal brain dysfunction. *New York Academy of Science Annals*, **205,** 310–20.
Snyder, S. H., Banerjee, S. P., Yamamura, H.-I. & Greenburg, D. (1974). Drugs neurotransmitters and schizophrenia. *Science*, **184,** 1243–53.
Tant, J. L. & Douglas, V. I. (1982). Problem solving in hyperactive, normal and reading disabled boys. *Journal of Abnormal Child Psychology*, **10,** 285–306.
Teicher, M. H., Shaywitz, B. A. & Kootz, H. L. (1981). Differential effects of maternal and sibling presence on hyperactivity of 6-hydroxydopamine-

treated developing rats. *Journal of Comparative and Physiological Psychology*, **95,** 134–45.
Thieme, R. E., Dijkstra, H. & Stoof, J. C. (1980). An evaluation of the young DA lesioned rat as an animal model for MBD. *Psychopharmacology*, **67,** 165–9.
Weldon, D. A., Wool, R. S., Teicher, M. H., Shaywitz, B. A. Cohen, D. J. & Anderson, G. M. (1982). Effects of apomorphine on appetitive conditioning in 6-hydroxydopamine treated rat pups. *Pharmacology, Biochemistry and Behavior*, **17,** 1281–4.
Wender, P. H. (1971). *Minimal Brain Dysfunction in Children.* New York: John Wiley & Sons.
Wender, P., Epstein, R. S., Kopin, I. J. & Gordon, E. K. (1971). Urinary monoamne metabolites in children with minimal brain dysfunction. *American Journal of Psychiatry*, **127,** 147–51.
Whalen, C. K. & Henker, B. (1976). Psychostimulants and children: a review and analysis. *Psychological Bulletin*, **83,** 1113–30.
Whalen, C. K. & Henker, B. (1980). The social ecology of psychostimulant treatment: a model for conceptual and empirical analysis. In *Hyperactive Children*, ed. C. K. Whalen & B. Henker. New York: Academic Press.
Zametkin, J. J., Brown, G. L., Karoum, F., Rapoport, J. L., Langer, D. H., Chuang, L. W. & Wyatt, R. J. (1948). Urinary phenethylamine response to d-amphetamine in 12 boys with attention deficit disorder. *American Journal of Psychiatry*, **141,** 1055–8.

13

Receptor studies in sleep and sleep disorders

Mortimer Mamelak

13.1 Introduction

Receptor studies in sleep research in man have had two objectives. The first has been to describe the regulation of the sleep–wakefulness cycle and has been achieved by documenting the effects of agonists and antagonists at brain receptor sites for noradrenaline, dopamine, serotonin and acetylcholine. The second objective has been to develop therapeutically useful agents for the disorders of sleep. Compounds active at benzodiazepine, adenosine and γ-hydroxybutyrate recognition sites, for example, are now being tested for this purpose. More recently studies on the number and binding characteristics of brain receptors in relation to certain sleep disorders have been initiated. These issues, receptor-mediated regulation of the sleep–wakefulness cycle in man, receptor changes in disease, and the treatment of sleep disorders with agents active at specific receptor sites, are the subject of this review.

13.2 Regulation of the sleep wakefulness cycle

Hobson and McCarley have proposed a neuronal model for the regulation of the three vigilance states, wakefulness, NREM sleep and REM sleep, which is based upon the reciprocal interaction of excitatory and inhibitory neurones (Hobson *et al.*, 1975; McCarley & Hobson, 1975). According to this model, cholinergic neurones in the pontine giganto-cellular tegmental field (FTG) are inhibited during wakefulness by the activity of noradrenergic neurones in the locus coerulens (LC). The sleep cycle starts when the LC neurones decrease their firing rates and release FTG neurones from inhibition. LC neurones achieve their lowest firing rates towards the end of NREM sleep and the beginning of REM sleep. At this point, FTG neurones, through self-excitation, reach maximal firing rates and firmly establish REM sleep. But activation of the FTG neurones triggers reciprocal excitation of the neurones in the LC. These neurones, in turn, reciprocally inhibit the FTG cells, terminating REM sleep. The cycle is now ready to start again. Serotonergic neurones, situated in the dorsal raphe, have inhibitory effects on the FTG cells comparable to LC neurones. Some of these neurones, too, show their lowest firing rates during REM sleep, suggesting that they work in tandem with the noradrenergic LC neurones. According to the Hobson–McCarley model, then, the vigilance states are cyclically elaborated by shifts in the balance between the activities of different neuronal systems and are not dependent upon the activity of a single system or the release of a single neurotransmitter. This multiply-determined control mechanism must be kept in mind when the actions of receptor agonists and antagonists on sleep are considered.

It must also be considered that agents active at receptor sites vary in their specificity, and that the receptors themselves often exist in multiple forms and in diverse locations where they mediate different actions. These issues often make it difficult to interpret the significance of the changes produced in the sleep cycle by a compound active at a receptor site.

13.2.1 *Adrenergic receptors*

Studies in man on the effects on sleep of agents active at adrenergic receptor sites indicate that alpha receptors are more closely involved in the regulation of the sleep cycle than are beta receptors. Although clinical reports indicate that beta blockers like propranolol promote arousal and can produce insomnia (Simpson, 1980), indeed this drug has been reported to alleviate daytime drowsiness in narcolepsy (Kales *et al.*, 1979; Meier-Ewart *et al.*, 1985), sleep laboratory studies have not demonstrated any changes in sleep morphology, for example, with 120 mg of propranolol at bedtime for one week (Dunleavy *et al.*, 1971). Nor have any consistent effects been found with metoprolol, acebutolol or satolol (Kayed & Gotlibsen, 1971; Bender *et al.*, 1979). Sleep efficiency was slightly, and then only transiently, decreased with 400 mg of metoprolol, and slight, and again transient, increases in REM sleep percentage were found with 200 mg of acebutolol (Kayed & Gotlibsen, 1977).

In contrast, agents acting at both α_1- and α_2-receptors effect significant changes in the sleep cycle (Monti, 1982, 1983). Clonidine, in a low dose, acts as an α_2-agonist and produces feedback inhibition of noradrenaline synthesis and release. Sleep laboratory studies reveal that 300 μg/kg or less of clonidine decreases REM sleep, increases stage 1 and stage 2 sleep and has no effect on slow wave sleep (Autre *et al.*, 1977; Gaillard & Kafi, 1979). Yohimbine, an α_2-antagonist, can block the actions of clonidine in 10 mg doses which have no effect on sleep; in cats, 2 mg/kg of yohimbine promotes wakefulness (Putkonen *et al.*, 1977). D-amphetamine, which stimulates α_1-adrenergic receptors indirectly through the release of norepinephrine, increases wakefulness and decreases NREM and REM sleep (Rechtschaffen & Maron, 1963; Lewis, 1970). The effects of D-amphetamine are complicated by the concomitant release of dopamine. In rats, however, where the effects of a specific α_1-adrenergic agonist, methoxamine, have been tested, an increase in wakefulness and a decrease in NREM and REM sleep have also been demonstrated (Pellejero *et al.*, 1984). In man, the α_1-antagonist thymoxamine, given intravenously in a dose of 150 mg/kg, increases wakefulness and suppresses slow wave sleep in the first part of the night but it also prolongs REM sleep at this time (Oswald *et al.*, 1975). In all, then, studies at α-adrenergic receptor sites suggest that noradrenaline promotes both REM sleep and wakefulness but that REM requires an optimal level of noradrenaline for its elaboration. REM is suppressed by agents which prevent the release of noradrenaline, but is replaced by wakefulness when noradrenaline is present in excess (Putkonen, 1979).

13.2.2 *Cholinergic receptors*

A substantial body of work implicates acetylcholine in the regulation of the sleep cycle and particularly in the regulation of REM sleep (Gillin *et al.*, 1983; Gillin & Siteram, 1984). In man, significant changes in sleep parameters have been observed with agents active at muscarinic receptor sites, but not with agents like piperidine, which may be active at nicotinic receptor sites (Mendelson *et al.*, 1981). For example, 1.0–1.5 mg of the muscarinic agonist, arecoline, given intravenously, shortens the latency to REM sleep when given during the first or second NREM sleep periods (Siteram *et al.*, 1978). The onset of subsequent REM sleep periods is reset but the duration of each REM period and the REM cycle time are unchanged. The net effect is to increase the number of REM periods and the overall duration of REM sleep. Arecoline has little effect on the total sleep time or on the other stages of sleep. Scopolamine, a muscarinic receptor antagonist given in a dose of 0.5 mg, delays the onset of REM sleep and blocks the effects of arecoline. These findings suggest that cholinergic mechanisms play a role in the induction and timing of REM sleep, but not in its maintenance. For this reason, the recent findings with RS86, an orally active muscarinic agonist are noteworthy. RS86, in a dose of 0.75–1.50 mg not only decreased the latency to the first REM sleep period but increased its duration as well, indicating that cholinergic mechanisms may both initiate and maintain REM sleep (Spiegel, 1984). Studies in cats also support this dual role (Bagdoyan *et al.*, 1984). The neuronal processes mediating REM sleep in this animal are presently actively being defined by the use of cholinergic agonists (Shiromani & McGinty, 1986).

In man, tolerance develops to the REM suppressing effects of scopolamine when this agent is given repeatedly at bedtime. This has been attributed to the development of muscarinic supersensitivity, (Sagales *et al.*, 1975), and indeed, in rats, repeated treatment with scopolamine has been shown to enhance the binding of [H^3]quinuclidinyl-benzylate (QNB) a muscarinic antagonist (Majocha & Baldessarini, 1980). Scopolamine has a duration of action of about six hours. An attempt was made to observe the consequences on sleep in man of muscarinic supersensitivity by administering the drug in the morning for three days (Siteram *et al.*, 1979). A decrease in the total sleep time and in the REM latency was observed as well as an increase in the REM density. Sensitivity to the REM inducing effects of arecoline was also increased.

Reduced sleep, with a short REM sleep latency and a high REM density, is typically found in patients with mental depression (Gillin & Siteram, 1984). Studies in these patients reveal that they are also unusually sensitive to the REM inducing effects of arecoline (Siteram *et al.*, 1980). This suggests that muscarinic supersensitivity develops in this condition. The metabolic balance between brain cholinergic and catecholaminergic activity may be tilted in favour of cholinergic neurotransmission in depression and the effectiveness of the tricyclic antidepressants may depend upon their capacity to restore this balance by inhibiting both the reuptake of noradrenaline and the activation of muscarinic receptors (Snyder & Yamamura, 1977).

The decrease in total sleep time with muscarinic supersensitivity suggests that cholinergic mechanisms promote wakefulness as well as REM sleep. The effects of the cholinesterase inhibitor physostigmine, in man, provide further evidence for this. Intravenous infusion of 0.25 mg of physostigmine during the second NREM period induces REM sleep, but a higher dose, 0.5 mg, induces wakefulness. RS86 produces a decrease in slow wave sleep in the first part of the night as well as an increase in REM sleep at this time (Spiegel, 1984). And in cats, in comparison with NREM sleep, a significant and almost identical increase in the release of acetylcholine from the cerebral cortex occurs during wakefulness and REM sleep (Jasper & Tessier, 1974).

13.2.3 *Serotogenic receptors*

Numerous studies have explored the role of serotonin in the regulation of the vigilance states (Gillin *et al.*, 1978). Most of these studies have documented the effects of serotonin precursors, and serotonin synthesis inhibitors on these states. Studies utilizing agents specifically active at serotonin recognition sites have been fewer in number. Methysergide, for example, a serotonin receptor blocker, given in a dose of 8 mg/day for two days reduced REM sleep, and slightly but significantly increased NREM sleep (Mendelson *et al.*, 1975). Overall sleep time was unchanged. These actions of methysergide, however, may not have been specifically due to serotonin receptor blockade, since this agent has other effects as well (Douglas, 1985). Lysergic acid diethylamide, a putative pre-synaptic serotonin agonist appears to act by inhibiting the activity of serotonin containing neurones but many of its effects belie this mechanism of action (Cooper *et al.*, 1982). When given to normal volunteers at bedtime, or one hour after falling asleep, in doses which produce psychological effects (0.08–0.73 μg/kg), LSD promoted arousal and increased the duration of the first and second REM periods (Muzio *et al.*, 1966).

These observations are insufficient to describe the role of serotonin in the regulation of the sleep cycle and additional studies with agents specifically active at serotonin receptor sites in man appear necessary. This requirement may not be easy to fulfil given the multiplicity of serotonin receptor subtypes (Douglas, 1985). An appealing view of serotonin's role, at least one which is in keeping with the predictions of the Hobson–McCarley model, comes from studies in rats. Here, quipazine, a serotonin receptor agonist, suppresses both slow wave and REM sleep (Fornal & Radulovacki, 1981). This might be expected if serotonergic neurones in the rat, as in the cat, decreased their firing rates during NREM sleep to reach their lowest levels during REM sleep (McGinty & Harper, 1976; Trulson & Jacobs, 1979; Cespuglio *et al.*, 1981).

13.2.4 *Dopaminergic receptors*

The role of dopamine in the regulation of the sleep–wakefulness cycle has been the subject of extensive research, yet its functions remain uncertain (Gillin *et al.*, 1981). Pimozide, for example, a fairly specific dopamine receptor blocker in low doses (1–4 mg) has no effect on sleep patterns in normal volunteers (Sagales & Erill, 1975). Neither are any consistent changes found in the sleep patterns of patients with Parkinson's disease in which dopamine neurotransmission is deficient (Gillin *et al.*, 1981). Dopamine receptors, like α-adrenergic receptors, occur both pre-synaptically and post-synaptically (Cooper *et al.*, 1982). These receptors have also been divided into two subtypes D_1 and D_2, depending on their capacity to mediate increased or decreased adenylate cyclase activity (Stoof & Kebabian, 1981). Although the traditional view has been that pre-synaptic receptors effect inhibition of dopamine release and post-synaptic receptors effect cell action, the physiological effect of dopamine may depend upon the specific receptor subtype which has been stimulated as much as on its location (Corsini *et al.*, 1977; Gessa *et al.*, 1985). The discovery of dopamine receptors on neurones which release other neurotransmitters, further complicates the definition of dopamine's role in the regulation of the sleep cycle (Fuxe *et al.*, 1977; Jouvet, 1981).

Apomorphine, a dopamine agonist, produces sleepiness when given during the day. Thus, nearly two hours of NREM sleep was induced in all subjects when a group of normal volunteers was given 1.5 mg of apomorphine subcutaneously (Bassi *et al.*, 1979). REM sleep was not observed but slow wave sleep occupied 30% of the sleep record. Sedation and sleep were also observed in a second study in which 1 mg of apomorphine was given intramuscularly (Corsini *et al.*, 1977). Dopamine receptor blockers like haloperidol and sulpiride prevented these sleep inducing effects. However, infusion of low and non-emetic doses of apomorphine (0.20–0.26 μg/kg/min) at bedtime for three to four hours, abolished REM sleep and decreased NREM stage 4 sleep. A compensatory increase in fragmented stage 2 sleep was observed at the time of infusion and a rebound increase in NREM stage 4 sleep and REM sleep occurred following the infusion. If the infusion was continued all night, slow wave sleep and REM sleep continued to be suppressed but wakefulness was increased (Cianchetti *et al.*, 1980, 1981). Again, these effects could be blocked by haloperidol and sulpiride. Almost the same effects on sleep were found with piribedal, another dopamine agonist. Infusion of 0.4–0.5 μg/kg/min. at bedtime abolished REM sleep and reduced slow wave sleep. These effects too could be blocked by haloperidol and sulpiride (Cianchetti *et al.*, 1981). Depressed patients given an average of 175 mg/day of piribedal by mouth also showed a significant reduction in REM sleep (Post *et al.*, 1978). Thus, some of the apomorphine and piribedal studies suggest that these drugs promote arousal rather than sleep. On the other hand, bromocriptine, another dopamine agonist, had little effect on sleep patterns when given in doses of 10–20 mg/day to patients with Parkinson's disease (Passouant, 1981) or in doses of up to 40 mg/day to patients with chronic schizophrenia (Brambilla *et al.*, 1983). Numerous investigations with the dopamine precursor, l-DOPA have also demonstrated variable effects depending on the dose, the target population and the route of administration (Mendelson *et al.*, 1977).

Dopamine's role in the regulation of sleep and wakefulness may become clearer when agents specific for the dopamine receptor subtypes are developed. A recent study in rats, for example, demonstrated that high doses of apomorphine which normally produce wakefulness and stereotypy produce sleep when given to animals pretreated with SCH 23390, a specific D_1-blocker. Sleep could be prevented if these animals, in turn, were treated with (−)sulpiride, a specific D_2-receptor blocker. Thus, the inconsistent effects observed in man with agents active at dopamine receptor sites may reflect the variable activation of dopamine receptor subtypes at different sites.

13.3 Receptor and sleep disorders

13.3.1 *The benzodiazepine receptor*

The benzodiazepines have become amongst the most widely used drugs since their introduction in 1960 when chlordiazepoxide, or Librium, was introduced (Greenblatt *et al.*, 1983). These agents have been marketed for their anxiolytic, muscle relaxant, anti-convulsant and hypnotic properties. In Canada, six benzodiazepine compounds are currently on the market as hypnotics, while others are in the testing stage. Still other benzodiazepines, prescribed for their anxiolytic or muscle relaxant properties, are used interchangeably by patients as hypnotics. The great popularity of these drugs has been attributed to their efficacy and safety (Harvey, 1985). Tolerance is slow to develop and side effects are minimal with low doses. Effects on EEG-sleep patterns are also minimal although these drugs tend to suppress REM sleep, and by decreasing the amplitude of delta activity, they also suppress NREM stages 3 and 4 sleep. Slow wave activity is tranferred to stage 2 sleep, and the duration of this sleep stage is reliably increased (Feinberg *et al.*, 1977). The major distinction between the different benzodiazepine hypnotics lies in their half-life. Compounds with long half-lives tend to accumulate when given repetitively. This may produce drowsiness and interfere with daytime performance, a problem which may be acute for the older patient (Oswald *et al.*, 1979). Compounds with short half-lives tend to produce rebound anxiety and rebound insomnia on withdrawal (Kales *et al.*, 1983).

In 1977 specific membrane binding sites for the benzodiazepines were found in the nervous system using radiolabeled diazepam. These sites bound benzodiazepines with an affinity which correlated well with their pharmacological effects. The receptor site was found to be part of a macromolecular complex consisting of a receptor for γ-aminobutyric acid as well as binding sites for benzodiazepines and barbiturates. The common site of action of the barbiturates and benzodiazepines offered an explanation for their many common pharmacological effects (Study & Barker, 1982).

Recently a number of newer compounds have been developed which bind tightly to the benzodiazepine receptor. One agonist, the pyrrolopyrazine derivative, zopiclone, is now being tested as a short acting hypnotic (Nicholson *et al.*, 1983). Other compounds, imidazodiazepines, pyrazoloquinolines and beta-carbolines have a spectrum of actions from partial agonist to competitive antagonist (Ashton, 1985). The distinct effects of these newer compounds suggest that the different clinical actions of the benzodiazepines may be separable. Of the benzodiazepine antagonists, the best studied in man has been the imidazodiazepine RO 15–1788. Sleep studies indicate that 100 mg of this compound has little effect on sleep, but that it will counteract the increase in sleep time produced by flunitrazepam, as well as the REM suppressing effects of this hypnotic (Gaillard & Blois, 1983). Intravenous administration of RO 15–1788 can also rapidly reverse the deep coma produced by an overdose of benzodiazepines (Scollo-Lavizzari, 1983). In the rat, 3-hydroxymethyl-beta-carboline induces a dose dependent increase in the sleep latency, but a low dose which has no effects on sleep can block the hypnotic actions of flurazepam (Mendelson *et al.*, 1983).

A number of studies have been undertaken to determine if changes in the characteristics of the benzodiazepine receptor mediate the development of tolerance to these drugs or explain their more potent effects with age. For example, in rats, chronic benzodiazepine administration has been shown either to slowly decrease [H^3] diazepam binding (Rosenberg & Chiu, 1979) or not to have any effect (Braestrup *et al.*, 1979). Different experimental conditions may account for these discrepant findings. In another study, no change in diazepam receptor binding was found in rats with aging. (Tsang *et al.*, 1982). It has been proposed that benzodiazepine use suppresses the synthesis of an endogenous ligand, and that the anxiety and insomnia which occur following the withdrawal of short acting drugs reflects the inadequate compensatory synthesis of this ligand (Kales *et al.*, 1978). Indeed, Scharf & Feil (1983) in support of this thesis, have reported increased numbers of available receptor binding sites in rats after withdrawal of short and intermediate acting benzodiazepines, but not after withdrawal of long acting compounds.

13.3.2 *Adenosine receptors*

Caffeinated beverages are well known to disturb sleep (Snyder & Sklar, 1984). For example, 1.1–4.6 mg/kg of caffeine, equivalent to one to four cups of coffee was found to decrease the total sleep time and prolong the time to sleep onset in a dose-related manner (Karacan *et al.*, 1976). Impaired sleep and decreased sleep time were also found in a more recent study on the effects of 100–300 mg of caffeine (Nicholson & Stone, 1980). It is now accepted that the excitatory effects of the methylxanthines are due to adenosine receptor blockade (Rall, 1985) rather than to brain phosphodiesterase inhibition, since concentrations of caffeine and theophylline which stimulate behaviour only slightly inhibit this enzyme. Recently, investigators have examined the effects of certain adenosine analogues on sleep in rats (Radulovacki *et al.*, 1982, 1983). These analogues, N^6-L-(phenylisopropyl) adenosine, cyclohexyladenosine and adenosine 5′-*N*-ethylcarboxamide, were used in place of adenosine because this compound is metabolized too rapidly. In low nanomolar doses, these analogues increased slow wave sleep and the first two, increased REM sleep duration as well. These effects occurred at the expense of light sleep. As the dose was increased, the effects on sleep disappeared and wakefulness was promoted. It was proposed that low nanomolar doses acted as A_1-adenosine receptors to induce sleep, while higher micromolar doses activated A_2-receptors to produce wakefulness. Caffeine was shown to block the increase in slow wave sleep produced by N^6-L-(phenylisopropyl) adenosine as might have been expected if these agents have opposing actions at the same site. As a result of these findings it has been suggested that the adenosine analogues might be useful clinical hypnotics. In contrast to the benzodiazepines and barbiturates, they promote both REM and slow wave sleep and thus a more physiological sleep.

13.3.3 *The gammahydroxybutyrate receptor and narcolepsy*

Narcolepsy is a common disorder of sleep characterized by excessive daytime drowsiness, cataplexy, or attacks of muscle weakness precipitated by emotion, sleep paralysis and sleep related hallucinations (Zarcone, 1973). These symptoms stem from the progressive dissociation of sleep as it fragments and drifts around the 24 hour period. Diagnostic sleep studied in this condition demonstrate pathognomonic sleep onset REM periods at night or during daytime naps.

Narcolepsy has been described in dogs, and certain breeds, the Doberman pinscher, for example, have been bred for the disorder (Foutz *et al.*, 1979). The brains of these animals show increased numbers of muscarinic receptors in the pontine region where REM control mechanisms are located (Boehme *et al.*, 1984). The binding characteristics of these receptors are unaltered. Dopamine (D_2) and benzodiazepine receptor numbers and binding characteristics in the brains of these animals are unchanged (Bowersox *et al.*, 1985). But dopamine and 3,4-dihydroxy phenyl-acetic acid concentrations are elevated in many brain regions, suggesting that dopamine utilization is impaired (Mefford *et al.*, 1983). Thus, as in patients with depression, the early REM sleep periods in narcolepsy appear to be associated with enhanced cholinergic and deficient catecholaminergic neurotransmission (Gillin & Siteram, 1984). Indeed, in the dogs, arecoline can induce cataplexy, that is, it can further promote the dissociation of REM sleep, while atropine and scopolamine prevent these attacks (Delashaw *et al.*, 1976). Cholinergic systems appear to be sensitized in canine narcolepsy.

In man, anticholinergic drugs like trihexyphenidyl do not prevent cataplexy, nor can physostigmine induce this symptom (Gillin *et al.*, 1976). But γ-hydroxybutyrate (GHB) a naturally occurring metabolite of the central nervous system reliably induces sleep onset REM periods in patients with narcolepsy (Broughton & Mamelak, 1979, 1980) and, remarkably, induces these periods in patients with depression as well (Mamelak *et al.*, 1977). Studies in rats indicate that GHB increases brain acetylcholine levels (Giarman & Schmidt, 1983; Sethy *et al.*, 1976) and promotes acetylcholine release (Stadler *et al.*, 1974) but inhibits dopamine release (Roth *et al.*, 1973). Thus, GHB augments the metabolic shift which occurs naturally in narcolepsy and depression. Narcoleptics and depressives appear to be particularly sensitive to the actions of GHB since this agent cannot dissociate REM sleep in normal individuals. For this reason, the discovery of central binding sites with high affinity for GHB in nerve ending fragments rich in acetylcholine and acetylcholinesterase is of great interest (Maitre *et al.*, 1983). It suggests that cholinergic and γ-hydro butyric mechanisms are closely allied and that supersensitivity at these sites may promote sleep dissociation.

References

Ashton, C. (1985). Benzodiazepine overdose: are specific antagonists useful? *Br. Med. J.*, **290**, 805–6.

Autret, A., Minz, M., Beillevaire, T., Cathala, H. P. & Schmitt, H. (1977). Effect of clonidine on sleep patterns in man. *Eur. J. Clin. Pharmacol.*, **12,** 319–22.

Baghdoyan, H., Monaco, A., Rodrigo-Angulo, M., Assens, F., McCarley, R. & Hobson, J. (1984). Microinjection of neostigmine into the pontine reticular formation of cats enhances desynchronized sleep signs. *J. Pharmacol. and Exp. Ther.*, **231,** 173–80.

Bassi, S., Albizzati, M., Frattola, L., Passerini, D. & Trabucchi, M. (1979). Dopamine receptors and sleep induction in man. *J. Neurol. Neurosurg. Psychiatry*, **42,** 458–60.

Bender, W., Greil, W., Ruther, E. & Schnelle, K. (1979). Effects of the beta-adrenoceptor blocking agent sotalol on CNS: sleep, EEG and psychophysiological parameter. *J. Clin. Pharmacol.*, **19,** 505–12.

Boehme, R., Baker, T., Mefford, I., Barchas, J., Dement, D. & Ciaranello, R. (1984). Narcolepsy: Cholinergic receptor changes in an animal model. *Life Sci.*, **34,** 1825–8.

Bowersox, S., Kilduff, T., Dement, W. & Ciaranello, R. (1985). Dopamine and benzodiazepine receptor characteristics in canine narcolepsy (Abstract). Second International Symposium on Narcolepsy, Palo Alto, California.

Braestrup, C., Neilsen, M. & Squires, R. (1979). No changes in rat benzodiazepine receptors after withdrawal from continuous treatment with lorazepam and diazepam. *Life Sci.*, **24,** 347–50.

Brambilla, F., Scarone, S., Pugnetti, L., Massironi, R., Penati, G. & Nobile, P. (1983). Bromocriptine therapy in chronic schizophrenia: Effects on symptomatology, sleep patterns and prolactin response to stimulation. *Psychiatry Res.*, **8,** 159–69.

Broughton, R. & Mamelak, M. (1979). The treatment of narcolepsy-cataplexy with nocturnal gammahydroxybutyrate. *Can. J. Neurol. Sci.*, **6,** 1–6.

Broughton, R. & Mamelak, M. (1980). Effects of gammahydroxybutyrate on sleep-waking patterns in narcolepsy-cataplexy. *Can. J. Neurol. Sci.*, **7,** 23–31.

Cespuglio, R., Faradji, H., Gomez, M. & Jouvet, M. (1981). Single Unit recordings in the nuclei raphe dorsalis and magnus during the sleep-waking cycle of semi-chronic prepared cats. *Neurosci. Lett.*, **24,** 133–8.

Cianchetti, C., Masala, C., Mangoni, A. & Gessa, G. (1980). Suppression of REM and delta sleep by apomorphine in man: A dopaminomimetic effect. *Psychopharmacology*, **67,** 61–5.

Cianchetti, C., Masala, C., Olivari, P., Marro, G. & Gessa, L. (1981). Sleep Pattern Modifications by Dopamine Agonist in Man. In *Apomorphine and Other Dopaminominmetics, Clinical Pharmacology*, vol. 2, ed. G. Corsini & G. Gessa, pp. 173–81. New York: Raven Press.

Cooper, J., Bloom, F. & Roth, R. (1982). *The Biochemical Basis of Neuropharmacology*. New York and Oxford: Oxford University Press.

Corsini, G., Del Zompo, M., Manconi, S., Piccardi, M., Onali, P. & Mangoni, A. (1977). Evidence for dopaminic receptors in the human brain mediating sedation and sleep. *Life Sci.*, **20,** 1613–18.

Delashaw, J., Foutz, A., Guilleminault, C. & Dement, W. (1979). Cholinergic mechanisms and cataplexy in dogs. *Exp. Neurol.*, **66,** 745–57.

Douglas, W. (1985). Histamine and 5-hydroxytryptamine (Serotonin) and their antagonists. In *The Pharmacological Basis of Therapeutics*, ed. A. Gilman, L. Goodman, T. Rall & F. Muradi, pp. 604–38. New York: MacMillan Publishing Co. Inc.

Dunleavy, D., MacLean, A. & Oswald, I. (1971). Debrisoquine, quanethidine, propranolol and human sleep. *Psychopharmacologia*, **21,** 101–10.

Feinberg, I., Fein, G., Walker, J., Price, L., Floyd, T. & March, J. (1977). Flurazepam effects on slow wave sleep; stage 4 suppressed but number of delta waves constant. *Science*, **198,** 847–8.

Fornal, C. & Radulovacki, M. (1981). Sleep suppressant action of quipazine: Relation to central serotogenic stimulation. *Pharmacol. Biochem. Behav.*, **15,** 937–44.

Foutz, A., Mitler, M., Cavalli-Sforza, L. & Dement, W. (1979). Genetic factors in canine narcolepsy. *Sleep*, **1,** 413–22.

Fuxe, K., Agnati, L., Everitt, B., Hokfelt, T., Ljungdahl, A. & Perez de la Mona, M. (1977). Action of beta (4-chlorphenyl) GABA, gamma-hydroxybutyrolactone and apomorphinic on central/dopamine neurones. In *Advances in Biochemical Psychopharmacology*, ed. E. Costa & G. Gessa, pp. 489–94. New York: Raven Press.

Gaillard, J. & Blois, R. (1983). Effect of the benzodiazepine antagonist RO15–1788 on flunitrazepam-induced sleep changes. *Br. J. Clin. Pharmacol.*, **15,** 529–36.

Gaillard, J. & Kafi, S. (1979). Involvement of pre-and post-synaptic receptors in catecholaminergic control of paradoxical sleep in man. *Eur. J. Clin. Pharmacol.*, **15,** 83–9.

Gessa, G., Porceddu, M., Collu, M., Mereu, G., Serr, M., Ongini, E. & Biggio, G. (1985). Sedation and sleep induced by high doses of apomorphine after blockade of D1 receptor by SCH 23390. *Eur. J. Pharmacol.*, **109,** 269–74.

Giarman, N. J. & Schmidt, K. F. (1963). Some neurochemical aspects of the depressant action of *υ* butyrolactone on the central nervous system. *Br. J. Pharmacol.*, **20,** 563–8.

Gillin, J., Horwitz, D. & Wyatt, K. (1976). Pharmacologic studies of narcolepsy involving serotonin, acetylcholine and monoamine oxidase. *Advances in Sleep Research*, **3,** 585–603.

Gillin, J., Mendelson, W., Sitaram, N. & Wyatt, R. (1978). The neuropharmacology of sleep and wakefulness. *Annu. Rev. Pharmacol. Toxicol.*, **18,** 563–79.

Gillin, J. & Sitaram, N. (1984). Rapid eye movement (REM) sleep; cholinergic mechanisms. *Psychol. Med.*, **14,** 501–6.

Gillin, J., Sitaram, N. & Mendelson, W. (1982). Acetylcholine, sleep and depression. *Hum. Neurobiol.*, **1,** 211–19.

Gillin, J., vanKammen, D., Post, R., Sitaram, N., Wyatt, R. & Bunney, W. (1981). What is the role of dopamine in the regulation of sleep-wake activity? In *Apomorphine and other dopaminomimetics, Clinical Pharmacology*, vol. 2, ed. G. Corsini & G. Gessa, pp. 157–64. New York: Raven Press.

Greenblatt, D., Shader, R. & Abernethy, D. (1983). Current status of benzodiazepines. *New Engl. J. Med.*, **309,** 354–8.

Harvey, S. (1985). Hypnotics and sedatives. In *The Pharmacological Basis of Therapeutics*, ed. A. Gilman, R. Goodman, T. Rall & F. Murad, pp. 339–71. New York: MacMillan Publishing Co.

Hobson, J., McCarley, R. & Wyzinski, P. (1975). Sleep Cycle Oscillation: Reciprocal discharge by two brainstem neuronal groups. *Science*, **189,** 55–8.

Jasper, H. & Tessier, J. (1971). Acetylcholine liberation from cerebral cortex during paradoxical (REM) sleep. *Science*, **172,** 601–2.

Jouvet, M., (1981). Dopamine and sleep – A neurophysiologist's introduction. In *Apomorphine and other dopaminomimetics, Clinical Pharmacology*, vol. 2, pp. 153–6. New York: Raven Press.

Kales, A., Scharf, M. & Kales, J. (1978). Rebound insomnia: A new clinical syndrome. *Science* **201,** 1039–41.

Kales, A., Soldatos, C., Bixler, E. & Kales, J. (1983). Rebound insomnia and rebound anxiety. A review. *Pharmacology*, **26,** 121–37.

Kales, A., Soldatos, C., Cadieux, R., Bixler, E., Tan, T. & Scharf, M. (1979). Propranolol in the treatment of narcolepsy. *Ann. Intern. Med.*, **91,** 742–3.

Karacan, I., Thornby, J., Anch, M., Booth, G., Williams, R. & Salis, P. (1976). Dose related sleep disturbances induced by coffee and caffeine. *Clin. Pharmacol. Ther.*, **20,** 682–9.

Kayed, K. & Godtlibsen, O. (1977). Effects of beta adreno receptor antagonists, acebutolol and metoprotol on sleep pattern in normal subjects. *Eur. J. Clin. Pharmacol.*, **12,** 323–6.

Lewis, S. (1970). Comparative effects of some amphetamine derivatives on human sleep. In *International Symposium on amphetamine and related compounds*, ed. E. Costa & S. Garratini, pp. 873–88. New York: Raven Press.

Maitre, M., Rumigny, J., Cash, C. & Mandel, P. (1983). Subcellular distribution of gammahydroxybutyrate binding sites in rat brain. Principal localization in synaptosomal fraction. *Biochem. Biophys. Res. Commun.*, **110,** 262–5.

Majocha, R. & Baldessarini, R. (1980). Increased muscarinic receptor binding in rat forebrain after scopolamine. *Eur. J. Pharmacol.*, **67,** 327–8.

Mamelak, M., Escriu, J. & Stokan, O. (1977). The effects of gamma-hydroxybutyrate on sleep. *Biol. Psychiatry*, **12,** 273–88.

Mefford, J., Baker, T., Boehme, R., Foutz, A., Ciaranello, R., Barchas, J. & Dement, W. (1983). Narcolepsy: Biogenic amine deficits in an animal model. *Science*, **220,** 629–32.

Meier-Ewert, K., Matsubayashi, K. & Benter, L. (1985). Propranolol: Long term treatment in narcolepsy-cataplexy. *Sleep*, **8,** 95–104.

Mendelson, W., Cain, M., Cook, J., Paul, S. & Skolnick, P. (1983). A benzodiazepine receptor antagonist decreases sleep and reverses the hypnotic actions of flurazepam. *Science*, **219,** 414–16.

Mendelson, W., Gillin, J. & Wyatt, R. (1977). *Human Sleep and Its Disorders*. New York and London: Plenum Press.

Mendelson, W., Lantigua, R., Wyatt, R., Gillin, J. & Jacobs, L. (1981). Piperidine enhances sleep-related and insulin-induced growth hormone secretion: Further evidence for a cholinergic secretory mechanism. *J. Clin. Endocrinol. & Metab.*, **52,** 409–15.

Mendelson, W., Reichman, J. & Othmer, E. (1975). Serotonin inhibition and sleep. *Biol. Psychiatry*, **10,** 459–64.

McCarley, R. & Hobson, J. (1975). Neuronal excitability modulation over the sleep cycle: A Structural and Mathematical Model. *Science*, **189,** 58–60.

McGinty, D. & Harper, R. (1976). Dorsal raphe neurons: Depression of firing during sleep in cats. *Brain Res.*, **101,** 569–75.

Monti, J. (1982). Mini review: Catecholamines and the sleep wake cycle. I. EEG and behavioural arousal. *Life Sci.*, **30,** 1145–57.

Monti, J. (1983). Mini review: Catecholamines and the sleep wake cycle. II. REM. sleep. *Life Sci.*, **32,** 1401–15.

Muzio, J., Roffwarg, H. & Kaufman, E. (1966). Alterations in the nocturnal sleep cycle resulting from LSD. *Electroencephalogr. Clin. Neurophysiol.*, **21,** 313–24.

Nicholson, A., Schlosberg, A. & Dreyfus, J. (1983). Zopiclone: A third generation of hypnotics. *Pharmacology*, **27,** *Suppl. 2*, 1–250.

Nicholson, A. & Stone, B. (1980). Heterocyclic amphetamine derivatives and caffeine on sleep in man. *Br. J. Clin. Pharmacol.*, **9**, 195–203.

Oswald, I., Adam, K., Borrow, S. & Idzikowski, C. (1979). The effects of two hypnotics on sleep, subjective feelings and skilled performance. In *Pharmacology of the States of Alertness*, ed. P. Passouant & I. Oswald, pp. 51–63. New York: Pergamon Press.

Oswald, I., Thacore, V., Adam, K., Brezinova, V. & Burack, R. (1975). Alpha-adrenergic receptor blockade increases human REM sleep. *Br. J. Clin. Pharmacol.*, **2**, 107–10.

Passouant, P. (1981). Effect of sleep on dopaminomimetics agonists. In *Apomorphine and other dopamine mimetics, Clinical Pharmacology*, vol. 2, ed. G. Corsini & L. Gessa, pp. 165–72. New York: Raven Press.

Pellejero, T., Monte, J., Baglietto, J., Jantos, H., Pazos, S., Cichevski, V. & Hawkins, M. (1984). Effects of methoxamine and alpha adrenoceptor, antagonists, prazosin and yohimbine on the sleep wake cycle of the rat. *Sleep*, **7**, 365–72.

Post, R., Gerner, R., Carman, J., Gillin, J., Jimerson, D., Goodwin, F. & Bunney, W. (1978). Effects of a dopamine agonist piribedil in depressed patient; relationship of pre-treatment homovanillic acid to antidepressant response. *Arch. Gen. Psychiatry*, **35**, 609–15.

Putkonen, P., Leppävuori, A. & Stenberg, D. (1977). Paraxodical sleep inhibition by central alpha-adrenoceptor stimulant clonidine antagonized by alpha-receptor blocker yohimbine. *Life Sci.*, **21**, 1059–66.

Putkonen, P. (1979). Alpha and beta adrenergic mechanisms in the control of the sleep stages. In *Sleep Research*, ed. R. Priest, A. Pletscher & J. Ward, pp. 19–34. Lancaster: MTP Press.

Radulovacki, M., Miletich, R. & Green, R. (1982). N^6 (L-phenylisopropyl) adenosine (L-PIA) increases slow-wave sleep (S_2) and decreases wakefulness in rats. *Brain Res.*, **246**, 178–80.

Radulovacki, M., Virus, R., Djuricic-Nedelson, M. & Green, R. (1983). Adenosine analogues and sleep in rats. *J. Pharmacol. Exp. Therp.*, **228**, 268–74.

Rall, T. (1985). Central nervous system stimulants: The Xanthines In *Pharmacological Basis of Therapeutics*, ed. A. Gilman, L. Goodman, T. Rall & F. Murad, pp. 589–603. New York: MacMillan Publishing Co.

Rechtschaffen, A. & Maron, L. (1964). The effect of amphetamine on the sleep cycle. *Electroencephalogr. Clin. Neurophysiol.*, **16**, 438–45.

Rosenberg, H. & Chiu, T. (1979). Decreased 3H-diazepam binding in a specific response to chronic benzodiazepine treatment. *Life Sci.*, **24**, 803–8.

Roth, R., Walters, J. & Aghajanian, G. (1973). Effect of impulse flow on the release and synthesis of dopamine in the rat striatum. In *Frontiers in Catecholamine Research*, ed. E. Usdin & S. Snyder, pp. 567–74. Oxford: Pergamon Press.

Sagalés, T. & Erill, S. (1975). Effects of central dopaminergic blockade with pimozide upon the EEG states of sleep in man. *Psychopharmacologia*, **41**, 53–6.

Sagalés, T., Erill, S. & Domino, E. (1975). Effects of repeated doses of scopolamine on the electroencephalographic stages of sleep in normal volunteers. *Clin. Pharmacol. Ther.*, **18**, 727–32.

Scharf, M. & Feil. P. (1983). Acute effects of drug administration and withdrawal on the benzodiazepine receptor. *Life Sci.*, **32**, 1771–7.

Scollo-Lavizzari, G. (1983). First clinical investigation of the benzodiazepine antagonist RO-1788 in comatose patients. *Eur. Neurol.*, **22**, 7–11.

Sethy, V., Roth, R., Walters, J., Marini, J. & VanWoert, M. (1976). Effect of anesthesia doses of gammahydroxybutyrate on the acetylcholine content of rat brain. *Naunyn-Schmiedeberg's Arch. Pharmacol.*, **295**, 9–14.
Shiromani, P. & McGinty, D. (1986). Pontine neuronal response to local cholinergic infusion: relation to REM sleep. *Brain Res.*, **386**, 20–31.
Simpson, F. (1980). Hypertensive disease. In *Drug Treatment Principles and Practice of Clinical Pharmacology*, ed. G. Avery, pp. 638–82. Sydney and New York: Adis Press.
Sitaram, N., Mendelson, W., Wyatt, R. & Gillin, J. (1977). The time dependent induction of REM sleep and arousal by physostigmine infusion during normal human sleep. *Brain Res.* **122**, 562–7.
Sitaram, N., Moore, A. & Gillin, J. (1978). Induction and resetting of REM sleep rhythm in normal man by arecholine blockade by scopolamine. *Sleep*, **1**, 83–90.
Sitaram, N., Moore, A. & Gillin, J. (1979). Scopolamine induced muscarinic supersensitivity in normal man: changes in sleep. *Psychiatry Res.*, **1**, 9–16.
Sitaram, N., Nunberger, J., Gershon, E. & Gillin, J. (1980). Faster cholinergic REM sleep induction in euthymic patients with primary affective illness. *Science*, **208**, 200–2.
Snyder, S. & Sklar, P. (1984). Behavioural and molecular actions of caffeine: Focus on adenosine. *J. Psychiatr. Res.*, **18**, 91–106.
Snyder, S. & Yamamura, H. (1977). Antidepressants and the muscarinic acetylcholine receptor. *Arch. Gen. Psychiatry*, **34**, 236–9.
Stadler, H., Lloyd, K. & Bartholini, I. (1974). Dopaminergic inhibition of striatal cholinergic neurons: Synergistic blocking action of gamma-butyrolactones and neuroleptic drugs. *Naunyn-Schmiedeberg's Arch. Pharmacol.*, **283**, 129–34.
Stoof, J. & Kebabian, J. (1981). Opposing roles for D1 and D2 dopamine receptors in efflux of cyclic AMP from rat neostriatim. *Nature*, **294**, 366–8.
Study, R. & Barker, J. (1982). Cellular mechanisms of benzodiazepine action. *J. Am. Med. Assoc.*, **247**, 2147–51.
Trulson, M. & Jacobs, B. (1979). Raphe unit activity in freely moving cats: Correlation with level of behavioural arousal. *Brain Res.*, **163**, 135–50.
Tsang, C., Speeg, K. & Wilkinson, G. (1981). Aging and benzodiazepine binding in the rat cerebral cortex. *Life Sci.*, **30**, 343–6.
Zarcone, V. (1973). Narcolepsy. *New Engl. J. Med.*, **288**, 1156–66.

14

Receptor localization in neuropsychiatry

James K. Wamsley and Ted M. Dawson

14.1 Introduction

A versatile and widely applicable technique for receptor localization was developed in 1979 by Michael Kuhar (Young & Kuhar, 1979). This *in vitro* technique makes it possible to analyze, under the microscope, the density and distribution of binding sites for various radioactively tagged compounds (Kuhar *et al.*, 1980, 1982). Further refinements of the techniques have included the availability of tritium-sensitive film to produce the autoradiograms from the labeled tissue sections and the development of standards for quantitating the actual receptor density on the basis of the density of associated autoradiographic grains (Palacios *et al.*, 1981a; Penny *et al.*, 1981; Unnerstall *et al.*, 1982; Rainbow *et al.*, 1982b). Localizations of this nature have been applied to a wide variety of neurotransmitter and drug receptors and the field continues to expand as new radioactively labeled compounds become available (Wamsley & Palacios, 1983; Kuhar *et al.*, 1986).

Receptor localization and quantitation are useful as a means of analyzing receptor alterations which occur in response to chronic drug treatments or to various lesions of the central nervous system. Since the technique is performed *in vitro*, it is not necessary for the investigators to concern themselves with the distribution or possible metabolic changes of the ligand, and it is possible to reduce the non-specific binding of the ligand to non-receptor sites by performing carefully monitored rinsing intervals. It is also possible to analyze the density and distribution of receptors in tissues derived from human postmortem cases. Using appropriate standards, for instance, it is possible to quantitate receptor alterations associated with human postmortem brain of patients who had Parkinson's disease with that from a normal postmortem brain of patients who had no neuropsychiatric disorder. Studies of this nature are still in their infancy, but their utility and importance is already apparent. A wealth of information on the involvement of receptor subtypes in the primary or secondary receptor changes accompanying the disease process may be analyzed by combining the study of receptor alterations in animal models with those performed in human postmortem tissues. These types of studies may also be useful in screening various pharmaceutical agents which might be efficacious in alleviating some of the symptomatology which accompanies various human maladies.

14.2 Autoradiographic methods of receptor localization

As pointed out earlier, the receptor autoradiographic technique has been applied to the localization of many different neurotransmitter and drug receptor populations within the central nervous system. For example, the differentiation of dopamine type 1 and type 2 receptors is possible using autoradiographic techniques and the appropriate parameters used in a typical experiment are shown in Table 14.1.

Animals are usually prepared for autoradiographic procedures by perfusing with an ice-cold isotonic buffered saline solution in order to rinse away the vascular contents and initiate an efficient and rapid cooling of the brain. The brain tissues are then dissected and frozen on dry ice or isopentane maintained at −70 °C. The frozen tissues can be stored in a −70 °C freezer for varying periods of time; however, the frozen tissue should be used as soon as possible, in order to minimize potential problems from prolonged storage of tissue sections.

Human postmortem tissues are obtained from freshly dissected brains at autopsy. The postmortem time to autopsy is critical and has been studied in certain cases in order to define the actual receptor alterations involved. The reader is referred to the paper by Whitehouse *et al.* (1984) for further consideration of this aspect. Frozen samples of sections of human brain are also available from various neurological specimen banks in several countries. The handling of these tissues, however, is not always performed in a fashion which is optimal for maintaining tissue morphology as is necessary for precision autoradiography. Thus, the best tissues would probably be obtained by the investigators themselves from their own pathology facility. These freshly dissected brains are further subjected to dissection of individual regions of brain which are subsequently frozen in a manner similar to that described for the animal tissues. Anatomical relationships, however, are maintained and more easily discernible when larger pieces of human brain are utilized for sectioning. Presumably, sections of an entire hemisphere of human brain could be

Table 14.1. *Incubation conditions for autoradiographic localization of DA receptors*

Ligand	Concentration (nM)	Buffer	Incubation procedure	Rinse procedure	Exposure time	References
(a) Conditions used for the labeling of D_1 receptors						
[^{3}H]SCH 23390	1	50 mM Tris-HCl, 120 mM NaCl, 5 mM KCl, 2 mM $CaCl_2$, 1 mM $MgCl_2$ (pH 7.4)	30 min (room temp.)	2 × 5 min (4 °C)	21 days	Dawson *et al.* (1985b, 1986b)
[^{3}H]SKF 38393	1	50 mM Tris-HCl (pH 7.4)	60 min (room temp.)	2 × 5 min (4 °C)	21 days	Scatton & Dubois (1985)
[^{125}I]SCH 23982	0.1	50 mM Tris-HCl, 120 mM NaCl, 5 mM KCl, 2 mM $CaCl_2$, 1 mM $MgCl_2$ (pH 7.4)	30 min (room temp.)	2 × 5 min (4 °C)	18–24 h	Dawson *et al.* (1986a)
(b) Conditions used for the labeling of D_2 receptors						
[^{3}H]Spiperone	0.4	0.17 M Tris-HCl, 120 mM NaCl, 5 mM KCl, 2 mM $CaCl_2$, 1 mM $MgCl_2$, 0.001% ascorbic acid (pH 7.7)	30 min (room temp.)	2 × 5 min (4 °C)	60 days	Palacios *et al.* (1981b)
[^{3}H](−)-sulpiride	15	0.17 M Tris-HCl, 120 mM NaCl, 5 mM KCl, 0.01% ascorbic acid (pH 7.4)	20 min (room temp.)	4 × 1 min (4 °C)	60 days	Gehlert & Wamsley (1984, 1985), Jastrow *et al.* (1984)

[^{3}H](−)-DO 710	5	50 mM Tris-HCl, 120 mM NaCl, 5 mM KCl, 1 mM $CaCl_2$, 1 mM $MgCl_2$, 5.7 mM ascorbic acid and 5×10^{-5} M hydroxyquinoline (pH 7.4)	30 min (room temp.)	2 × 2 min (4 °C)	14 days	Sokoloff *et al*. (1985)
[^{125}I]-iodosulpiride	0.3	50 mM Tris-HCl, 120 mM NaCl, 5 mM KCl, 1 mM $CaCl_2$, 1 mM $MgCl_2$, 5.7 mM ascorbic acid, 10 μM hydroxyquinoline (pH 7.4)	30 min (25 °C)	2 × 2 min (4 °C)	5 days	Martres *et al*. (1985)

obtained and used to perform receptor localization by autoradiography (Cortes *et al.*, 1986). However, the esoteric expertise involved in obtaining such large sections and the exorbitant cost involved in the labeling of these sections make such experiments almost impossible for many investigators. Most studies involving human brain have utilized the labeling of small dissected areas.

Thin sections of the tissues are cut in a cryostat maintained at −20 °C. These sections vary in thickness according to the investigator's preference but ten microns in thickness seems to be optimal. This thickness allows for most of the beta rays emitted from the tritium to expose the overlying film. The thinness of the section does not contribute any untoward amount of non-specific binding and at this thickness, the autoradiographic grains appearing on the surface of the tissue section can be easily associated with other underlying structures which may show up in the stained tissue section. The sections are thaw-mounted onto cold chrome/alum gelatin-coated (subbed) microscope slides and stored, in a refrigerator overnight, in the presence of desiccant in order to allow the sections to adhere more strongly to the slide.

The appropriate incubation time, rinse time, incubation temperature, buffer, pH, concentration of radioactive ligand, concentration of displacer and the appropriate displacer to utilize are determined in preliminary experiments aimed at defining these various parameters in order to obtain optimal labeling of the tissue sections and provide high specific to non-specific binding ratios.

After determining the optimal conditions for labeling slide-mounted tissue sections, another set of tissue sections is labeled under the previously determined parameters. This usually involves a preincubation in buffer in order to dissociate any endogenous ligand which may be present in the tissue sections and interfere with the subsequent labeling procedure. These endogenous substances are then rinsed away and the tissue sections are placed in Coplin jars containing buffer plus an appropriate concentration of the radioactive ligand. At the same time, an adjacent set of tissue sections is exposed, under the same conditions and to the same amount of radioactive ligand, in the added presence of a displacer. The displacer is a compound which is specific for the receptor of interest (preferably a compound that is different structurally from the labeled compound, but pharmacologically similar) and is present in excess so as to compete successfully for the specific binding of the radioactive ligand to the receptor being studied. Comparison of these two sets of tissue sections then allows the specific to non-specific binding ratio to be determined. All of the tissue sections are then rinsed in fresh buffer to wash away as much of the unbound radioactivity as possible without sacrificing too much of the specifically bound radioactive compound. The sections are next dried under a stream of cool, dry, filtered air before being stored in a sealed box in the presence of desiccant and maintained in a refrigerator overnight. The dry labeled tissue sections are then placed in an x-ray cassette in apposition to tritium-sensitive film and stored at −4 °C for an appropriate exposure period. Following this interval, the x-ray cassettes are opened in the darkroom and the tritium-sensitive films are developed so that the latent images on the film, as generated by the bound radioactive ligand, become visible.

By including appropriate standards along with labeled tissue sections on the exposure of each film, it is possible to associate certain concentrations of radioactivity with related densities of the generated autoradiographic grains. A standard curve can then be plotted, enabling the direct correlation of optical density with concentration of radioactivity. These standard curves can be utilized to analyze the data from the labeled tissue sections, thereby allowing one to quantitate the actual femtomoles of ligand bound per mg tissue in individual microscopic regions of the brain. By incubating serial sections in varying concentrations of the radioactive ligand and by comparing the optical density with the concentration of radioactivity in the tissue section area, a saturation curve can be obtained. A Scatchard plot of the data or analysis of the data by various computer curve fitting programs may be used to calculate the affinity and maximal binding density of receptors in each individual region of brain. Thus, it is possible to calculate the actual femtomoles of receptor per mg tissue in these discrete microscopic regions of brain. This provides a very powerful method to uncover subtle alterations in receptor distribution, density and/or affinity which might be taking place in response to chronic drug exposure or to a pathologic disease process.

Analysis and quantitation of the autoradiograms are usually performed under a microscope using some sort of microdensitometry apparatus. The very simplest of these systems involves only a microphotometer which can be used to obtain optical densities from both the microscopic regions of brain and the autoradiographic grains associated with the tritium standards. Much more elaborate systems are available which combine the microphotometry system with a computer in order to obtain more sophisticated receptor analyses. These computer-based microdensitometry systems can utilize either the optics of a microscope or a video-based camera to obtain the individual optical density readings. The computer can then color-code the varying degrees of optical density present in the autoradiogram thereby allowing the investigator to define quickly where potential alterations in receptors have taken place and how the distribution of receptor associated autoradiographic grains varies from region to region within the tissue section. Both the software and hardware available for microdensitometric analysis of receptor autoradiogram, have become quite sophisticated and a very rapid and accurate analysis of receptor alterations can be accomplished. These types of studies have been utilized to analyze receptor alterations associated with various animal models of human disease states and they have been employed to a lesser extent to analyze the actual receptor alterations associated with human disorders as determined in postmortem tissues.

14.3 Animal models

14.3.1 *Dopamine receptors*

Several lines of investigation point to the existence of two subtypes of dopamine receptors, the dopamine type 1 receptor (D_1) and the dopamine type 2 receptor (D_2). The dopamine type 1 receptor is thought to be associated with activation of adenylate cyclase whereas dopamine type 2 receptor stimulation is thought to either not be involved with adenylate cyclase or to have an inhibitory effect on this enzyme (Kebabian & Calne, 1979; Stoof & Kebabian, 1984). Original localizations of dopamine receptors employed the radiolabeled neuroleptic compound spiperone (Creese *et al.*, 1977; Leysen *et al.*, 1978). Autoradiographic studies using this compound showed the presence of dopamine receptors within various brain regions (Palacios *et al.*, 1981b; Palacios & Wamsley, 1983, 1984). However, the localization of tritiated spiperone binding was complicated by the fact that this ligand also labels 5-HT_2 receptors (serotonin type 2 receptors), α_1-adrenergic receptors and a nondescript site known as the spirodecanone site (Peroutka *et al.*, 1977; Leysen *et al.*, 1978; Howlett *et al.*, 1979; Peroutka & Snyder, 1979). More recent autoradiographic studies have employed the specific dopamine$_2$ receptor antagonist sulpiride to localize this dopamine receptor subtype in the central nervous system (Gehlert & Wamsley, 1984, 1985; Jastrow *et al.*, 1984). A recently discovered selective dopamine$_1$ antagonist SCH 23390 has been employed to localize autoradiographically this particular receptor subtype in the CNS (Dawson *et al.*, 1985, 1986b). Iodinated forms of these two selective ligands are currently available and have been employed for autoradiographic localization of dopamine receptor subtypes (Martres *et al.*, 1985; Dawson *et al.*, 1986a). These ligands circumvent the problems associated with tritium quenching by white matter as described by Kuhar & Unnerstall (1985) and do not require tissue defatting as recommended by Herkenham & Sokolof (1984). The iodinated ligands also require less time on film and therefore the receptor autoradiograms are much more easily obtained, however some anatomical resolution is sacrificed with iodinated compounds. Dopamine receptors show a widespread localization throughout various parts of the brain and spinal cord. Alterations in these receptors, whether they be the primary cause or secondary to another derangement in the CNS, are thought to be intimately involved in such disorders as Parkinson's disease, schizophrenia, tardive dyskinesia and attention deficit disorder, to name a few.

Both dopamine type 1 and dopamine type 2 receptors are found in high densities in such structures as the caudate–putamen, nucleus accumbens and the olfactory tubercle. D_1 receptors predominate in regions such as the cerebral cortex, claustrum, suprachiasmatic nucleus, zona incerta and the substantia nigra pars reticulata. D_2 receptors predominate in such structures as the intermediate lobe of the pituitary gland, the hypothalamus, habenula, inferior colliculus, nucleus of the solitary tract and the substantia nigra pars compacta.

Dopamine type 1 and 2 receptors show a similar localization in both rat and human brain (Gehlert *et al.*, 1986a; Dawson *et al.*, 1986b) (see Fig. 14.1). Thus, there are many areas of overlap between these two receptor subtypes and yet there are areas where the two exist quite independently. These types of studies raise the possibility that we may be able to design pharmaceutical compounds which will stimulate or block one receptor without affecting the other receptor subtype. This could be very important in developing new treatment modalities for the neuropsychiatric disorders which potentially are the result of altered dopamine receptors within the central nervous system. Drugs more specifically targeted for certain receptor sites would presumably be better therapeutic agents and would probably have reduced side effects associated with the treatment.

There are few animal models which exist for the study of schizophrenia and the most potentially serious associated side effect of treatment, namely tardive dyskinesia (Baldessarini & Tarsy, 1980; Rupniak *et al.*, 1983). Clinically, amphetamine abuse can lead to the development of a syndrome in a patient which is very difficult to distinguish from paranoid schizophrenia (Bell, 1974). Thus, chronic amphetamine treatment may be a useful means of attempting to study receptor alterations which may be associated with amphetamine abuse and possibly related to schizophrenia. Recent autoradiographic studies have determined that dopamine receptors are significantly down-regulated in specific regions of

Fig. 14.1. Autoradiographic localization of dopamine type 1 (D_1) and dopamine type 2 (D_2) receptors in sections of rat and human brain. (*A*) A photomicrograph of an autoradiogram is shown. The autoradiographic grains (black dots against a white background) were generated from a section taken at the level of the midbrain of a rat which was subsequently labeled with [^{3}H]SCH 23390. The grains under these conditions reflect the density and distribution of dopamine type 1 receptors in this region. Note the dense labeling of the substantia nigra zona reticulata (SNR) and the lower level of labeling in the ventral tegmental area (VTA). The presence of D_1 receptors is also indicated in the dentate gyrus (DG), superficial gray layer of the superior colliculus (SuG) and in lamina VI of the cerebral cortex (VI). (*B*) The labeling of [^{3}H]SCH 23390 associated with a section through the human substantia nigra (SN) is shown in this photomicrograph. Note the very dense labeling indicating a high concentration of dopamine type 1 receptors is associated with this structure in the human brain. (*C*) The autoradiogram shown in this photomicrograph is from a section of rat brain similar to that shown in A but which was labeled with [^{3}H]sulpiride to demonstrate the localization of dopamine type 2 (D_2) receptors in the rat brain. In this instance, the dopamine type 2 receptors are found principally in the substantia nigra zona compacta (SNC). Labeling of both D_1 and D_2 receptors occurs in the ventral tegmental area and in the superficial gray layer of the superior colliculus. Dopamine type 2 receptors are found in the lacunosum moleculare of the hippocampus (LMol) as opposed to the labeling of the dentate gyrus found with the D_1 receptor. (*D*) This autoradiogram reflects the density and distribution of dopamine type 2 receptors in the substantia nigra of the human brain. Note the labeling here is associated with the more dorsal aspects of the substantia nigra indicating a predominance of the receptor in the substantia nigra zona compacta as seen with the rat brain. Bar = 1 mm.

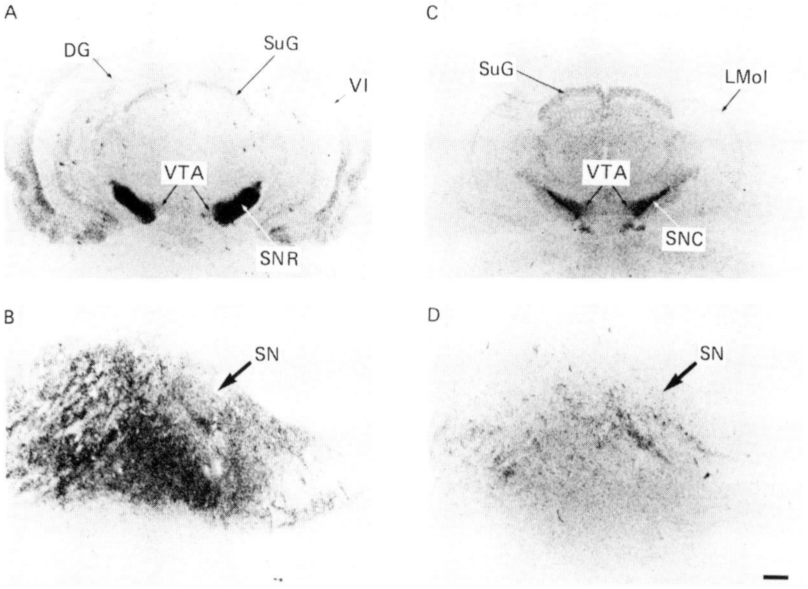

the brain following repeated amphetamine treatment (Schmidt *et al.*, 1985; McCabe *et al.*, 1987a). Amphetamine, which is a dopamine reuptake blocker, presumably results in accumulation of dopamine within the synaptic cleft. This continued stimulation of the dopamine receptors results in the cell down-regulating its receptor density. The studies quoted above have shown that the receptor down-regulation response to amphetamine treatment is an actual change in density (B_{max}) as opposed to an alteration in receptor affinity. Following cessation of the amphetamine exposure, the dopamine receptors not only returned to normal but actually overshot their normal density. This supersensitivity following amphetamine withdrawal could be important in interpreting how the system is influenced by suddenly stopping drugs of this nature. The receptor alterations noted occurred both in dopamine type 1 and dopamine type 2 receptor populations in such regions as the caudate–putamen and substantia nigra. The most predominant changes took place in the nucleus accumbens, olfactory tubercle and entorhinal cortex. Both of these receptor sites are thus probably involved in the functional response to chronic amphetamine exposure.

Tardive dyskinesia is a movement disorder which quite often accompanies antipsychotic treatment (Klawans, 1973). This debilitating disorder is probably the most devastating and one of the more frequent adverse effects of chronically treating schizophrenics with antipsychotics (DeVeaugh-Geiss, 1982) or for that matter any patient subjected to chronic neuroleptic therapy. Many different chemical compounds have been shown to be effective antipsychotics. The one common characteristic these various compounds share is their ability to block the dopamine receptor (Anderson & Kuehnle, 1980). Thus, it would seem to be appropriate that an animal model of tardive dyskinesia would involve chronic neuroleptic or antipsychotic treatment (Klawans *et al.*, 1983). Studies of this nature have recently been undertaken using the autoradiographic technique to analyze the brain tissue from animals subjected to chronic neuroleptic therapy (Filloux *et al.*, 1987). Previous studies in membrane homogenates have indicated that a potent up-regulatory response has been initiated in the animals chronically exposed to antipsychotics (Burt *et al.*, 1977; Clow *et al.*, 1979). With autoradiography, it was possible to discern that not only did up-regulation of the D_2 receptor take place in many regions of the brain including the caudate–putamen but, down-regulation and up-regulation of the D_1 receptor occurred in certain areas of the brain. These observations of up-regulation of receptors are in keeping with the hypothesis that tardive dyskinesia may develop as a consequence of chronic dopamine receptor blockade, in that the dopamine receptors in the basal ganglia may become supersensitive in response to this type of drug exposure. This supersensitivity may become manifest in many other regions of the brain as well. However, because of the high content of dopamine in the basal ganglia, the supersensitivity may eventually override the receptor blockade induced by the antipsychotic, thereby leading to the symptoms of tardive dyskinesia. Furthermore, antipsychotic efficacy would be maintained if one postulated that the receptors being chronically down-regulated were involved in psychotic symptomatology. In any event, it would be necessary to treat tardive dyskinesia by increasing the concentration of the antipsychotic and thereby contribute to a further up-regulation developing in the future. Alternatively, one could treat the movement disorder by administering an anticholinergic for instance, or by withdrawal of the agent. The most effective means of controlling the tardive dyskinesia is to increase the antipsychotic. Perhaps by studying the receptor response, a treatment regime could be worked out where intermittent drug holidays would be utilized to interrupt the development of this receptor supersensitivity while maintaining antipsychotic efficacy. This could, quite possibly, cause a down-regulation of the supersensitive dopamine receptors in such a way that the antipsychotic treatment when reinitiated would be effectively enhanced.

Following Langston's discovery of MPTP (*N*-methyl-4-phenyl-1,2,3,6-tetrahydropyridine) as the causative agent underlying the development of a severe Parkinsonian-like syndrome in a few isolated cases of Californians ingesting synthetic heroin (Langston *et al.*, 1983), many questions have arisen as to the actual involvement of MPTP in the development of Parkinsonism in patients. Apparently, there are certain instances when this compound can be found within the natural environment. MPTP, however, is quite valuable in producing a dopaminergic impairment very similar to Parkinson's disease when laboratory animals are treated with the substance. MPTP lesions of the animal brain may be a suitable model for the study of receptor alterations associated with Parkinson's disease in human patients. Binding sites for a tritiated form of MPTP have been localized by autoradiography (Wieczorek *et al.*, 1984). Receptor autoradiographic techniques have also recently been applied to the localization of dopamine receptor subtypes in MPTP-treated animals (Gupta *et al.*, unpublished data). These studies have shown that dramatic alterations in the density and distribution of dopamine receptors have occurred in response to the lesion. These alterations took place in many brain areas and severe alterations were well defined in the caudate–putamen. Thus, the dopaminergic projection from the substantia nigra to the caudate–putamen was impaired.

Recent studies have demonstrated that the D_2 receptors within the substantia nigra are on catecholamine-containing neurons (Dawson *et al.*, 1986b). When animals are lesioned with the neurotoxin 6-hydroxydopamine, the D_2 receptors diminish within the substantia nigra zona compacta. Ibotenic acid lesions of the striatum (which destroys cell bodies while leaving terminals intact) causes a dramatic loss of dopamine receptor binding within the striatum. These same lesions, however, also cause a loss of dopamine D_1 receptor binding in the substantia nigra. This observation, coupled with the fact that transport of dopamine receptors has been characterized within the striatal-nigral pathway, indicates that there may be pre-synaptic D_1 receptors in the substantia nigra as well. These pre-synaptic receptors are associated with axons emanating from cells within the caudate–putamen. There is some evidence that these pre-synaptic dopamine receptors may be on GABAergic neurons. These types of studies will provide further insight into the wiring of the dopaminergic system, and give us a better appreciation of how and where dopamine receptors may be influencing the nervous system.

It is difficult to define an animal model for which to study attention deficit disorder (ADD), although attempts have been made using selective lesions (Shaywitz *et al.*, 1976). The hyperactive component which often accompanies ADD may be studied, however, in certain animal strains bred for this characteristic (Helmeste & Seeman, 1983). The Fisher 344 rat has been reported to be such a model since these rats apparently have a genetically induced hyperactivity when compared with a Buffalo strain of rats. Studies of membrane homogenates have demonstrated that the dopamine receptors in these animals are supersensitive (Wolfe *et al.*, 1980; Helmeste *et al.*, 1981; Helmeste, 1983; Spirduso *et al.*, 1984). This up-regulation may be in response to a dopamine deficit and thus explain why treating with a stimulant such as amphetamine preferentially affects this system and causes the animals to relax.

Autoradiographic studies of dopamine receptor alterations in ADD are still in progress. However, autoradiographic localization of binding sites for one of the drugs used to treat ADD has been accomplished (Unis, *et al.*, 1985). This compound, methylphenidate (Ritalin), presumably labels a select group of dopaminergic neurons which are involved in ADD. The compound is a dopamine reuptake inhibitor and tritiated methylphenidate was shown to label neurons within the caudate–putamen, olfactory tubercle, nucleus accumbens, the bed nucleus of the stria terminalis and the median eminence. Lower amounts of specific binding were also demonstrated in the frontal cortex and in the dentate gyrus of the hippocampal formation. Studies such as these will provide more insight into possible receptor alterations involved in ADD and hopefully help define an appropriate animal model of the disorder.

14.3.2 *GABA and associated receptors*

γ-aminobutyric acid (GABA) is one of the most widespread inhibitory neurotransmitters in the central nervous system. GABA's most predominant effect is to cause the opening of chloride channels allowing chloride influx into the cell creating a hyperpolarization in the affected neuron (Olsen, 1982). This chloride-sensitive effect is thought to involve only one of the two subtypes of GABA receptor. GABA's chloride-sensitive effect is mediated through a $GABA_A$ receptor whereas a non-chloride-sensitive effect (thus presumably not involving an action at the chloride channel) is mediated through a $GABA_B$ receptor. The $GABA_A$ sites are bicuculline sensitive/baclofen insensitive whereas the $GABA_B$ sites are baclofen sensitive/bicuculline insensitive. The $GABA_A$ sites can be further subdivided into high affinity $GABA_A$ and a low affinity $GABA_A$ sites. Agonists such as muscimol preferentially act on the high affinity $GABA_A$ receptor since their off rate at the low affinity $GABA_A$ receptor is quite rapid. At high enough concentrations and under appropriate conditions, however, muscimol can very effectively label these low affinity sites.

All three of the subtypes of GABA receptors have been localized using autoradiographic techniques (Wamsley *et al.*, 1986, 1987b). Tritiated muscimol was utilized to analyze the density and distribution of high affinity $GABA_A$ sites using conditions which limited the binding of this agonist to the low affinity $GABA_A$ sites (Palacios *et al.*, 1981c). These receptors were widespread throughout the central nervous system being most prevalent in areas such as the superficial laminae of the cerebral cortex, the medial and lateral geniculate bodies, the granule layer of the cerebellum and many thalamic nuclei. Low levels were seen in the caudate–putamen, substantia nigra, zona incerta, the molecular layer of the cerebellum and in the brainstem.

Autoradiographic localization of the low affinity $GABA_A$ sites were accomplished with tritiated bicuculline in the presence of high concentrations of thiocyanate (Olsen *et al.*, 1984a). The anion effectively interfered with the binding of tritiated bicuculline to the high affinity sites, thus revealing the presence of the low affinity sites in the incubated sections. High densities of low affinity $GABA_A$ sites were found in lamina IV of the cerebral cortex, in the cingulate cortex, in the molecular layer of the dentate gyrus, the superficial laminae of the superior colliculus, the hippocampus, the periaqueductal gray matter and the molecular layer of the cerebellum. Lower densities of this $GABA_A$ receptor subtype were found in the granule cell layer of the cerebellum. Thus, there are only a few areas of the brain where the high affinity $GABA_A$ receptors overlap with the low affinity $GABA_A$ receptors. This is in further contrast to the distribution of the $GABA_B$ sites which have been localized using $[^3H]$baclofen (Gehlert *et al.*, 1985b). This receptor subtype is found in the superficial layer of the cerebral cortex, the molecular layer of the cerebellum, interpeduncular nucleus, and the superficial layer of the superior colliculus. Somewhat lower levels were found in many thalamic nuclei, including the medial and lateral geniculate bodies, with only low levels being found in the caudate–putamen, nucleus accumbens, hypothalamus, substantia nigra and the molecular layer of the dentate gyrus. Thus, there appears to be layers where $GABA_B$ receptors exist independently, although there are many areas where both $GABA_A$ and $GABA_B$ receptor subtypes can be found.

Allosteric interactions at the GABA receptor site are thought to involve complex interactions with benzodiazepine, barbiturate and convulsant sites (Olsen, 1981; Supavilai & Karobath, 1984). Thus, the GABA receptor may exist as a macromolecular receptor complex which involves many different components. The benzodiazepines are widely used anxiolytic, anticonvulsant, sedative/hypnotic and muscle relaxant compounds. These drugs are thought to act via their ability to enhance GABAergic inhibition of central nervous system neurons (Tallman *et al.*, 1980). Presence of GABA in the incubation medium can accentuate the binding of benzodiazepines to the receptor sites. Autoradiographic localization of the distribution of benzodiazepine receptors most closely overlaps with that of the low affinity $GABA_A$ site. Results from homogenate studies have also indicated that it appears to be the low affinity $GABA_A$ site which is affiliated with the benzodiazepine receptor action (Olsen & Snowman, 1983).

Two subtypes of benzodiazepine receptor (BZ_1 and BZ_2) have been defined based on several different criteria (Squires, 1983; Richards & Mohler, 1984). The most prevalent type of benzodiazepine receptor is that of the BZ_2 subtype which shows widespread distribution throughout many regions of the central nervous system (Wamsley & Palacios, 1984). The BZ_1 receptor shows a much more unique distribution (Young *et al.*, 1981; Wamsley *et al.*, 1985). The latter receptor is found in highest concentration in lamina IV of the cerebral cortex, the zona incerta and the molecular layer of the cerebellum. These BZ receptor subtypes may be playing different roles in mediating BZ effects. This could have very important pharmacological implications. Differential localization of these receptor subtypes pinpoints specific regions for further study in an attempt to define these potential roles.

The cage convulsant t-butylbicyclophosphorothionate (TBPS) has been labeled (Squires *et al.*, 1983) and successfully employed to analyze the density and distribution of the convulsant sites (Gee *et al.*, 1983; Wamsley *et al.*, 1983). Again, these sites are thought to exist in association with the GABA receptor chloride ionophore complex. The distribution of these sites was very similar to that of the low affinity $GABA_A$ and the benzodiazepine receptors except in the cerebellum where these sites seem to predominate in the granule cell layer as opposed to the molecular layer. Thus, there may be regions where subcomponents of the GABA receptor associated macromolecular receptor complex are not all present.

The presence of these receptor subtypes and their involvement in anxiety and sedation are difficult to study on the basis of animal models. However, chronic exposure to BZ compounds, for instance, does cause a dramatic down-regulation in the receptor density as defined in many different regions of the brain (McCabe *et al.*, 1987b). The role of the GABA receptor macromolecular complex in convulsions, and in animal models of epilepsy, is much more well defined (Olsen *et al.*, 1984b). An inbred strain of seizure-sensitive gerbils has been analyzed by autoradiography to determine how the $GABA_A$ receptors and benzodiazepine receptors respond to this seizure-sensitive state (Olsen *et al.*, 1985, 1986a). Receptor down-regulation of both the low affinity $GABA_A$ and benzodiazepine receptor sites appears to occur in many regions of the seizure-sensitive animal brain when compared to the seizure-resistant strain. This receptor down-regulation has been defined as an actual change in the number of receptors (B_{max}) as opposed to any alteration in receptor affinity. These receptor alterations were most predominant in the substantia nigra of these animals. This is important since GABA-ergic dysfunction in epilepsy has previously been hypothesized to involve the substantia nigra (Iadarola & Gale, 1982; McNamara *et al.*, 1984). Thus, in the seizure-sensitive animal the benzodiazepine receptors are becoming subsensitive and it is necessary to stimulate these receptors with a benzodiazepine compound in order to abort the seizure.

Various kindling models of epilepsy have also been used to define regions where GABAergic function has been altered (McNamara, 1984). Kindling appears to create an ectopic focus in the brain similar to that thought to be involved in epilepsy in humans. As the neurons are kindled to a certain stimulus, they begin to respond more easily to the repeated stimulus (reverse tolerance). Using this paradigm, GABA receptors have been shown to be altered, as determined by autoradiographic techniques, in the dentate gyrus of the hippocampal formation in the kindled vs unkindled animal (Shin et al., 1985). Another model of the convulsions similar to those seen in epilepsy is the audiogenic mice (Olsen *et al.*, 1986b). These genetically inbred mice show seizure activity in response to sound. Again, the receptor alterations that have occurred include down-regulation of the benzodiazepine receptors in the substantia nigra. A study of these models may provide some insight into convulsions and give us a better understanding of how benzodiazepine and GABAergic function are altered in epilepsy.

14.3.3 *Serotonin and norepinephrine receptors*

Both serotonergic and noradrenergic systems are thought to be involved in the etiology of depression (Murphy *et al.*, 1978; Schildkraut, 1978). This hypothesis stems from the fact that the drugs that are used to treat endogenous depression prevent the reuptake of serotonin or norepinephrine into their respective neurons. This increase of norepinephrine or serotonin in the synaptic cleft is thought to alleviate some deficit brought on by the mechanisms involved in depression and ultimately elevate the mood of the affected patient. Likewise, drugs such as Reserpine which deplete serotonin and norepinephrine from nerve terminals can cause a severe depression in the treated patient. The actual recognition sites for the tricyclic antidepressant imipramine (the prototype of the tricyclics) have been localized using the autoradiographic technique (Grabowsky *et al.*, 1983; Rainbow *et al.*, 1982a). These 'uptake inhibiting sites' have been found in many regions of the brain and correspond, in most cases, to areas of known serotonergic innervation. Lesion of the central nervous system with the neurotoxin 5,7-dihydroxytryptamine causes a loss of these imipramine binding sites as determined by autoradiography (Dawson & Wamsley, 1983). Furthermore, the imipramine binding site (or serotonin transport complex) was shown to undergo axonal transport within the medial forebrain bundle of the rat brain and it was also demonstrated that it was synthesized in the neuronal perikarya of dorsal raphe nucleus (Dawson *et al.*, 1985a). Thus, the parent compound imipramine seems to be specific for inhibiting the reuptake of serotonin and these sites are located pre-synaptically on serotonergic terminals. Administration of this compound *in vivo*, however, creates the demethylated form of imipramine known as desipramine.

The latter compound seems to be specific for noradrenergic neurons, since desipramine is a very potent norepinephrine reuptake inhibitor and localization of tritiated desipramine binding sites has allowed the demonstration of their association with noradrenergic terminals, since these sites are lost after 6-hydroxydopamine lesions (Biegon & Rainbow, 1983).

Chronic treatment with tricyclic antidepressants, atypical antidepressants or MAOIs is thought to cause a down-regulation of post-synaptic receptors due to the chronic presence of the neurotransmitter in the synaptic cleft (Charney *et al.*, 1981). This down-regulation has been hypothesized to be involved in the mode of action of the antidepressant compounds since the down-regulation effect very closely follows the time course of efficacy of these compounds. All forms of antidepressant treatment, including ECT (electroconvulsive therapy), appear to involve receptor down-regulation. Drugs which inhibit serotonin reuptake, down-regulate 5-HT_1 and 5-HT_2 receptors whereas drugs which inhibit the reuptake of norepinephrine, down-regulate β-adrenergic receptors. Interestingly, studies with the very potent and specific serotonin reuptake inhibitor fluoxetine have demonstrated that this compound may also be affecting β-adrenergic receptors (Wamsley *et al.*, 1987a). Thus, we may be seeing a 'downstream' phenomenon which involves serotonin affecting noradrenergic neurons which subsequently down-regulate their β-adrenergic receptors. Recent evidence would indicate that the down-regulation of β-adrenergic receptors may be the common denominator involved in the efficacy of antidepressant treatments.

14.3.4 *Muscarinic cholinergic receptors*

Acetylcholine effects in the central nervous system are mediated by two populations of receptors, the muscarinic and nicotinic cholinergic receptors (Krnjevic, 1974). Most of the behavioral effects of cholinergic stimulation in the central nervous system are thought to be mediated through the ubiquitous muscarinic cholinergic receptor subtype. This receptor subtype has been localized throughout the forebrain, brainstem and spinal cord of the mammalian nervous system (Rotter, 1984). Muscarinic receptor blockade has been shown to interfere with normal processing of memory function (Squire & Davis, 1981). Thus, muscarinic receptors may be involved in normal memory as well as being implicated in disorders of memory such as dementia (Bartus *et al.*, 1982; Price *et al.*, 1982).

Autoradiographic techniques have been used to analyze receptor alterations occurring in animals in response to chronic thiamine deficiency (Gehlert *et al.*, 1985a). This deficiency is thought to appear in patients following chronic alcohol abuse. Alcoholics show various symptoms in response to thiamine deficiency including memory loss. Muscarinic receptor up-regulation has been demonstrated in specific regions of the brain in animals made chronically thiamine deficient (animals were fed a thiamine-free diet). Many of these areas are thought to be involved in memory function including the cerebral cortex and the hippocampus. Likewise, other areas of the brain such as the ventromedial hypothalamus (the so-called satiety center) showed a dramatic down-regulation of muscarinic receptors in response to the thiamine deficient diet. Thus, there may be regions of the brain where receptors respond differently to the same stimulus.

Animal models of Alzheimer's disease involve ablation of the nucleus basalis and/or the medial septum (Mash *et al.*, 1985). Receptor autoradiographic techniques have been used to demonstrate dramatic alterations in muscarinic cholinergic receptors in response to these two lesion paradigms. Thus, in accord with the potential animal models, the memory effects associated with dementia may involve a pre-synaptic loss of muscarinic cholinergic receptors accompanied by a post-synaptic supersensitivity which may be transient in nature.

Muscarinic receptors may also be involved in the response of the central nervous system to spinal cord injury (Gehlert *et al.*, 1986). Cervical transection of the spinal cord results in an increase in muscarinic cholinergic receptor density in the ventral horn at lumbar levels. This supersensitivity becomes manifest within two days following the transection and diminishes over a period of 14 days (never quite returning to normal). This receptor supersensitivity then may be involved in the spasticity of lower motor neuron disorders.

14.4 Studies of human postmortem tissues

14.4.1 *Schizophrenia*

Membrane homogenate assays of brain tissues have demonstrated dramatic alterations in many different receptors when the brains of schizophrenic patients are compared to those from normal (patients having died of non-neurological causes) controls (Olsen *et al.*, 1980). These receptor measurements include the demonstration of dopamine receptor alteration as defined by tritiated spiperone binding. Several studies utilizing autoradiographic techniques to analyze these same tissues are currently being undertaken.

14.4.2 *Parkinson's disease*

Autoradiographic localization of dopamine receptors in the brains of Parkinson's disease patients have demonstrated a dramatic down-regulation of dopamine type 1 receptors in the frontal cortex (Dawson *et al.*, 1987). Previous studies in homogenate assays have demonstrated alterations of dopamine receptors in the Parkinsonian patient, however, some of these studies did not differentiate between the D_1 and D_2 receptor populations (Olsen *et al.*, 1980; Bokobza *et al.*, 1984). Other studies have shown no changes in the D_1 receptors of the putamen in Parkinsonian patients (Pimoule *et al.*, 1985); or supersensitive receptors have developed which can be reversed with 1-DOPA treatment (Raisman *et al.*, 1985). Thus, the demonstration of D_1 receptor down-regulation may be a novel finding either involved in the etiology of Parkinson's disease or may be a down-regulation effect in response to treatment of these patients with the precursor to dopamine, 1-DOPA. Very much insight into areas of the brain affected by this disorder or by the treatment of this disorder can be gained from such studies. Likewise, identification of regions affected in Parkinson's disease might be indicated by localization of MPTP binding sites. This has been accomplished in human brain (Javitch *et al.*, 1984).

14.4.3 *Epilepsy*

Binding studies performed in homogenates of brains from epileptic patients have demonstrated alterations in benzodiazepine and GABA receptors in various brain regions. Autoradiographic studies have been accomplished which show the presence of these sites in normal human brain (Young & Kuhar, 1979b; Wamsley *et al.*, 1985a). Other studies already initiated show a trend in down-regulation of benzodiazepine receptors in such regions of the brain as the substantia nigra in patients having suffered from status epilepticus, however, sufficient tissues have not been accumulated in order to show statistical significance (Olsen, McCabe & Wamsley, unpublished observations). Focal epilepsy, on the other hand, may involve specific changes in the temporal lobe of these patients, but these studies have not been performed to date.

14.4.4 *Depression*

Again, the results of binding studies using the autoradiographic technique to examine receptors in brains from chronically depressed patients have not appeared in the literature. Localization of serotonin sites, however, has been accomplished in the normal human brain (Palacios *et al.*, 1983) as have α_2-adrenergic receptors (Probst *et al.*, 1984).

Membrane studies have shown a decrease in imipramine binding sites in the frontal cortex of suicide patients (Stanley *et al.*, 1982). Thus, if one were to hypothesize the existence of an endogenous ligand for the imipramine binding site, the efficacy of this compound may be reduced due to receptor loss in the chronically depressed patient.

14.4.5 *ALS*

Amyotrophic lateral sclerosis (ALS) is a neurological disorder characterized by a progressive degenerative loss of neurons predominantly in the ventral horn of the spinal cord, although other areas of the central nervous system may be involved. Receptor autoradiographic techniques have been utilized to examine various receptor populations in the ventral horn of the spinal cord in the ALS patient vs normal controls (Whitehouse *et al.*, 1983). These studies have demonstrated that a loss of muscarinic cholinergic receptors as well as glycine and benzodiazepine receptors occurs in response to the progression of this disease. Again, these studies may indicate potential therapeutic agents to employ to alleviate some of the symptomatology associated with ALS. However, it is not clear whether the receptor alterations are involved in the disorder or if they are simply occurring secondarily in response to the progress of the disease. Thus, agents of this sort may be useful in treating the symptoms but not the disease. Hopefully, future studies may resolve these issues.

14.4.6 *Alzheimer's disease*

Alzheimer's disease tissues have been examined by autoradiography to show the presence of muscarinic cholinergic receptors associated with neurofibrillary plaques and tangles (Palacios, 1982). Localization of muscarinic receptors in the hippocampus of Alzheimer's disease patients shows that there was not a diminution or focus of muscarinic receptors in association with these plaques, indicating that the tissues involved show no alteration in cholinergic receptors associated with these particular membranes. Additional studies will be necessary to localize possible alterations in muscarinic receptor subtypes as reported in binding assay of membrane preparations (Mash *et al.*, 1985).

14.4.7 *Attention deficit disorder*

ADD with hyperactivity is a disorder predominantly of children which involves alterations in the dopamine system treated by drugs which accentuate dopamine function. Thus, it would be expected that receptor alterations associated with these dopaminergic systems are most likely taking place as the result of the disorder and in response to the treatment of the disorder. Studies with tissues derived from patients with ADD are just being initiated and again nothing has appeared in the literature to date.

14.5 Future directions

Much insight into the alterations in receptors associated with various animal models of human disorders can be gained through the use of autoradiographic techniques. These studies pinpoint regions of the brain for electrophysiologists to probe in order to determine the functional significance of these receptor alterations. Involvement of one receptor subtype over that of another may indicate potential therapeutic agents which could be useful in treating the disorders in human patients. Localization of these receptor alterations in human postmortem tissues also sets the stage for utilizing receptor imaging techniques in living human patients in order to verify various diagnoses. Thus, using positron emission tomography (PET) scanning techniques it may be possible to demonstrate these receptor alterations in patients suffering from the various associated disorders (Wagner *et al.*, 1983; Wong *et al.*, 1984; Frost *et al.*, 1985). Hopefully, further refinement of these receptor localization techniques may make it possible to diagnose the presence of the disorder prior to the development of the debilitating symptoms associated with the disease. This would allow initiation of drug therapy prior to the surfacing of the treatable symptoms and possibly reduce their severity or slow their progress.

Receptor autoradiography techniques have also been extended beyond the level of receptor localization. It is now possible to look within the cell at various populations of enzymes, proteins and other recognition sites. For instance, autoradiographic localization of adenylate cyclase has been accomplished using a tritiated form of the drug forskolin (Gehlert *et al.*, 1984, 1986b). This compound apparently recognizes activated forms of the enzyme adenylate cyclase and thus is useful for quantitating the density and distribution of this enzyme in cells within the central nervous system. It may thus be possible to analyze second messenger effects of various drug treatments and to define how potential enzymatic dysfunctions contribute to disease processes. It has also been possible to localize guanine nucleotide binding proteins using a tritiated form of guanosine triphosphate (GTP) or a tritiated form of the GTP analog guanylyl-5′-imidodiphosphate (Gehlert & Wamsley, 1986). These studies will help assess the regulation, transport, and turnover of receptor complexes within neurons in the central nervous system. Likewise, it has been possible to localize dopamine reuptake inhibiting binding sites using the potent dopamine reuptake inhibitor GBR-12935 (Dawson *et al.*, 1986c). These studies have provided a means of determining which neuronal populations have a potent dopamine reuptake inhibiting system which may be contributing to many neuropsychiatric disorders which involve dopamine dysfunction. This may also indicate regions where similar drugs may be useful in providing a treatment for disorders involving a deficiency in dopamine.

14.6 Conclusion

Autoradiographic methods of receptor localization provide a very powerful tool for the neuroscientist interested in determining the potential sites of drug action in the central nervous system. These studies also provide insight into how neurotransmitter receptors may be affected by various neuropsychiatric disorders and the pharmaceutical agents used to treat those disorders. A wealth of new information from studies accomplished using this methodology is currently available to present investigators. Extending these studies in the future should provide a continual expansion of our realm of understanding and hopefully provide a basis for new discoveries in our various fields of scientific and medical research endeavor.

References

Anderson, W. H. & Kuehnle, J. C. (1980). Treatment of psychosis by rapid neuroleptization: Update 1980. In *Haloperidol Update: 1958–60*, ed. F. J. Ayd, pp. 31–9. Baltimore, MD: Waverly Press, Inc.

Baldessarini, R. J. & Tarsy, D. (1980). Dopamine and the pathophysiology of dyskinesias induced by antipsychotic drugs. *Annu. Rev. Neurosci.*, **3,** 23–41.

Bartus, R. T., Dean, R. L., Beer, B. & Lippa, R. S. (1982). The cholinergic hypothesis of geriatric memory dysfunction. *Science*, **217,** 408–17.

Bell, D. S. (1974). The experimental reproduction of amphetamine psychosis. *Arch. Gen. Psychiatry*, **29,** 35–40.

Biegon, A. & Rainbow, T. C. (1983). Localization and characterization of [^{3}H]-desmethylimipramine binding sites in the rat brain by quantitative autoradiography. *J. Neurosci.*, **3,** 1069–76.

Bokobza, B., Ruberg, M., Scatton, B., Javoy-Agid, F. & Agid, Y. (1984). [^{3}H]-spiperone binding, dopamine and HVA concentrations in Parkinson's disease and supranuclear palsy. *Eur. J. Pharmacol.*, **99,** 167–9.

Burt, D. R., Creese, I. & Snyder, S. H. (1977). Antischizophrenic drugs: Chronic treatment elevates dopamine receptor binding in brain. *Science*, **196,** 326–8.

Charney, D. L., Menkes, D. B. & Heninger, G. R. (1981). Receptor sensitivity and the mechanism of action of antidepressant treatment. *Arch. Gen. Psychiatry*, **38,** 1160–80.

Clow, A., Jenner, P., Theodorou, A. & Marsden, C. D. (1979). Striatal dopamine receptors become supersensitive while rats are given trifluoperazine for six months. *Nature*, **278,** 56–61.

Cortes, R., Probst, A., Tobler, H.-J. & Palacios, J. M. (1986). Muscarinic cholinergic receptor subtypes in the human brain. II. Quantitative autoradiographic studies. *Brain Res.*, **362,** 239–53.

Creese, I., Schneider, R. & Snyder, S. H. (1977). [^{3}H]-SP labels dopamine receptors in pituitary and brain. *Eur. J. Pharmacol.*, **46,** 377–81.

Dawson, T. M., Barone, P., Sidhu, A., Wamsley, J. K. & Chase, T. N. (1986a). Quantitative autoradiographic localization of D-1 dopamine receptors in the rat brain: Use of the iodinated ligand [^{125}I]-SCH 23982. *Neurosci. Lett.*, **68,** 261–6.

Dawson, T. M., Gehlert, D. R., McCabe, R. T., Barnett, A. & Wamsley, J. K. (1986b). D-1 dopamine receptors in the rat brain: A quantitative autoradiographic analysis. *J. Neurosci.*, **6,** 2352–65.

Dawson, T. M., Gehlert, D. R., Snowhill, E. W. & Wamsley, J. K. (1985a). Quantitative autoradiographic evidence for axonal transport of imipramine receptors in the CNS. *Neurosci. Lett.*, **55,** 261–6.

Dawson, T. M., Gehlert, D. R. & Wamsley, J. K. (1986c). Quantitative autoradiographic localization of the dopamine transport complex in the rat brain: use of a highly selective radioligand: [^{3}H]-GBR 12935. *Eur. J. Pharmacol.*, **126,** 171–3.

Dawson, T. M., Gehlert, D. R., Yamamura, H. I., Barnett, A. & Wamsley, J. K. (1985b). D-1 dopamine receptors in the rat brain: Autoradiographic localization using [^{3}H]-SCH 23390. *Eur. J. Pharmacol.*, **108,** 323–5.

Dawson, T. M. & Wamsley, J. K. (1983). Autoradiographic localization of [^{3}H]-imipramine binding sites: Association with serotonergic terminals. *Brain Res. Bull.*, **11,** 325–34.

Dawson, T. M., Whitehouse, P. J., Filloux, F. M. & Wamsley, J. K. (1987). Dopamine D-1 receptors down-regulate in Parkinson's Disease. *Brain Res.*, in press.

DeVeaugh-Geiss, J. (1982). Tardive dyskinesia: Phenomenology, pathophysiology and pharmacology. In *Tardive Dyskinesia and Related Involuntary Movement Disorders*, ed. J. DeVeaugh-Geiss, pp. 1–19. Massachusetts: John Wright PSG, Inc.

Filloux, F. M., Dawson, T. M., Vine, D. & Wamsley, J. K. (1987). Chronic exposure to antipsychotics: alterations in dopamine receptor subtypes. *Brain Res.*, in press.

Frost, J. J., Wagner, H. N., Dannals, R. F., Ravert, H. T., Links, J. M., Wilson, A. A., Burns, H. D., Wong, D. F., McPherson, R. W., Rosenbaum, A. E., Kuhar, M. J. & Snyder, S. H. (1985). Imaging opiate receptors in the human brain by positron tomography. *J. Comput. Assist. Tomogr.*, **9,** 231–6.

Gee, K. W., Wamsley, J. K. & Yamamura, H. I. (1983). Light microscopic autoradiographic identification of picrotoxin/barbiturate binding sites in rat brain with [^{35}S]-t-butyl-bicyclophosphorothionate. *Eur. J. Pharmacol.*, **89,** 323–4.

Gehlert, D. R., Dawson, T. M., Barnett, A., Yamamura, H. I. & Wamsley, J. K. (1986a). Autoradiographic localization of dopamine type-1 receptors after labeling with [^{3}H]-SCH 23390 in the rat and human brain: Comparison with the distribution of D-2 receptors. In *Modulation of Central and Peripheral Transmitter Function*, ed. G. Biggio, P. F. Spano, G. Toffano

& G. L. Gessa, pp. 27–35. FIDIA Research Series, Liviana Press, Padova, Italy.

Gehlert, D. R., Dawson, T. M., Yamamura, H. I. & Wamsley, J. K. (1984). Localization of [^{3}H]-forskolin binding sites in the rat brain using quantitative autoradiography. *Eur. J. Pharmacol.*, **160,** 223–5.

Gehlert, D. R., Dawson, T. M., Yamamura, H. I. & Wamsley, J. K. (1986b). Quantitative autoradiography of [^{3}H]-forskolin binding sites in the rat brain. *Brain Res.*, **361,** 351–60.

Gehlert, D. R., Morey, W. A. & Wamsley, J. K. (1985a). Alterations in muscarinic cholinergic receptor densities induced by thiamine deficiency: Autoradiographic detection of changes in high and low affinity agonist sites. *J. Neurosci. Res.*, **13,** 443–52.

Gehlert, D. R., Yamamura, H. I., Roeske, W. R. & Wamsley, J. K. (1986). Autoradiographic localization of subtypes of muscarinic agonist and antagonist binding sites: Alterations following CNS lesions. In *Biology of Cholinergic Function*, ed. I. Hanin, pp. 65–78. New York: Plenum Press.

Gehlert, D. R., Yamamura, H. I. & Wamsley, J. K. (1985b). $GABA_B$ receptors in the rat brain: Autoradiographic localization using [^{3}H](−)-baclofen. *Neurosci. Lett.*, **56,** 183–8.

Gehlert, D. R. & Wamsley, J. K. (1986). In vitro autoradiographic localization of guanine nucleotide binding sites in sections of rat brain labeled with [^{3}H]-guanylyl-5′-imidodiphosphate. *Eur. J. Pharmacol.*, **129,** 169–74.

Gehlert, D. R. & Wamsley, J. K. (1985). Dopamine receptors in the rat brain: Autoradiographic localization using [^{3}H]-sulpiride. *Neurochem. Int.*, **7,** 717–23.

Gehlert, D. R. & Wamsley, J. K. (1984). Autoradiographic localization of [^{3}H]-sulpiride binding sites in the rat brain. *Eur. J. Pharmacol.*, **98,** 311–12.

Grabowsky, K. L., McCabe, R. T. & Wamsley, J. K. (1983). Localization of [^{3}H]-imipramine binding sites in rat brain by light microscopic autoradiography. *Life Sci.*, **32,** 2355–61.

Helmeste, D. M. (1983). Spontaneous and apomorphine-induced locomotor changes parallel dopamine receptor differences in two rat strains. *Pharmacol. Biochem. Behav.*, **19,** 153–5.

Helmeste, D. M. & Seeman, P. (1983). Genetic differences in brain dopamine receptors and amphetamine response: Possible model for hyperkinetic children. *Prog. Clin. Biol. Res.*, **135,** 401–3.

Helmeste, D. M., Seeman, P. & Coscina, D. V. (1981). Relation between brain catecholamine receptors and dopaminergic stereotypy in rat strains. *Eur. J. Pharmacol.*, **69,** 465–70.

Herkenham, M. & Sokolof, L. (1984). Quantitative receptor autoradiography: Tissue defatting eliminates differential self-absorption of tritium radiation in gray and white matter of brain. *Brain Res.*, **321,** 363–8.

Howlett, D. R., Morris, H. & Nahorski, S. R. (1979). Anomolous properties of ^{3}H-spiperone binding sites in various areas of the rat limbic system. *Mol. Pharmacol.*, **15,** 506–14.

Iadarola, M. J. & Gale, K. (1982). Substantia nigra: Site of anticonvulsant activity mediated by gamma-aminobutyric acid. *Science*, **218,** 1237–40.

Jastrow, T. R., Richfield, E. & Gnegy, M. E. (1984). Quantitative autoradiography of [^{3}H]-sulpiride binding sites in rat brain. *Neurosci. Lett.*, **51,** 47–53.

Javitch, J. A., Uhl, G. R. & Snyder, S. H. (1984). Parkinsonianism-inducing neurotoxin, *N*-methyl-4-phenyl-1,2,3,6-tetra-hydropyridine: Characterization and localization of receptor binding sites in rat and human brain. *Proc. Nat. Acad. Sci. USA*, **81,** 4591–5.

Kebabian, J. W. & Calne, D. B. (1979). Multiple receptors for dopamine. *Nature*, **277,** 93–6.

Klawans, H. W., Goetz, C. G. & Carvey, P. (1983). Animal models of tardive dyskinesia. *Clin. Pharmacol.*, **6,** 129–35.

Klawans, H. L. (1973). The pharmacology of tardive dyskinesias. *Am. J. Psychiatry*, **130,** 82–6.

Krnjevic, K. (1974). Chemical nature of synaptic transmission in vertebrates. *Physiol. Rev.*, **54,** 418–540.

Kuhar, M. J., De Souza, E. B. & Unnerstall, J. R. (1986). Neurotransmitter receptor mapping by autoradiography and other methods. *Annu. Rev. Neurosci.*, **9,** 27–59.

Kuhar, M. J. & Unnerstall, J. R. (1985). Quantitative receptor mapping by autoradiography: Some current technical problems. *Trends Neurosci.*, **8,** 49–53.

Kuhar, M. J., Wamsley, J. K., Palacios, J. M., Niehoff, D. L., Zarbin, M. A. & Unnerstall, J. (1982). Drug and neurotransmitter receptors: Anatomical localization in the brain. In *Pharmacological and Biochemical Aspects of Neurotransmitter Receptors*, ed. H. Yoshida & H. I. Yamamura, pp. 161–74. New York: John Wiley & Sons.

Kuhar, M. J., Young, W. S. III, Palacios, J. M. & Wamsley, J. K. (1980). Radiohistochemistry of drug and neurotransmitter receptors. In *Psychopharmacology and Biochemistry of Neurotransmitter Receptors*, ed. H. I. Yamamura, R. W. Olsen & S. Usdin, pp. 357–80. New York: Elsevier/North Holland.

Langston, J. W., Ballard, P., Tetrud, J. W. & Irwin, I. (1983). Chronic Parkinsonism in humans due to a product of meperidine-analog synthesis. *Science*, **219,** 979–81.

Leysen, J. E., Gommeren, W. & Laduron, P. (1978). Spiperone: A ligand of choice for neuroleptic receptors. No. 1. Kinetics and characteristics of in vitro binding. *Biochem. Pharmacol.*, **27,** 307–16.

Martres, M. P., Bouthenet, M. L., Sales, N., Sokoloff, P. & Schwartz, J. C. (1985). Widespread distribution of brain dopamine receptors evidenced with [^{125}I]-iodosulpride, a highly selective ligand. *Science*, **228,** 752–5.

Mash, D. C., Flynn, D. D. & Potter, L. T. (1985). Loss of M-2 muscarine receptors in the cerebral cortex in Alzheimer's disease in experimental cholinergic denervation. *Science*, **228,** 1115–17.

McCabe, R. T., Hanson, G. R., Dawson, T. M., Wamsley, J. K. & Gibb, J. W. (1987a). Methamphetamine-induced reduction in D-1 and D-2 receptors as evidenced by autoradiography: Comparison with tyrosine hydroxylase activity. *Neurosci.*, in press.

McCabe, R. T., Pulsipher, M. W. & Wamsley, J. K. (1987b). Chronic benzodiazepine (BZ) treatment down-regulates BZ receptors in the mouse brain. *Biochem., Pharmacol., Behav.*, in press.

McNamara, J. O. (1984). Kindling: An animal model of complex partial epilepsy. *Ann. Neurol.*, **16** (Suppl.), S72–6.

McNamara, J. O., Rigsbee, L. C., Galloway, M. T. & Shin, C. (1984). Evidence that activation of substantia nigra is necessary for limbic seizures. In *Neurotransmitters, Seizures and Epilepsy*, vol. 2, ed. R. G. Fariello, P. L. Morselli, K. G. Lloyd, L. F. Quesney & J.Engel, pp. 49–56. New York: Raven Press.

Murphy, D. L., Campbell, I. & Costa, J. L. (1978). Current status of the indoleamine hypothesis of the affective disorders. In *Psychopharmacology: A Generation of Progress*, ed. M. A. Lipton, A. DiMascio & K. F. Killam, pp. 1235–348. New York: Raven Press.

Olsen, R. W. (1981). GABA-benzodiazepine-barbiturate receptor interaction. *J. Neurochem.*, **37,** 1–21.

Olsen, R. W. (1982). Drug interaction at the GABA receptor ionophore complex. *Annu. Rev. Pharmacol. Toxicol.*, **22,** 245–70.

Olsen, R. W., Reisine, T. D. & Yamamura, H. I. (1980). Neurotransmitter receptors – biochemistry and alterations in neuropsychiatric disorders. *Life Sci.*, **27,** 801–8.

Olsen, R. W., Snowhill, E. W. & Wamsley, J. K. (1984a). Autoradiographic localization of low affinity GABA receptors with [^{3}H]-bicuculline methochloride. *Eur. J. Pharmacol.*, **99,** 247–8.

Olsen, R. W. & Snowman, A. M. (1983). [^{3}H]-bicuculline methochloride binding to low affinity GABA receptor sites. *J. Neurochem.*, **41,** 1653–63.

Olsen, R. W., Snowman, A. M., Lee, R., Lomax, P. & Wamsley, J. K. (1984b). Role of the gamma-aminobutyric acid receptor/ionophore complex in seizure disorders. *Annals Neurol.*, **16** (Suppl.), S90–7.

Olsen, R. W., Wamsley, J. K., Lee, R. J. & Lomax, P. (1986a). Benzodiazepine/barbiturate/GABA receptor-chloride ionophore complex in a genetic model for generalized epilepsy. In *Advances in Neurology*, vol. 44, ed. A. V. Delgado-Escueta, A. A. Ward, Jr., D. M. Woodbury & R. J. Porter, pp. 1–14. New York: Raven Press.

Olsen, R. W., Wamsley, J. K., McCabe, R. T., Lee, R. J., Lomax, P. (1985). Benzodiazepine/GABA receptor deficit in the midbrain of the seizure-susceptible gerbil. *Proc. Nat. Acad. Sci., USA*, **82,** 6701–5.

Olsen, R. W., Wamsley, J. K., McCabe, R. T., Lee, R. J., Lomax, P. & Seyfried, T. N. (1986b). Midbrain GABA receptor deficit in genetic animal models of epilepsy. In *Neurotransmitters, Seizures and Epilepsy*, vol. 3, ed. P. L. Morselli. New York: Raven Press. (In press.)

Palacios, J. M. (1982). Autoradiographic localization of muscarinic cholinergic receptors in the hippocampus of patients with senile dementia. *Brain Res.*, **243,** 173–5.

Palacios, J. M., Niehoff, D. L. & Kuhar, M. J. (1981a). Receptor autoradiography with tritium-sensitive film: Potential for computerized densitometry. *Neurosci. Lett.*, **25,** 101–5.

Palacios, J. M., Niehoff, D. L. & Kuhar, M. J. (1981b). ^{3}H-spiperone binding sites in brain: Autoradiographic localization of multiple receptors. *Brain Res.*, **213,** 277–89.

Palacios, J. M., Probst, A. & Cortes, R. (1983). The distribution of serotonin receptors in the human brain: High density of ^{3}H-LSD binding sites in the raphe nuclei of the brainstem. *Brain Res.*, **274,** 150–5.

Palacios, J. M. & Wamsley, J. K. (1983). Microscopic localization of adrenoceptors. In *Adrenoceptors and Catecholamine Action*, Part B, ed. G. Kunos, pp. 295–313. New York: John Wiley & Sons.

Palacios, J. M. & Wamsley, J. K. (1984). Catecholamine receptors. In *Handbook of Chemical Neuroanatomy*, vol. 3, *Classical Transmitters and Transmitter Receptors in the CNS*, Part II, ed. A. Bjorklund, T. Hokfelt & M. J. Kuhar, pp. 325–51. Amsterdam: Elsevier/North Holland.

Palacios, J. M., Wamsley, J. K. & Kuhar, M. J. (1981c). High affinity GABA receptors – autoradiographic localization. *Brain Res.*, **222,** 285–307.

Penney, J. B., Frey, K. & Young, A. B. (1981). Quantitative autoradiography of neurotransmitter receptors using tritium-sensitive film. *Eur. J. Pharmacol.*, **72,** 421–2.

Peroutka, S. J. & Snyder, S. H. (1979). Multiple serotonin receptors: Differential binding of ^{3}H-5-hydroxytryptamine, ^{3}H-lysergic acid diethylamide and ^{3}H-spiroperidol. *Mol. Pharmacol.*, **16,** 687–99.

Peroutka, S. J., U'Prichard, D. C., Greenberg, D. A. & Snyder, S. H. (1977). Neuroleptic drug interactions with norepinephrine alpha receptor binding sites in rat brain. *Neuropharmacol.*, **16,** 549–56.

Pimoule, C., Schoemaker, H., Reynolds, G. P. & Langer, S. Z. (1985). [^{3}H]-SCH 23390 labeled D_1 dopamine receptors are unchanged in schizophrenia and Parkinson's disease. *Eur. J. Pharmacol.*, **114,** 235–7.

Price, D. L., Whitehouse, P. J., Struble, R. G., Clark, A. W., Coyle, J. T., DeLong, M. R. & Hedreen, J. C. (1982). Basal forebrain cholinergic systems in Alzheimer's disease and related dementias. *Neurosci. Comm.*, **1,** 84–92.

Probst, A., Cortes, R. & Palacios, J. M. (1984). Distribution of alpha-2 adrenergic receptors in the human brainstem: An autoradiographic study using ^{3}H-p-amino-clonidine. *Eur. J. Pharmacol.*, **106,** 477–88.

Rainbow, T. C., Biegon, A. & McEwen, B. S. (1982a). Autoradiographic localization of imipramine binding in rat brain. *Eur. J. Pharmacol.*, **77,** 363–4.

Rainbow, T. C., Bleisch, W., Biegon, A. & McEwen, B. S. (1982b). Quantitative densitometry of neurotransmitter receptors. *J. Neurosci. Methods*, **5,** 127–38.

Raisman, R., Cash, R., Ruberg, M., Javoy-Agid, F. & Agid, Y. (1985). Binding of [^{3}H]-SCH 23390 to D-1 receptors in the putamen of control and Parkinsonian subjects. *Eur. J. Pharmacol.*, **113,** 467–8.

Richards, J. G. & Mohler, H. (1984). Benzodiazepine receptors. *Neuropharmacology*, **23,** 233–42.

Rotter, A. (1984). Cholinergic receptors. In *Handbook of Chemical Neuroanatomy*, vol. 3, ed. A. Bjorklund, T. Hokfelt & M. J. Kuhar, pp. 273–303. Amsterdam: Elsevier Science Publishers.

Rupniak, N. M. J., Jenner, P. & Marsden, C. D. (1983). The effect of chronic neuroleptic administration on cerebral dopamine receptor function. *Life Sci.*, **32,** 2289–311.

Scatton, B. & Dubois, A. (1985). Autoradiographic localization of D-1 dopamine receptors in the rat brain with [^{3}H]-SKF 38393. *Eur. J. Pharmacol.*, **111,** 145–6.

Schildkraut, J. J. (1978). Current status of the catecholamine hypothesis of affective disorders. In *Psychopharmacology: A Generation of Progress*, ed. M. A. Lipton, A. DiMascio & K. F. Killam, pp. 1223–34. New York: Raven Press.

Schmidt, C. J., Gehlert, D. R., Peat, M. A., Sonsalla, P. I., Hanson, G. R., Wamsley, J. K. & Gibb, J. W. (1985). Studies on the mechanism of tolerance to methamphetaminc. *Brain Res.*, **343,** 305–13.

Shaywitz, B. A., Yager, R. D. & Klopper, J. H. (1976). Selective brain dopamine depletion in developing rats: An experimental model of minimal brain dysfunction. *Science*, **191,** 305–7.

Shin, C., Pedersen, H. B. & McNamara, J. O. (1985). Gamma-aminobutyric acid and benzodiazepine receptors in the kindling model of epilepsy: A quantitative radiohistochemical study. *J. Neurosci.*, **5,** 2696–701.

Sokoloff, P., Brann, M., Redouane, K., Martres, M. P., Schwartz, J. C., Bouthenet, M. L., Sales, N., Mann, A., Hamdi, P., Wermuth, C. G., Roy,

J. & Morgat, J. L. (1985). The use of [^{3}H](−)-DO 710 as selective dopaminergic ligand for binding and autoradiographic studies. *Eur. J. Pharmacol.*, **107,** 243–51.

Spirduso, W. W., Gilliam, P. & Wilcox, R. E. (1984). Speed of movement initiation performance predicts differences in [^{3}H]-spiroperidol receptor binding in normal rats. *Psychopharmacology*, **83,** 205–9.

Squire, L. R. & Davis, H. P. (1981). The pharmacology of memory: A neurobiological perspective. *Annu. Rev. Pharmacol. Toxicol.*, **21,** 323–56.

Squires, R. F. (1983). Benzodiazepine receptor multiplicity. *Neuropharmacology*, **22,** 1443–50.

Squires, R. F., Casida, J. E., Richardson, M. & Saederup, E. (1983). [^{35}S]-t-butylbicyclophosphorothionate binds with high affinity to brain specific sites coupled to gamma-aminobutyric acid-A and ion recognition sites. *Mol. Pharmacol.*, **23,** 326–36.

Stanley, M., Virgilio, J. & Gershon, S. (1982). Tritiated imipramine binding sites are decreased in the frontal cortex of suicides. *Science*, **216,** 1337–9.

Stoof, J. C. & Kebabian, J. W. (1984). Two dopamine receptors: Biochemistry, physiology and pharmacology. *Life Sci.*, **35,** 2281–96.

Supavilai, P. & Karobath, M. (1984). [^{35}S]-t-butylbicyclophosphorothionate binding sites are constituents of the gamma-aminobutyric acid benzodiazepine receptor complex. *J. Neurosci.*, **4,** 1193–205.

Tallman, J. F., Paul, S. M., Skolnick, P. & Gallager, D. W. (1980). Receptors for the age of anxiety: Pharmacology of the benzodiazepines. *Science*, **207,** 274–81.

Unis, A. S., Dawson, T. M., Gehlert, D. R. & Wamsley, J. K. (1985). Autoradiographic localization of [^{3}H]-methylphenidate binding sites in rat brain. *Eur. J. Pharmacol.*, **113,** 155–7.

Unnerstall, J. R., Niehoff, D. L., Kuhar, M. J. & Palacios, J. M. (1982). Quantitative receptor autoradiography using [^{3}H]-Ultrofilm: Application to multiple benzodiazepine receptors. *J. Neurosci. Meth.*, **6,** 59–73.

Wagner, H. N., Burns, H. D., Dannals, R. F., Wong, D. F., Langstrom, B., Duelfer, T., Frost, J. J., Ravert, H. T., Links, J. M., Rosenbloom, S. B., Lukas, S. E., Kramer, A. V. & Kuhar, M. J. (1983). Imaging dopamine receptors in the human brain by positron tomography. *Science*, **221,** 1264–6.

Wamsley, J. K., Byerley, W. F., McCabe, R. T., McConnell, E., Dawson, T. M. & Grosser, B. I. (1987a). Receptor alterations associated with the use of serotonergic agents: An autoradiographic analysis. *J. Clin. Psychiatry*, **48,** 19–25.

Wamsley, J. K., Gee, K. W. & Yamamura, H. I. (1983). Comparison of the distribution of convulsant/barbiturate and benzodiazepine receptors using light microscopic autoradiography. *Life Sci.*, **33,** 2321–9.

Wamsley, J. K., Gehlert, D. R. & Olsen, R. W. (1986). The benzodiazepine/barbiturate-sensitive convulsant/GABA receptor-chloride ionophore complex: Autoradiographic localization of individual components. In *Benzodiazepine-GABA Receptors and Chloride Channels: Structural and Functional Properties*, ed. R. W. Olsen & J. C. Venter, pp. 299–313. New York: Alan R. Liss.

Wamsley, J. K., Golden, J. S., Yamamura, H. I. & Barnett, A. (1985a). Quazepam, a sedative-hypnotic selective for the benzodiazepine type-1 receptor: Autoradiographic localization in rat and human brain. *Clin. Neuropharmacology*, **8,** Suppl. 1, S26–40.

Wamsley, J. K., Golden, J. S., Yamamura, H. I. & Barnett, A. (1985b).

Autoradiographic demonstration of the selectivity of two 1-N-trifluoroethyl benzodiazepines for the BZD-1 receptors in the rat brain. *Pharmacol. Biochem. Behav.*, **23,** 973–8.

Wamsley, J. K., McCabe, R. T. & Gehlert, D. R. (1987b). Autoradiographic localization of GABA and related receptor subtypes. In *GABA and Benzodiazepine Receptors*, ed. R. F. Squires. New York: CRC Press. (In press.)

Wamsley, J. K., Gee, K. W. & Yamamura, H. I. (1983). Comparison of the distribution of convulsant/barbiturate and benzodiazepine receptors using light microscopic autoradiography. *Life Sci.*, **33,** 2321–9.

Wamsley, J. K. & Palacios, J. M. (1984). Amino acid and benzodiazepine receptors. In *Handbook of Chemical Neuroanatomy*, vol. 3, *Classical Transmitters and Transmitter Receptors in the CNS*, Part II, ed. A. Bjorklund, T. Hokfelt & M. J. Kuhar, pp. 352–85. Amsterdam: Elsevier/North Holland.

Wamsley, J. K. & Palacios, J. M. (1983). Apposition techniques of autoradiography for microscopic receptor localization. In *Current Methods in Cellular Neurobiology*, ed. J. L. Barker & J. F. McKelvy, pp. 241–68. New York: John Wiley & Sons.

Whitehouse, P. J., Lynch, D. & Kuhar, M. J. (1984). Effects of postmortem delay in temperature on neurotransmitter receptor binding in a rat model of the human autopsy process. *J. Neurochem.*, **43,** 553–9.

Whitehouse, P. J., Wamsley, J. K., Zarbin, M. A., Price, D. L., Tourtellotte, W. W. & Kuhar, M. J. (1983). Amyotrophic lateral sclerosis: Alteration in neurotransmitter receptors. *Ann. Neurol.*, **14,** 8–16.

Wieczorek, C. M., Parsons, B. & Rainbow, T. C. (1984). Quantitative autoradiography of [^{3}H]-MPTP binding sites in rat brain. *Eur. J. Pharmacol.*, **98,** 453–4.

Wolfe, M. D., Wilcox, R. E., Riffee, W. H. & Abraham, L. D. (1980). Strain difference in dopamine receptor function in the initiation of movement. *Pharmacol. Biochem. Behav.*, **13,** 5–7.

Wong, D. F., Wagner, H. N., Dannals, R. F., Links, J. M., Frost, J. J., Ravert, H. T., Wilson, A. A., Rosenbaum, A. E., Gjedde, A., Douglass, K. H., Petronis, J. D., Folstein, M. F., Toung, J. K. T., Burns, H. D. & Kuhar, M. J. (1984). Effects of age on dopamine and serotonin receptors measured by positron tomography in the living human brain. *Science*, **226,** 1393–6.

Young, W. S. & Kuhar, M. J. (1979a). A new method for receptor autoradiography: [^{3}H]-opioid receptors in the rat brain. *Brain Res.*, **179,** 255–70.

Young, W. S. & Kuhar, M. J. (1979b). Autoradiographic localization of benzodiazepine receptors in brains of humans and animals. *Nature*, **280,** 393–5.

Young, W. S., Niehoff, D. L., Kuhar, M. J., Beer, B. & Lippa, A. S. (1981). Multiple benzodiazepine receptor localization by light microscopic radiohistochemistry. *J. Pharmacol. Exp. Ther.*, **216,** 425–30.

15

Brain tissue transplantation: applications to neurological research

Stephen B. Dunnett and Anders Björklund

15.1 Introduction

The transplantation of nervous tissue into the adult central nervous system has been attempted sporadically since the 1870s (see Table 15.1), but a hundred years passed before the conditions for the achievement of reliable graft survival and growth were determined (Olson & Malmfors, 1970; Das & Altman, 1971, 1972; Björklund & Stenevi, 1971; Olson & Seiger, 1972; Stenevi *et al.*, 1976). The key factors for graft viability in the CNS of adult recipants appeared to be:

(i) The use of CNS tissue taken from embryonic or neonatal donors within a limited ontogenetic time 'window', which needs to be determined experimentally for any particular population of graft neurons (Seiger, 1985).

(ii) The selection or artificial creation of a host CNS target site which is adequately vascularized for the rapid incorporation of the graft tissue into the host vascular and cerebrospinal fluid circulation (Stenevi *et al.*, 1980).

(iii) Immunological factors appear to be of lesser importance than is the case for peripheral organ transplants into sites outside the CNS. The brain has been described as an 'immunologically privileged site', and although this privilege is not complete, rejection of neuronal grafts taken from animals of the same species is generally weak in the CNS (Mason *et al.*, 1985). Thus, at least in studies of transplants between rats of the same strain, the occasional failures of graft survival are more likely to be attributable to infection introduced in surgery or a failure of adequate vascularization of the grafts rather than a specific immunological rejection.

Based on these principles, a variety of grafting procedures have been used in the mammalian CNS, which are well reviewed in the methodological chapters 2–8 of Björklund & Stenevi (1985a).

In the decade from 1970 to 1980, an increasing number of studies used these techniques to study growth and regenerative processes in the CNS (see Björklund & Stenevi, 1979a) confirming that neuronal regeneration is not inevitably abortive in the adult mammalian brain (Cajal, 1928). However, the widespread current interest in intracerebral transplantation techniques for the study of processes underlying neurological damage and recovery probably began with the first demonstrations, in 1979, that grafts of embryonic dopamine-rich tissue could have beneficial functional consequences for animals with dopamine-depleting lesions (Björklund & Stenevi, 1979b; Perlow *et al.*, 1979).

Applications of CNS transplantation to neurological research have essentially been concerned with several related issues:

Table 15.1. *Early history of neural grafting in the mammalian CNS*

Date	Author	Location	Observation
1890	W. G. Thompson	New York, USA	First attempt to graft adult CNS tissue to the brain
1898	J. Forssman	Lund, Sweden	First report of neurotrophic effects of grafted tissue
1907	G. Del Conte	Naples, Italy	First attempt to graft embryonic tissues to the brain
1909	W. Ranson	Chicago, USA	First successful grafting of spinal ganglia to the brain
1911	F. Tello	Madrid, Spain	First successful grafting of peripheral nerve to the brain
1917	E. Dunn	Chicago, USA	First successful grafting of neonatal CNS to the brain
1921	Y. Shirai	Tokyo, Japan	First demonstration of brain as an immunologically privileged site
1924	G. Faldino	Pisa, Italy	First successful grafting of foetal CNS to the anterior eye chamber
1940	W. E. LeGros Clark	Oxford, UK	First successful grafting of foetal CNS to the neonatal brain
1957	B. Flerko and J. Szentagothai	Pecs, Hungary	First successful intraventricular grafting of endocrine tissue
1970 & 1971	Olson & Seiger, Das & Altman, Björklund & Stenevi		First reports of conditions for reliable transplantation to the brain and anterior eye chamber

From Björklund & Stenevi (1985b).

(i) What is the extent and limitations of regenerative capacity in the adult mammalian CNS?
(ii) Under what conditions can intracerebral grafts ameliorate functional impairments, whether as a consequence of genetic defect, trauma or disease?
(iii) The use of transplantation to develop and refine animal models of neurological disorders.
(iv) The determination of conditions under which transplants might provide a viable clinical treatment of neurological disorders.

15.2 Application to CNS regeneration

Following the detailed studies by Cajal (1928) of the morphological changes that take place in neurons following damage, it became widely accepted that effective regeneration does not take place in the adult mammalian brain. Whereas severed axons might initially give rise to growth cones, the process was generally abortive and no effective reconnection of deafferented targets could be demonstrated.

This pessimistic conclusion was challenged by Raisman (1969), who showed that the phenomenon of axonal sprouting and synaptogenesis, which is well known in the periphery, can also be demonstrated in the CNS. Thus, lesion of one major set of afferents to the septum, in either the fimbria or the medial forebrain bundle, resulted in acute degeneration of synaptic connections onto the soma and dendrites of septal neurons. However, connections reformed over subsequent months, as demonstrated by counting the distribution and type of synapses in the septum, which could be best attributed to sprouting of collateral terminals into vacated post-synaptic sites from axons of the unlesioned set of afferents. This was then confirmed by mapping the pattern of degeneration following further lesions to the previously spared axons.

So is the limited regeneration generally seen in the CNS related to limitations in the sprouting capacity of central neurons, an inability of central tissue to support extensive axonal elongation, an absence of trophic and growth factors in the CNS, or some more general influence such as susceptibility to the formation of astrocytic or other glial barriers following injury? Considerable information on these topics has been derived from CNS transplantation studies in mammals.

In one influential series of studies, Olson & Malmfors (1970) found that peripheral sympathetic neurons implanted into the anterior eye chamber would readily reinnervate the iris if denervated of its adrenergic input from host ciliary ganglion. They went on to show that (central) locus coeruleus neurons had a similar capacity if the grafts were taken from embryonic donors (Olson & Seiger, 1972). Moreover, adult central adrenergic neurons have a similar sprouting capacity following damage. Intracerebral grafts of iris or smooth muscle tissues (Björklund & Stenevi, 1971; Stenevi *et al.*, 1973) placed into the medial forebrain bundle attract an extensive reinnervation from the ascending noradrenergic fibres. Thus the limited regeneration seen in adult mammalian CNS does not appear to be due primarily to a lack of growth potential of central neurons *per se*.

Perhaps then CNS tissue provides poor support for regenerating axons in the CNS, in contrast to the support and guidance provided by the Schwann cells of the peripheral nervous system. Evidence for such a view comes from the studies of Aguayo and colleagues. Thus, David & Aguayo (1981) used a sciatic nerve graft to provide a peripheral nerve 'bridge' between the medulla and lower cervical or upper thoracic spinal cord. Central axons were seen to grow extensively (up to 3 cm) through this peripheral nerve environment, but on re-entry to CNS at the far end of the graft only limited further growth was seen (no more than 2 mm). Although in these studies the spinal cord was intact, similar observations were made by Richardson *et al.* (1982) when the sciatic graft was inserted between the two stumps of the transected cord.

However, the limited regrowth potential of central axons in the adult mammalian CNS is not absolute: the key development in intracerebral grafting techniques was the observation that foetal CNS tissue had a much greater survival and growth capacity (Olson & Seiger, 1972; Das, 1974; Stenevi *et al.*, 1976). Thus embryonic adrenergic or cholinergic neurons grafted to a cavity adjacent to the hippocampus can provide an extensive reinnervation of the host brain (Björklund & Stenevi, 1977). In particular, the regrowing fibres establish a terminal laminar distribution in the hippocampus that is fully appropriate for the particular transmitter-specific populations of grafted neurons (Björklund *et al.*, 1976).

An intriguing feature of graft-derived reinnervation is that rather than always taking place, its extent and pattern is determined by the status of the intrinsic host innervation and a variety of host-derived trophic and growth factors. Thus, for example, although the pattern of noradrenergic fibres reinnervating hippocampal targets mimics the normal noradrenergic innervation, extensive growth is only achieved following additional cholinergic deafferentation, suggesting a separate regulation of the extent of growth and its guidance (Björklund *et al.*, 1976; Björklund & Stenevi, 1981).

The mechanisms by which this and other trophic and guidance

influences are exerted in the CNS is currently an area of active research in which most of the relevant factors are yet to be identified. Thus, nerve growth factor appears to have a stimulatory effect on the differentiation and outgrowth of peripheral adrenergic graft tissues (chromaffin cells) in the CNS (Strömberg *et al.*, 1985) or of the extent of growth of central adrenergic fibres into grafts (Stenevi *et al.*, 1974), and can influence the pre-synaptic biochemical activity in grafted central cholinergic neurons (Toniolo *et al.*, 1985), but it does not appear to be crucial for the survival or growth of most other CNS graft tissues. Similarly, the ganglioside GM_1, which has been suggested to inhibit degeneration and stimulate sprouting of lesioned nigrostriatal dopamine neurons (Agnati *et al.*, 1983), does not appeared to have any detectable stimulatory effect on dopamine fibre outgrowth from grafted nigral neurons (Freed, 1985).

Rapid progress might be expected in the identification of diffusable factors important in CNS regeneration. Nieto-Sampedro *et al.* (1983) have extracted fractions from wound fluids and adjacent tissues after making aspirative cavities in the rat entorhinal cortex that have a marked survival influence on peripheral ganglionic cells maintained in culture. This 'neuronotrophic' activity reaches a peak 1–2 weeks following the lesion, which was also seen to correlate with the optimal time course for survival and growth of striatal cholinergic neurons implanted into the adult rat hippocampus. It is likely that many rather than a single such factor will be shown to be of importance. Thus, Lindsay (1979) found that astrocytes taken from the lesioned rat brain can enable the *in vitro* survival of both sensory and sympathetic neurons, which was blocked by anti-NGF treatment in the latter but not the former population of cells, suggestisng the influence of at least two diffusible factors.

15.3 Application to functional recovery

As indicated above, functionally beneficial effects of intracerebral grafts for the host animal were first demonstrataed in rats with nigrostriatal dopamine lesions, made with the neurotoxin 6-hydroxydopamine (6-OHDA). A unilateral lesion of these neurons produces a marked behavioural asymmetry, in which the rat has a spontaneous postural bias to the ipsilateral side and a neglect of contralateral stimuli of all sensory modalities (Ungerstedt, 1971a; Marshall *et al.*, 1974). A major advantage of this model system is that the motor asymmetry can be enhanced by dopaminergic drugs producing a 'rotation' response in which the rat turns in tight head-to-tail circles at a high rate, which is easily quantified (Ungerstedt, 1971a,b).

Perlow *et al.* (1979) showed that embryonic dopamine cells implanted in the lateral ventricle adjacent to the deafferented neostriatum reduced the contralateral rotation following injections of the agonist apomorphine by about 40%, which was attributed to a reduction of receptor supersensitivity in the host neostriatum following reinnervation from the grafts. More directly, (Björklund & Stenevi (1979b), working with nigral grafts placed in a cortical cavity on the dorsal surface of the denervated striatum, found that the ipsilateral turning induced by the presynaptic stimulant amphetamine was also reversed, and in some animals completely so. These results have been amply confirmed subsequently (Freed *et al.*, 1980; Björklund *et al.*, 1980; Dunnett *et al.*, 1981a, 1983a; Freed, 1983). Moreover, graft-derived recovery is not restricted to drug-induced behaviours, since postural bias, ipsilateral turning while activated by stressors such as tail pinch, side bias in T-maze exploration and contralateral sensory neglect can all be ameliorated by dopamine-rich grafts (Björklund *et al.*, 1980; Dunnett *et al.*, 1981a,b, 1983a).

How might such behavioural recovery following transplantation take place? We have recently proposed a hierarchy of potential levels of reorganization that might take place following introduction of a neural transplant into the damaged CNS (see Table 15.2), against which any particular model system might be assessed (Dunnett *et al.*, 1987).

It is unlikely that the functionally beneficial effects of dopamine grafts is mediated by a completely non-specific action (level 1) since the pattern of recovery is dependent on graft placement and mimics the intrinsic topographic organization of the intact striatal system (Dunnett *et al.*, 1981b, 1983a). However, it has been suggested that the grafts do exert a pharmacological (level 2) action on the host brain, by diffuse release of the transmitter into the denervated neostriatum (Freed *et al.*, 1980). This view gains support from the great compensatory plasticity seen in the intrinsic nigrostriatal system following damage (Stricker & Zigmond, 1976), and the pharmacological amelioration of symptoms that can be induced by dopaminergic drugs such as l-DOPA or apomorphine (Marshall & Ungerstedt, 1976; Ungerstedt & Ljungberg, 1976; Marshall & Gotthelf, 1979), and might well apply to the diffuse release of dopamine from adrenal chromaffin cell grafts implanted into the denervated neostriatum (Freed *et al.*, 1981; Strömberg *et al.*, 1985). However, there are strong indications that grafts of embryonic nigral dopamine cells not only provide a tonic reinnervation (level 3) such that the extent of behavioural recovery correlates well with the extent of fibre ingrowth (Björklund *et al.*, 1980; Schmidt *et al.*, 1983), but also they become reciprocally influenced (level 4) by host brainstem systems, including the ascending monoaminergic systems originating in the locus coeruleus and raphe nucleus (Arbuthnott *et al.*, 1985). Nevertheless, functional recovery is not complete in the grafted rats, and in particular there has been a repeated failure to reverse with dopamine-rich grafts the regulatory eating and drinking impairments induced by bilateral dopamine denervation (Dunnett *et al.*, 1981c, 1983b).

Since the studies in rats with nigrostriatal dopamine lesions suggest a degree of reorganization beyond the level which might be sufficient to achieve functional amelioration of the lesion symptoms, it is instructive to consider other model systems, involving different levels of intrinsic organization and requiring different levels of reorganization for functional recovery. Perhaps, the simplest type of reorganization might be expected to be provided by neuroendocrine systems where some amelioration could be achieved by diffuse release of neurohormones and other active substances into the host parenchyma, blood or cerebrospinal fluid circulation. In one such model, Gash *et al.* (1980) have reported that vasopressin-rich hypothalamic tissue grafted to the third ventricle can,

Table 15.2. *Levels of anatomical reorganization by intracerebral grafts*

Level	Definition
1. Non-specific consequences	Transplantation provokes changes in the host brain of a nature unrelated to the graft tissue or its location, e.g. the trophic stimulation of host reorganization
2. 'Pharmacological' action	The grafts secrete biologically active molecules into host parenchyma, vasculature or cerebro spinal fluid circulation, which exert their effects by diffuse action
3. 'Tonic' reinnervation	The grafts establish a partial or complete reinnervation of denervated host targets, and restore a tonic but unregulated activation of those targets
4. Reciprocal reinnervation	In addition to reinnervation of the host, the grafts come under host influence, either by diffuse hormonal regulation or by collateral reinnervation
5. Full reconstruction	The grafts not only establish full reciprocal connections with the host brain, but additionally develop an internal organization and physiological activity appropriate for the populations of intrinsic cells they replace

After Dunnett *et al.* (1987).

at least temporarily, ameliorate the polyuria and polydipsia of the diabetes insipidus Brattleboro rat which has a genetic vasopressin deficiency. Even in this case, the grafts undergo a degree of appropriate reorganization, in that fenestrated portal capilliaries invade ventral portions of the grafts and establish neurovascular zones (Scott & Sherman, 1984), suggesting that graft–host interactions may be quite specific rather than functioning at a completely diffuse level.

Even though a degree of caution must be applied to interpreting the functioning changes taking place in the Brattleboro graft model (Scott & Sherman, 1984; Richards *et al.*, 1985), there are other reports of even more dramatic functional effects of grafts in conditions of neuroendocrine deficiency. For example, mice of the mutant hypogonadal (hpg) strain have an autosomal genetic deficiency of hypothalamic gonadotrophin-releasing hormone (GnRH), resulting in a failure of gonadal development. The hypogonadism of hpg mice has been reversed not only by systemic injections of GnRH, but also by hypothalamic implantation of foetal GnRH-rich preoptic neurons (Krieger *et al.*, 1982). The grafts not only re-establish normal development of the ovaries and uterus in females and of the testicles in males, but reinstate normal mating behaviour, at least in females, to the point of pregnancy and normal birth (Gibson *et al.*, 1984). Although it might be possible to achieve such effects by diffuse secretion of GnRH into host CSF, in this case also the grafts were seen to give rise to GnRH-positive fibres innervating the normal host targets in the lateral median eminence (Silverman *et al.*, 1985).

Thus, although neuroendocrine grafts might be able to exert functional effects via some diffuse release mechanism, in fact in those cases which have been studied this does not seem to be the case: rather the grafts appear to re-establish appropriate specialized connections with the host capillary network, suggesting at least a level 3 pattern of reorganization.

At the other end of the spectrum of complexity are several recent studies of functional effects following transplantation in more precisely organized neuronal systems. Thus grafted retinae which survive and establish connections with the host brain show appropriate graded physiological responses to light (Freed & Wyatt, 1980; Lund & Simons, 1985) and elicit specific responses in cells of the host susperior colliculus (Lund & Simons, 1985), although there are as yet no suggestions that such grafts can restore any features of normal vision.

In another series of experiments, Isacson *et al.*, (1984, 1986) have demonstrated the capacity of embryonic striatal cells to emeliorate both conditioned and unconditioned impairments that follow neurotoxic lesions of the neostriatum. As part of the 'prefrontal system' (Rosvold, 1972; Divac *et al.*, 1978), striatal lesions disconnect the cortical control of complex performance of tasks such as T-maze alternation from motor, in particular pallidal, output systems, Thus, the recovery of alternation impairments in the host animals with striatal grafts, and the indication that the grafts may receive inputs from host thalamus and substantia nigra as well as reforming some efferent connections with the host pallidum and substantia nigra (Pritzel *et al.*, 1985), suggests that the grafts may be providing a more extensive reconstruction of damaged host circuitries than previously was suspected to be possible.

15.4 Application to the development of animal models

In addition to the recent interest in the extent and limitations of functional recovery that can be achieved with intracerebral grafts, there has been an increasing use of the technique as a complement to lesions in the development of animal models of brain function and pathology. In certain situations, the use of intracerebral transplants can yield a degree of specificity that is difficult to achieve with lesion procedures alone. This application can be illustrated with three examples.

Since the phenomenon was first described by Olds & Milner (1954), intracranial self-stimulation (ICSS) has been widely studied as a potential means of direct access to the central mechanisms of motivation and reward (Hall *et al.*, 1977). One consistent theme has been the suggestion that ascending catecholamine pathways can provide a sufficient substrate for ICSS, and yet the direct demonstration of this hypothesis has proved extremely difficult. Thus, although the effective central sites for ICSS are distributed along the major ascending catecholamine pathways of the brain, many other ascending and descending axons run together in the medial forebrain bundle with those catecholamine systems. Moreover, whereas lesions or drugs which disrupt ascending dopamine pathways do block ICSS, this could be attributable to the motor impairments produced by the treatment. Fray *et al.* (1982) grafted embryonic substantia nigra to a site in the dorsal parietal cortex, from which an extensive striatal reinnervation of dopamine fibres was established. Electrodes were implanted into the graft, which was found to be an effective site for ICSS, whereas control grafts of non-nigral tissue were ineffective. Since the electrodes in this artificial 'nigro'-striatal pathway were distant from any effective ICSS site in the host brain, and the rate of responding in individual animals was directly related to the proximity between the electrode tip and dopamine neurons in the grafts, this study provides strong evidence in support of the hypothesis that dopamine neurons in the brain can provide a sufficient substrate for self-stimulation.

A second example comes from aging research. The aging brain manifests a decline in many different neurotransmitters, including the monoaminergic and cholinergic systems (McGeer, 1981), which may underlie some aspects of the declining sensory, motor or cognitive capacities of aged animals. And yet most information of the involvement of individual transmitter systems, in particular patterns of impairment, is correlative and indirect. A number of studies have recently treated aging as providing an implicit lesion, and then investigated whether grafts rich in individual transmitter-specific neuronal types can ameliorate any of the aged animals' impairments (Gage *et al.*, 1983a). Thus Gage and colleagues have shown that dopamine-rich nigral grafts innervating the aging neostriatum provide a significant amelioration of the host animals' motor coordination impairments (Gage *et al.*, 1983b), whereas acetylcholine-rich septal grafts innervating the hippocampus restore aspects of cognitive (spatial maze) learning abilities (Gage *et al.*, 1984). This dissociation was specific to the task, cell type and transplantation site, supporting hypotheses of the aged animals' impairments that could be suggested from lesion studies in young animals.

A related application to the interpretation of correlations in aging rats is the interpretation of the effects of lesions in young animals. Thus, recent interest in aging, and in particular the neuropathological presenile dementia of Alzheimer's disease, has focused on a potential decline in forebrain cholinergic systems as underlying the cognitive impairments of dementia (Drachman & Leavitt, 1974; Bartus *et al.*, 1982; Coyle *et al.*, 1983). The extrinsic cholinergic innervation of the neocortex arises from the diffuse nucleus basalis magnocellularis (NBM) cell group in the ventral forebrain. in agreement with the cholinergic hypothesis of aging, lesions of this nucleus in rats produce a range of learning and memory impairments in rats that might be considered to mimic the cognitive disruption seen in demented patients. However, the major difficulty with this line of reasoning is that, in the absence of any specific cholinergic neurotoxin, it is not possible to achieve destruction of the NBM cell group without also sustaining extensive damage of cell groups in the ventral pallidum and lateral diencephalon. This non-specific damage might fully account for the impairments manifested by the lesioned rats. However, it has recently been shown that grafts of ventral forebrain cholinergic cells implanted into the deafferented neocortex can ameliorate many of the lesioned rats' impairments, not just in passive avoidance tests of their memory capacity but also in the precision of their spatial learning abilities and in some aspects of sensorimotor performance (Fine *et al.*, 1985; Dunnett *et al.*, 1985). Control grafts of non-cholinergic tissue into the neocortex or of cholinergic tissue into subcortical sites did not produce any similar recovery, suggesting that several aspects of the lesion syndrome are indeed attributable to disruption of the cholinergic innervation of the neocortex. However, this system appears to be implicated not simply in the rats' memory performance but also in a wide range of cortical functions.

15.5 Potential application to clinical practice

In the six years since the first reports of functional benefits for the host animal (Perlow *et al.*, 1979; Björklund & Stenevi, 1979b), the functional consequences of intracerebral grafts has been investigated in a wide range of animal models of neurological disease, some of which have been described above. Even in the first of these studies, Perlow *et al.* (1979) suggested that intracerebral transplantation might provide a radical new clinical treatment for neurodegenerative conditions such as Parkingson's disease, and recently the first such clinical trials, using autografts of the patients' own adrenal chromaffin cells, have been attempted (Backlund *et al.*, 1985). In these two patients, some acute benefits were seen in the reduction both of symptoms and of the maintenance doses for pharmacological therapy. However, the effects were not as dramatic or sustained as might have been hoped, and there is no evidence that the grafts showed long-term survival. As emphasized by Freed (1984), a number of theoretical and practical issues need to be resolved before it can be determined whether such procedures have the potential for continuing clinical application:

(i) Is the aetiology of Parkinson's disease, or other neurodegenerative conditions in which clinical transplantation might be considered, such that grafted tissues might be expected to survive and reverse the symptoms?
(ii) What might be a socially and ethically acceptable source of viable donor tissue?
(iii) What immunological constraints are imposed on alternative sources of donor tissue?
(iv) What practical techniques are required to achieve effects in the primate or human brain comparable to those achieved in rodent studies?

Although these questions are all unresolved at the present time, each is an area of active investigation and potentially amenable to solution.

Firstly, it is not yet clear whether aetiological factors might preclude transplantation as a viable approach. Although post-encephalitic parkinsonism is of viral origin, and the recent description of a similar disease state following injection of the heroin analogue 1-methyl-4-phenyl-1,2,5,6-tetrahydropyridine (Langston *et al.*, 1983) is clearly also due to an external toxic agent, the cause of idiopathic Parkinson's disease remains unidentified. This raises two problems. It may turn out to be the case that grafted dopamine cells are subject to the same assault as the patient's intrinsic dopamine system. Additionally, although parkinsonism is characterized by a specific dopaminergic decline in the early stages of the disease, it progressively involves more widespread neuronal degeneration in the forebrain. If this generalized degeneration is independent of, rather than secondary to, the primary dopaminergic deficit, then specific replacement of dopamine neurons would not be expected to halt the progressive course of the disease. This issue remains unsolved, and indeed further insights might first be derived from the viability of transplantation therapy itself.

Secondly, if Parkinson's disease or another neurological disorder is amenable to clinical transplantation, appropriate sources of donor tissue need to be identified. From animal studies, it seems that the optimal source would be the homotypic populations of cells lost in the disease taken from embryonic donors of the same species. However, the use of human foetal material for transplantation purposes remains an ethically controversial issue in most countries, and the social acceptability of such an approach is not yet clear. With this in mind, several studies have investigated alternative peripheral sources of catecholaminergic neurons, in particular the chromaffin cells of the adrenal medulla, and demonstrated some success in ameliorating impairments induced by central dopamine depletions in rats (Freed *et al.*, 1982; Strömberg *et al.*, 1985). Since peripheral nervous tissue will survive grafting in adulthood, it might then be possible to use autografts of the patient's own adrenal tissue, avoiding both the ethical difficulties and overcoming potential problems of immunolgical rejection. This was the procedure adopted by Backlund *et al.* (1985) in the first clinical trials. However, adrenal tissue does not provide as extensive growth or functional recovery as embryonic nigral tissue, and the degree of phenotypic plasticity in mature, as opposed to young adult, adrenal tissue may have been overemphasized (Freed. 1983).

Other alternatives, such as use of cross-species foetal cells, might also be considered, and embryonic mouse tissue has been shown to survive in rats and to be functional in some behavioural tests (Björklund *et al.*, 1982; Daniloff *et al.*, 1985). However, transplantation across such histocompatibility barriers does induce substantial, even if not complete, immunological rejection (Mason *et al.*, 1985), and again the functional effects are weaker than can be achieved with allografts. These studies highlight the importance of determining with greater precision the extent and limitations of immunological privilege in the CNS, in primates as well as in rodents.

In addition to these theoretical considerations, a number of practical issues are likely to be encountered in transferring data derived from rodent studies to the primate or human brain, including the selection of appropriate cell distribution in the host brain and 'scaling' factors (Freed, 1984). Most immediately, there is now the need for the detailed consideration of the functional effects of alternative sources of donor tissue and graft placements in primate models of dopamine denervation (Morihisa *et al.*, 1984; Patel-Vaidya *et al.*, 1985).

Although many practical questions remain, it is plausible that the biological principles underlying viable transplantation of neural tissues in the human brain may be explicated during the next decade, making available a radically new therapeutic approach to some previously-intractable neurological disorders.

References

Agnati, L. F., Fuxe, K., Calza, L., Benfenati, F., Cavicchioli, L., Toffano, G. & Goldstein, M. (1983). Gangliosides increase the survival of lesioned nigral dopamine neurons and favour the recovery of dopaminergic synaptic function in striatum of rats by collateral sprouting. *Acta Physiol. Scand., suppl.*, **119,** 347–63.

Arbuthnott, G., Dunnett, S. B. & MacLeod, N. (1985). Electrophysiological recording from nigral transplants in the rat. *Neurosci. Lett.*, **57,** 205–10.

Backlund, E.-O., Granberg, P.-O., Hamberger, B., Knutson, E., Martensson, A., Sedvall, G., Seiger, Å. & Olson, L. (1985). Transplantation of adrenal medullary tissue to striatum in parkinsonism. First clinical trials, *J. Neurosurg.*, **62,** 169–73.

Bartus, R. T., Dean, R. L., Beer, B. & Lippa, A. S. (1982). The cholinergic hypothesis of geriatric memory dysfunction. *Science*, **217,** 408–17.

Björklund, A. & Stenevi, U. (1971). Growth of central catecholamine neurons into smooth muscle grafts in the rat mesencephalon. *Brain Res.*, **31,** 1–20.

Björklund, A. & Stenevi, U. (1977). Reformation of the severed septohippocampal cholinergic pathway in the adult rat by transplanted septal neurons. *Cell Tissue Res.*, **185,** 289–302.

Björklund, A. & Stenevi, U. (1979a). Regeneration of monoaminergic and cholinergic neurons in the mammalian central nervous system. *Physiol. Rev.*, **59,** 62–100.

Björklund, A. & Stenevi, U. (1979b). Reconstruction of the nigrostriatal dopamine pathway by intracerebral nigral transplants. *Brain Res.*, **177,** 555–60.

Björklund, A. & Stenevi, U. (1981). In vivo evidence for hippocampal adrenergic neurotrophic factor specifically released on septal deafferentation. *Brain Res.*, **229,** 403–28.

Björklund, A. & Stenevi, U. (ed.) (1985a). *Neural Grafting in the Mammalian CNS.* Amsterdam: Elsevier.

Björklund, A. & Stenevi, U. (1985b). Intracerebral neural grafting: a historical perspective. In *Neural Grafting in the Mammalian CNS*, ed., A. Bjorklund & U. Stenevi, pp. 3–14. Amsterdam: Elsevier.

Björklund, A., Dunnett, S. B., Stenevi, U., Lewis, M. R. & Iversen, S. D. (1980). Reinnervation of the denervated striatum by substantia nigra transplants: functional consequences as revealed by pharmacological and sensorimotor testing. *Brain Res.*, **199,** 307–33.

Björklund, A., Stenevi, U., Dunnett, S. B. & Gage, F. H. (1982). Cross-species neural grafting in a rat model of Parkinson's disease. *Nature*, **298,** 652–4.

Björklund, A., Stenevi, U. & Svendgaard, N.-Aa. (1976). Growth of transplanted monoaminergic neurones into the adult hippocampus along the perforant path. *Nature*, **262,** 787–90.

Cajal, S. Ramón y (1928). *Degeneration and Regeneration in the Nervous System.* London: Oxford University Press.

Coyle, J. T., Price, D. L. & DeLong, M. R. (1983). Alzheimer's disease: a disorder of cortical cholinergic innervation. *Science*, **219,** 1184–90.

Daniloff, J. K., Bodony, R. P., Low, W. C. & Wells, J. (1985). Cross-species embryonic septal transplants: restoration of conditioned learning behavior. *Brain Res.*, **346,** 176–80.

Das, G. D. (1974). Transplantation of embryonic neural tissue in the mammalian brain. I. Growth and differentiation of neuroblasts from various regions of the embryonic brain in the cerebellum of neonate rats. *T.I.T. J. Life Sci.*, **4,** 93–124.

Das, G. D. & Altman, J. (1971). Transplanted precursors of nerve cells: their fate in the cerebellums of young rats. *Science*, **173,** 637–8.

Das, G. D. & Altman, J. (1972). Studies on the transplantation of developing neural tissue in the mammalian brain. I. Transplantation of cerebellar slabs into the cerebellum of neonate rats. *Brain Res.*, **38,** 233–49.

David, S. & Aguayo, A. J. (1981). Axonal elongation into PNS 'bridges' after CNS injury in adult rats. *Science*, **214,** 931–3.

Divac, I., Markowitsch, H. J. & Pritzel, M. (1978). Behavioural and anatomical consequences of small intrastriatal injections of kainic acid in the rat. *Brain Res.*, **151,** 523–32.

Drachman, D. A. & Leavitt, J. (1974). Human memory and the cholinergic system – a relationship to aging? *Arch. Neurol.*, **30,** 113–21.

Dunnett, S. B., Björklund, A., Isacson, O. & Brundin, P. (1987). Nigral and striatal grafts to the lesioned neostriatum: models of graft function. In *Movement Disorders II: Neurology of the Extrapyramidal Systems*, ed. L. Findlay, M. Gresty & R. Capildeao, London: Macmillan Press. (In press.)

Dunnett, S. B., Björklund, A., Schmidt, R. H., Stenevi, U. & Iversen, S. D. (1983a). Intracerebral grafting of neuronal cell suspensions. IV. Behavioural recovery in rats with unilateral implants of nigral cell suspensions in different forebrain sites. *Acta Physiol. Scand., suppl.*, **522,** 29–37.

Dunnett, S. B., Björklund, A., Schmidt, R. H., Stenevi, U. & Iversen, S. D. (1983b). Intracerebral grafting of neuronal cell suspensions. V. Behavioural recovery in rats with bilateral 6-OHDA lesions following

implantation of nigral cell suspensions. *Acta Physiol. Scand. suppl.*, **522,** 39–47.
Dunnett, S. B., Björklund, A., Stenevi, U. & Iversen, S. D. (1981a). Behavioural recovery following transplantation of substantia nigra in rats subjected to 6-OHDA lesions of the nigrostriatal pathway. I. Unilateral lesions. *Brain Res.*, **215,** 147–61.
Dunnett, S. B., Björklund, A., Stenevi, U. & Iversen, S. D. (1981b). Grafts of embryonic substantia nigra reinnervating the ventrolateral striatum ameliorate sensorimotor impairments and akinesia in rats with 6-OHDA lesions of the nigrostriatal pathway. *Brain Res.*, **229,** 209–17.
Dunnett, S. B., Bjorklund, A., Stenevi, U. & Iversen, S. D. (1981c). Behavioural recovery following transplantation of substantial nigra in rats subjected to 6-OHDA lesions of the nigrostriatal pathway. II. Bilateral lesions. *Brain Res.*, **229,** 457–70.
Dunnett, S. B., Toniolo, G. Fine, A., Ryan, C. N., Björklund, A. & Iversen, S. D. (1985). Transplantation of embryonic ventral forebrain neurons to the neocortex of rats with lesions of nucleus basalis magnocellularis. II. Sensorimotor and learning impairments. *Neurosci.*, **16,** 787–97.
Fine, A., Dunnett, S. B., Björklund, A. & Iversen, S. D. (1985). Cholinergic ventral forebrain grafts into the neocortex improve passive avoidance memory in a rat model of Alzheimer's disease. *Proc. Nat. Acad. Sci. USA*, **82,** 5227–30.
Fray, P. J., Dunnett, S. B., Iversen, S. D., Bjorklund, A. & Stenevi, U. (1983). Nitral transplants reinnervating the dopamine-depleted neostriatum can sustain intracerebral self-stimulation. *Science*, **219,** 416–9.
Freed, W. J. (1983). Functional brain tissue transplantation: reversal of lesion-induced rotation by intraventricular substantia nigra and adrenal medulla grafts, with a note on intracranial retinal grafts. *Biol. Psychiatry*, **18,** 1205–67.
Freed, W. J. (1984). Application of brain tissue transplantation to the nigrostriatal dopamine system. *Intern. Med.*, **4,** 17–23.
Freed, W. J. (1985). GM_1 ganglioside does not stimulate reinnervation of the striatum by substantia nigra grafts. *Brain Res. Bull.*, **14,** 91–5.
Freed, W. J., Morihisa, J. M., Spoor, E., Hoffer, B. J., Olson, L., Seiger, Å. & Wyatt, R. J. (1981). Transplanted adrenal chromaffin cells in rat brain reduce lesion-induced rotational behaviour. *Nature*, **292,** 351–2.
Freed, W. J., Perlow, M. J., Karoum, F., Seiger, Å., Olson, L., Hoffer, B. J. & Wyatt, R. J. (1980). Restoration of dopaminergic function by grafting of fetal rat substantia nigra to the caudate nucleus: long-term behavioural, biochemical, and histochemical studies. *Ann. Neurol.*, **8,** 510–9.
Freed, W. J. & Wyatt, R. J. (1980). Transplantation of eyes to the adult rat brain: histological findings and light-evoked potential responses. *Life Sci.*, **27,** 503–10.
Gage, F. H., Björklund, A., Stenevi, U. & Dunnett, S. B. (1983a). Intracerebral grafting in the mammalian brain. In *Aging of the Brain*, ed. W. H. Gispen & J. Traber, pp. 125–37. Amsterdam: Elsevier.
Gage, F. H., Björklund, A., Stenevi, U., Dunnett, S. B. & Kelly, P. H. (1984) Intrahippocampal septal grafts ameliorate learning impairments in aged rats. *Science*, **225,** 533–6.
Gage, F. H., Dunnett, S. B., Björklund, A. & Stenevi, U. (1983b). Aged rats: recovery of motor coordination impairments by intrastriatal nigral grafts. *Science*, **221,** 966–9.
Gash, D. M., Sladek, J. R. & Sladek, C. D. (1980). Functional development of grafted vasopressin neurons. *Science*, **210,** 1367–9.

Gibson, M. J., Krieger, D. T., Charlton, H. M., Zimmerman, E. A., Silverman, A. J. & Perlow, M. J. (1984). Mating and pregnancy can occur in genetically hypogonadal mice with preoptic area brain grafts. *Science*, **255,** 949–51.

Hall, R. D., Bloom, F. E. & Olds, J. (1977). Neuronal and neurochemical substrates of reinforcement. *Neurosci. Res. Program Bull.*, **15,** 133–314.

Isacson, O., Brundin, P., Kelly P. A. T., Gage, F. H. & Björklund, A. (1984). Functional neuronal replacement by grafted striatal neurones in the ibotenic acid-lesioned rat striatum. *Nature*, **311,** 458–60.

Isacson, O., Dunnett, S. B. & Björklund, A. (1986). Graft-induced behavioral recovery in an animal model of Huntington disease. *Proc. Nat. Acad. Sci. USA*, **83,** 2728–32.

Krieger, D. T., Perlow, M. J., Gibson, M. J., Davies, T. F., Zimmerman, E. A., Ferin, M. & Charlton, H. M. (1982). Brain grafts reverse hypogonadism of gonadaotropin releasing hormone deficiency. *Nature*, **298,** 468–71.

Langston, J. W., Ballard, P., Tetrud, J. W. & Irwin, I. (1983). Chronic parkinsonism in humans due to a product of meperidine-analog synthesis. *Science*, **219,** 979–80.

Lindsay, R. M. (1979). Adult rat brain astrocytes support survival of both NGF-dependent and NGF-insensitive neurones. *Nature*, **282,** 80–2.

Ljungberg, T. & Ungerstedt, U. (1976). Reinstatement of eating by dopamine agonists in aphagic dopamine denervated rats. *Physiol. & Behav.*, **16,** 277–83.

Lund, R. D. & Simon, D. J. (1985). Retinal transplants: structural and functional interrelations with the host brain. In *Neural Grafting in the Mammalian CNS*, ed. A. Björklund & U. Stenevi, pp. 345–54. Amsterdam: Elsevier.

Marshall, J. F. & Gotthelf, T. (1979). Sensory inattention in rats with 6-hydroxydopamine-induced lesions of ascending dopaminergic neurons: apomorphine induced reversal of deficits. *Exp. Neurol.*, **65,** 389–411.

Marshall, J. F. & Ungerstedt, U. (1976). Apomorphine-induced restoration of drinking to thirst challenges in 6-hydroxydopamine-treated rats. *Physiol. & Behav.*, **17,** 817–22.

Marshall, J. F., Richardson, J. S. & Teitelbaum, P. (1974). Nigrostriatal bundle damage and the lateral hypothalamic syndrome. *J. comp. physiol. Psychol.*, **87,** 808–80.

Mason, D. W., Charlton, H. M., Jones, A., Parry, D. M. & Simmonds, S. J. (1985). Immunology of allograft rejection in mammals. In *Neural Grafting in the Mammalian CNS*, ed. A. Björklund & U. Stenevi, pp. 91–8. Amsterdam: Elsevier.

McGeer, E. G. (1981). Neurotransmitter systems in aging and senile dementia. *Prog. Neuro-psychopharmacol*, **5,** 435–45.

Morihisa, J. M., Nakamura, R. K., Freed, W. J., Mishkin, M. & Wyatt, R. J. (1984). Adrenal medulla grafts survive and exhibit catecholamine specific fluorescence in the primate brain. *Exp. Neurol.*, **84,** 643–53.

Nieto-Sampedro, M., Manthorpe, M., Barbin, G., Varon, S. & Cotman, C. W. (1983). Injury-induced neuronotrophic activity in adult rat brain: correlation with survival of delayed implants in the wound cavity. *J. Neurosci.*, **3,** 2219–29.

Olds, J. & Milner, P. M. (1954). Positive reinforcement produced by electrical stimulation of septal area and other regions of rat brain. *J. comp. physiol. Psychol.*, **47,** 419–27.

Olson, L. & Malmfors, T. (1970). Growth characteristics of adrenergic nerves in the adult rat. Fluorescence histochemical and ^{3}H-noradrenaline uptake studies using tissue transplantation to the anterior chamber of the eye. *Acta Physiol. Scand.*, **348,** 1–112.

Olson, L. & Seiger, Å. (1972). Brain tissue transplanted to the anterior chamber of the eye. 1. Fluorescence histochemistry of immature catecholamine and 5-hydroxytryptamine neurons innervating the iris. *Z. Zellforsch.*, **195,** 175–94.

Patel-Vaidya, U., Wells, M. R. & Freed, W. J. (1985). Survival of dissociated adrernal chromaffin cells of rat and monkey transplanted into rat brain. *Cell Tissue Res.*, **240,** 281–85.

Perlow, M. J., Freed, W. J., Hoffer, B. J., Seiger, Å., Olson, L. & Wyatt, R. J. (1979). Brain grafts reduce motor abnormalities produced by destruction of nigrostriatal dopamine system. *Science*, **204,** 643–7.

Pritzel, M., Isacson, O., Brundin, P., Wiklund, L. & Björklund, A. (1985). Fibre connections of grafted caudate-putamen in the rat: a WGA-HRP study. *Neurosci. Lett., suppl.*, **22,** 531.

Raisman, G. (1969). Neuronal plasticity in the septal nuclei of the adult brain. *Brain Res.*, **14,** 25–48.

Richards, S. J., Morris, R. & Raisman, G. (1985). Solitary magnocellular neurones in the homozygous Brattleboro rat have vasopressin and glycopeptide immunoreactivity. *Neurosci.*, **16,** 617–23.

Richardson, P. M., McGuinness, U. M. & Aguayo, A. J. (1982). Peripheral nerve autografts to the rat spinal cord: studies with axonal tracing methods. *Brain Res.*, **237,** 147–62.

Rosvold, H. E. (1972). The frontal lobe system: cortical–subcortical interrelationships. *Acta Neurobiol. Exp.*, **32,** 439–60.

Schmidt, R. H., Björklund, A., Stenevi, U., Dunnett, S. B. & Gage, F. H. (1983). Intracerebral grafting of neuronal cell suspensions. III. Activity of intrastriatal nigral suspension implants as assessed by measurements of dopamine synthesis and metabolism. *Acta Physiol. Scand., suppl.*, **522,** 19–28.

Scott, D. E. & Sherman, D. M. (1984). Neuronal and neurovascular integration following transplantation of the fetal hypothalamus into the third cerebral ventricle of adult Brattleboro rats. Neurological transplants: I. *Brain Res. Bull.*, **12,** 453–67.

Seiger, Å. (1985). Preparation of immature central nervous system regions for transplantation. In *Neural Grafting in the Mammalian CNS*, ed. A. Björklund & U. Stenevi, pp. 71–7. Amsterdam: Elsevier.

Silverman, A. J., Zimmerman, E. A., Gibson, M. J., Perlow, M. J., Charlton, H. M., Kokoris, G. J. & Krieger, D. T. (1985). Implantation of normal fetal preoptic area into hypogonadal mutant mice: temporal relationships of the growth of gonadotropin-releading hormone neurons and the development of the pituitary/testicular axis. *Neurosci.*, **16,** 69–84.

Stenevi, U., Bjerre, B., Björklund, A. & Mobley, W. (1974). Effects of localized intracerebral injections of nerve growth factor on the regenerative growth of lesioned central noradrenergic neurones. *Brain Res.*, **69,** 217–34.

Stenevi, U., Björklund, A. & Dunnett, S. B. (1980). Functional reinnervation of the denervated neostriatum by nigral transplants. *Peptides* **1,** *suppl.* 1, 111–6.

Stenevi, U., Björklund, A. & Moore, R. Y. (1973). Morphological plasticity of central adrenergic neurons. *Brain Behav. Evol.*, **8,** 110–34.

Stenevi, U., Björklund, A. & Svendgaard, N.-Aa. (1976). Transplantation of central and peripheral monoaminergic neurons to the adult rat brain: techniques and conditions for survival. *Brain Res.*, **114,** 1–20.
Stricker, E. M. & Zigmond, M. J. (1976). Recovery of function following damage to central catecholamine-containing neurons: a neurochemical model for the lateral hypothalamic syndrome. in *Progress in Physiological Psychology*, ed. J. M. Sprague & A. N. Epstein, pp. 121–89. New York: Academic Press.
Strömberg, I., Herrera-Marschitz, M., Ungerstedt, U., Ebendal, T. & Olson, L. (1985). Chronic implants of chromaffin tissue into the dopamine-denervated striatum. Effects of NGF on graft survival, fiber growth and rotational behavior. *Exp. Brain Res.*, **60,** 335–49.
Toniolo, G., Dunnett, S. B., Hefti, F. & Will, B. (1985). Acetylcholine-rich transplants in the hippocampus: influence of intrinsic growth factors and application of nerve growth factor on choline acetyltransferase activity. *Brain Res.*, **345,** 141–6.
Ungerstedt, U. (1971a). Striatal dopamine release after amphetamine or nerve degeneration revealed by rotational behavior. *Acta Physiol. Scand., suppl.*, **367,** 49–68.
Ungerstedt, U. (1971b). Post-synaptic supersensitivity after 6-hydroxydopamine induced degeneration of the nigro-striatal dopamine system. *Acta Physiol. Scand., suppl.*, **367,** 69–93.

INDEX